Clinics in Developmental Medicine No. 176
NEUROLOGICAL ASSESSMENT IN THE
FIRST TWO YEARS OF LIFE

© 2007 Mac Keith Press
30 Furnival Street, London EC4A 1JQ

Editor: Hilary M. Hart
Managing Editor: Michael Pountney
Project Manager: Sarah Pearsall

The views and opinions expressed herein are those of the authors and do not necessarily
represent those of the publisher

First published in this edition 2007

British Library Cataloguing-in-Publication data
A catalogue record for this book is available from the British Library

ISBN: 978-1-898683-54-4

Typeset by Keystroke, 28 High Street, Tettenhall, Wolverhampton
Printed by The Lavenham Press Ltd, Water Street, Lavenham, Suffolk
Mac Keith Press is supported by Scope

Clinics in Developmental Medicine No. 176

Neurological Assessment in the First Two Years of Life

Instruments for the follow-up of high-risk newborns

Edited by

GIOVANNI CIONI
Stella Maris Scientific Institute and University of Pisa, Pisa

and

EUGENIO MERCURI
Catholic University of Rome, Rome and Hammersmith
Hospital, London

2007
Mac Keith Press

CONTENTS

AUTHORS' APPOINTMENTS

Enrico Biagioni   Department of Developmental Neuroscience,
                           Stella Maris Scientific Institute, Pisa; Child
                           Neuropsychiatric Service, ASL 3, Toscana Region,
                           Italy

Suzann Campbell   Department of Physical Therapy, University of
                           Illinois at Chicago, USA

Anna Chilosi   Department of Developmental Neuroscience,
                           Stella Maris Scientific Institute, Pisa, Italy

Giovanni Cioni   Department of Developmental Neuroscience,
                           Stella Maris Scientific Institute, Pisa; Division of
                           Child Neurology and Psychiatry, University of Pisa,
                           Italy

Paola Cipriani   Department of Developmental Neuroscience,
                           Stella Maris Scientific Institute, Pisa; Division of
                           Child Neurology and Psychiatry, University of Pisa,
                           Italy

Frances Cowan   Department of Paediatrics and Neonatal
                           Medicine, Hammersmith Hospital, London, UK

Lilly Dubowitz   Department of Paediatrics and Neonatal
                           Medicine, Hammersmith Hospital, London, UK

Christa Einspieler   Department of Systems Physiology, Medical
                           University of Graz, Graz, Austria

Janet Eyre   Department of Child Health, University of
                           Newcastle, UK

Elisabetta Genovese   Audiology and Foniatry Service, University of
                           Modena and Reggio Emilia, Italy

Andrea Guzzetta   Department of Developmental Neuroscience,
                           Stella Maris Scientific Institute, Pisa, Italy

Francesco Guzzetta   Pediatric Neurology and Child Psychiatry Unit,
                           Catholic University, Rome, Italy

Leena Haataja   Department of Paediatric Neurology, University
                           Hospital of Turku, Turku, Finland

Samantha Johnson   Division of Child Health, Queen's Medical
                           Centre, Nottingham, UK

Sandra Maestro   Department of Developmental Neuroscience,
                           Stella Maris Scientific Institute, Pisa, Italy

Neil Marlow   Division of Child Health, Queen's Medical Centre, Nottingham, UK

Eugenio Mercuri   Department of Child Neurology and Psychiatry, Catholic University of Rome, Rome, Italy; Department of Paediatrics and Neonatal Medicine, Hammersmith Hospital, London, UK

Michael Msall   Developmental and Behavioral Pediatrics, University of Chicago, Chicago, USA

Anthony Norcia   Smith-Kettlewell Eye Research Institute, San Francisco, USA

Paola Paolicelli   Department of Developmental Neuroscience, Stella Maris Scientific Institute, Pisa, Italy

Francesca Pei   Associazione Italiana di Scienze della Visione, Pisa, Italy

Daniela Ricci   Department of Child Neurology and Psychiatry, Catholic University of Rome, Rome, Italy

Mary Rutherford   Department of Paediatrics and Neonatal Medicine, Hammersmith Hospital, London, UK

Francesca Tinelli   Department of Developmental Neuroscience, Stella Maris Scientific Institute, Pisa; Division of Child Neurology and Psychiatry, University of Pisa, Pisa, Italy

Chiara Veredice   Department of Child Neurology and Psychiatry, Catholic University of Rome, Rome, Italy

Laura Zawacki   Department of Physical Therapy, University of Illinois at Chicago, Chicago, USA

1
INTRODUCTION

Giovanni Cioni and Eugenio Mercuri

The advent of neonatal intensive care units in the 1950s dramatically changed the spectrum of survival and outcome of high-risk newborns, and raised the need to identify appropriate instruments for the assessment of these infants.

Several methods for the neurological examination of the newborn have been developed, including assessments of tone and reactions (Saint-Anne Dargassies 1977), behaviour (Brazelton 1973), movements (Prechtl 1990), and methods integrating the different approaches (Dubowitz et al 1999). In contrast, less attention has been devoted to the assessment of neurological function after the neonatal period and, more generally, in the first years after birth. Some neurological examinations suitable for infants have been developed and used in clinical and research studies (Touwen 1976, Amiel-Tison and Grenier 1986, Haataja et al 1999).

More attention has been devoted to developmental scales. Over the years it has become obvious that the development of the infant's brain is not just related to motor function and that different aspects of development, such as perceptual and cognitive function, should be systematically investigated. From the pioneering work of Gesell in the 1940s a number of scales have been developed over the years. This has made it possible to obtain not only a global measure of development but also subscores for the main domains. Moreover, neuropsychological tests are also available, mainly in the research setting, for the assessment of specific aspects of behaviour.

The advent of sophisticated neurophysiological and neuroimaging techniques has provided further evidence of the complexity of the developing brain and of the onset and maturation of different neural functions. Until recently, however, some of these techniques, although widely used in older children and adults, had not been used in infants because of the lack of age-appropriate normative data. Using an integrated approach, recent studies in high-risk infants have described the maturation of specific aspects of function and their correlation with the maturation of brain structures on imaging.

This book is the result of collaborative work among three groups (in Pisa, London and Rome), and their collaboration with other European and American centres.

The aim of the book is to provide a review of the state of the art of the clinical application of various techniques for the neurological assessment in the first two years of life. After a brief description of the neurophysiological basis of development in the first years, and of brain reorganization after early lesions, we critically review various methods used for

1

neurological assessment in young infants, providing details of our own experience using two different approaches (classical neurological examination and assessment of general movements) in normal infants, and assess their value in identifying infants at risk of neurological sequelae and predicting outcome.

Chapters 2–7 describe the value of neuroimaging and neurophysiological techniques, reporting the changes observed on brain MRI in normal preterm and full-term infants in the first two years, the main types of abnormal MRI findings and their prognostic value, and the predictive value of neurophysiological findings (EEG and evoked potentials) in relation to brain lesions.

Chapters 8–12 describe neuropsychological and perceptual/communication assessment techniques for use in the follow-up, with a systematic review of the methods of multi-domain assessment (developmental scales) and other techniques assessing specific aspects of cognitive, perceptual and sensory abilities. Special attention is given to hearing, language and communication and to development of vision and visual attention both in normal infants and in those with neonatal brain lesions.

The final two chapters are devoted to intervention, describing how the identification of specific profiles of impairment can lead to the development of appropriate plans for early intervention, and to the potential contribution of data from multicentre longitudinal follow-up studies to the identification of major risk factors, and the validation of new diagnostic and treatment protocols.

REFERENCES

Amiel-Tison C, Grenier A (1986) *Neurological Assessment during the First Years of Life*. New York: Oxford University Press.

Brazelton TB (1973) *Neonatal Behavioral Assessment Scale*. Clinics in Developmental Medicine 50. Philadelphia, PA: JB Lippincott.

Dubowitz L, Dubowitz V, Mercuri E (1999) *The Neurological Assessment of the Preterm and Full Term Newborn Infant, 2nd edn*. Clinics in Developmental Medicine 148. London: Mac Keith Press.

Haataja L, Mercuri E, Regev R, Cowan F, Rutherford M, Dubowitz V, Dubowitz L (1999) Optimality score for the neurologic examination of the infant at 12 and 18 months of age. *J Pediatr* 135: 153–161.

Prechtl HFR (1990) Qualitative changes of spontaneous movements in fetus and preterm infants are a marker of neurological dysfunction. *Early Hum Dev* 23: 151–158.

Saint-Anne Dargassies S (1977) *Neurological Development in the Full-Term and Premature Neonate*. Amsterdam: Elsevier.

Touwen B (1976) *Neurological Development in Infancy*. Clinics in Developmental Medicine 58. London: Heinemann

2
NEUROPHYSIOLOGICAL BASIS OF DEVELOPMENT

Janet Eyre

Introduction

Older views of developmental plasticity focused on the protective effect of a young age at the time of the brain damage. A younger rather than an older age at onset was thought to produce fewer and/or less severe symptoms and a more rapid recovery. It is now clear that quite specific effects of early brain damage persist and produce complex and often severe patterns of impairment which are different from those observed following lesions in the adult brain.

Although an understanding of the nature of neural plasticity in response to damage is critical to those attempting to augment recovery from neurological insults, it is misleading to treat the underlying mechanisms as self-reparative. An appreciation that these mechanisms evolved as an expedient for fine-tuning neurological circuitry during *normal* development by taking advantage of contextual information, and that they may only be available for response to damage as an incidental side effect, can help us to focus on how best to augment desirable, and avoid any undesirable, effects.

Seminal studies in the early 1960s by Wiesel and Hubel on the organization of ocular dominance columns signified the starting point of extensive basic research on developmental brain plasticity (Wiesel and Hubel 1965). Investigation of neuroplasticity has expanded rapidly over the past ten years and has uncovered the remarkable capacity of the developing brain to be shaped by activity and environmental input. Reorganization of developmental systems occurs not only within modalities but can even extend across different modalities (Rauschecker and Korte 1993) and lead to transfer of functions between cerebral hemispheres (Eyre 2003b 2004, 2005).

Knowledge of the time course and processes of normal development is essential both for a better understanding of current rehabilitation treatments and for the design of new strategies for the treatment of children who sustain brain damage early in life.

Development of the cortex

NEUROGENESIS AND THE DEVELOPMENT OF CORTICAL LAYERS
Cortical neurons are generated in the ventricular zone of the cortical wall and in the subcortical ganglionic eminence and reach their destination by both radial and tangential migration (Rakic 1972, Anderson et al 2002). The first postmitotic neurons accumulate superficial to

the neuroepithelium immediately beneath the pial surface at five weeks postconceptional age (PCA), forming the preplate (Rickmann and Wolff 1981). The largest of the preplate neurons already have dendritic processes and also axons which course into the intermediate zone and give rise to the first efferent connections of the cortex by 7 weeks PCA.

Although preplate cells are also neurons, they are distinct from those that will populate the definitive cellular layers 2–6 of the mature adult cortex. Layers 2–6 emerge from the neurons of the cortical plate. The cortical plate first emerges within the preplate at 8 weeks PCA (Meyer et al 2000). As the cortical neurons become postmitotic, they migrate to split the preplate into two zones: a superficial marginal zone, which will later become layer 1, and a deeper subplate, a transient structure present only during development. At this time subplate neurons have already assumed a pyramidal shape, and have complex dendritic trees and axons which form a clearly visible fibre tract within the intermediate zone (Meyer et al 2000). The subplate neurons therefore have a high degree of maturity in comparison to the immature morphology and tight compaction of the cortical plate neurons at this early stage of development. An intermediate zone also develops above the ventricular zone but below the subplate, comprising migrating neurons and efferent and afferent fibres (Fig. 2.1) (Marin-Padilla 1971, 1972).

After the arrival of the first cortical plate neurons, formation of the layers within the cortical plate proceeds by progressive adjunction of new immigrant neurons in an inside-out gradient; thus layers 6 and 5 are generated early and layers 2 and 3 are generated last (Rakic 1974). The marginal zone will eventually form layer 1 of the cortex.

The peak of cell proliferation in the germinal epithelium occurs at the end of the first trimester in humans. The neuronal migration period occurs between 8 and 16 weeks PCA. Cell proliferation in the ventricular zone is evident until 16 weeks. From this time the volume and thickness of the ventricular zone decreases until 22–24 weeks, when only a few rows of sparse cells can be recognized in the germinal epithelium (Zecevic et al 1999). There is a 50 per cent increase in the volume of the cortical grey matter between 28 weeks PCA and term (Hüppi et al 1998). This is associated with growth and differentiation of cortical neurons, the arrival of a massive contingent of afferent fibres relocating from the subplate into the cortical plate, and the growth of callosal and long associative corticocortical fibre systems (Kostovic and Judas 2002).

The subplate

The subplate comprises a heterogeneous population of neurons located directly under the cortical plate, which is only present during development. There is structural, immuno-cytochemical and electrophysiological evidence that subplate neurons are integrated in a functioning synaptic circuit with extensive axonal projections within the developing cortical plate (Kanold 2004). Thalamocortical axons initially form temporary synapses on subplate neurons (Kostovic and Judas 2002). Deletion of the subplate (Ghosh and Shatz 1992) or its improper differentiation (Zhou et al 1999) causes inappropriate thalamocortical innervation and prevents the accurate formation of layer 4. These data indicate that molecular markers as well as electrical activity patterns in the subplate may influence the in-growing thalamocortical axons.

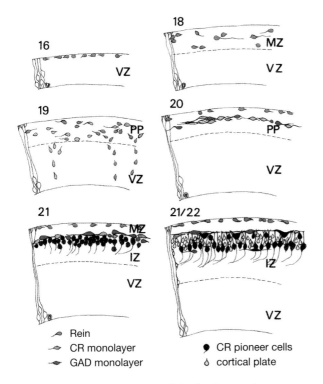

Fig. 2.1 Diagrammatic representation of the developmental events proposed by Meyers and her colleagues for the early development of the human neocortex. All figures were drawn at the same magnitude with the aid of a camera lucida. The first Reln immunoreactive neurons appear at Carnegie stage 16 (5 weeks PCA) and increase in number from Carnegie stages 17 to 19 (6 to 6.5 weeks PCA). The first CR immunoreactive neurons appear at Carnegie stage 19 (6.5 weeks PCA) in what could now be called the preplate. GAD immunoreactive neurons first appear at stage 20 (7 weeks PCA). Concurrently, Reln immunoreactive neurons settle in the subpial compartment. At stage 21 (7 weeks PCA), the pioneer cells send the first corticofugal fibres. The preplate is split apart into a minor superficial component and a large deep component, the subplate, through the first cohorts of the cortical plate, at stages 21 and 22 (8 weeks PCA). (IZ, intermediate zone; MZ, marginal zone; PP, preplate; VZ, ventricular zone.)

Source: Meyer et al 2000.

Finally subplate neurons also extend the first corticofugal axons from the neocortex into the internal capsule, before many of the neurons of layer 5 and 6 have become post-mitotic and begun migration from the ventricular zone (Fig. 2.1) (Meyer et al 2000). The observation that subplate neurons send the first axons into the internal capsule led to the intriguing suggestion that these axons may play a pioneering role in establishing the corticofugal projections of layer 5 and 6 neurons (McConnell 1988, Shatz et al 1990). In rats, however, the subcortical distribution of subplate axons is restricted to the internal capsule and thalamus; subplate neurons do not project to the superior colliculus nor extend from the internal capsule into the cerebral peduncle (De Carlos and O'Leary 1992), suggesting that the axons of the subplate do not have a central role in pioneering deep subcortical projections such as the corticospinal tract.

The generalization of these observations to other species, especially man, must be made with caution since the population of subplate neurons in rodents, and in rats in particular, is relatively small. The subplate structure is very much larger and more highly developed in phylogenetically more advanced species. The maximum subplate to cortical plate ratio during development in the mouse and rat is only 1:2; in the cat, 1:1; in the monkey, 3:1; and in humans it reaches a ratio of 4:1 at approximately 25 weeks PCA. Not only is the subplate larger in extent in human and subhuman primates than in cats and rats, but it also persists for a much longer period during development. In man the subplate is discernible but progressively decreasing in size up until soon after birth (Mrzljak et al 1988, Meyer et al 2000, Kostovic and Judas 2002).

It has been proposed that subplate neurons are required for the development of a complex cortical organization, since the size of subplate and the extent of its synaptic linkages are more prominent in species with increased radial and tangential cortical connectivity, such as cats, monkeys and humans (Kostovic and Rakic 1990, Mrzljak et al 1992). The relevance of this proposal to human development lies in the observation that in a neonatal rat model of hypoxic-ischaemic injury which produces the characteristic pattern of subcortical injury associated with human periventricular leucomalacia, selective subplate neuron death is seen. This may provide an explanation for the high frequency of cognitive, motor and sensory deficits observed in babies with periventricular leucomalacia, and for the fact that, with decreasing gestational age, periventricular leucomalacia is associated with more pervasive abnormalities of cortical development (Inder et al 1999).

Differentiation of the neocortex
The adult neocortex is composed of six major layers, which are distinguished by differences in the morphology and density of neurons that constitute them (Brodmann 1909). The developing cortical plate lacks many features that distinguish neocortical areas in the adult, even after all the neurons have been generated and layers begin to differentiate within it. During corticogenesis the laminar destination of cortical neurons appears to be determined early in the life of the neuron, potentially prior to the final mitosis in the ventricular zone (McConnell 1995). Although neurons in different layers have unique dendritic con- figurations and axonal projections, most, if not all, types of cortical pyramidal neuron initially develop with a common morphology and only later develop the dendritic shape characteristic of their class and layer, by developmental sculpting (Koester and O'Leary 1992).

Different regions of the developing cortex may initially be interchangeable in terms of the axonal connections they develop and maintain, and even in their capacity to form complex and highly organized neuronal assemblies (O'Leary et al 1992). Thus, the neo- cortical neuroepithelium generates populations of neurons which rely on interactions with intrinsic and extrinsic patterning information, acting both separately and synergistically at different stages of neocortical development, to generate their characteristic area-specific features. Intrinsic and extrinsic cortical patterning information includes: molecular factors

6

intrinsic to the ventricular zone, to the subplate and to the maturing neocortex; spontaneous activity patterns in the subplate or neocortex; later arriving molecular factors extrinsic to the cortex, such as derived anterogradely from afferent pathways or retrogradely from efferent pathways; and extrinsically driven activity patterns, either sensory inputs or spontaneous activity extrinsic to the cortex (O'Leary and Nakagawa 2002).

The timing and pattern of development of efferent projections from and afferent projections to the cortex is important in understanding this activity-dependent phase of cortical development.

Development of afferent somatosensory projections

The arrival and entry of the first complement of dorsal root fibres occurs by 2.5 weeks PCA and these axons bificate into ascending and descending projections by 3 weeks PCA. According to Okado the first synapses appear in the primordial dorsal horn at 4.5 weeks PCA and at this time a few axons also project into the ventral motor pools (Okado 1981). The growth of the long ascending branches of the dorsal root axons to form the cuneate and gracile fasciculi occurs between 6.5 and 8 weeks PCA. Myelination of dorsal root fibres and some ascending fibres begins by 24 weeks PCA and by 31 weeks the entire cuneate and gracile fasciculi are well myelinated (Konstantinidou et al 1995).

The structural and functional development of cutaneous sensory synaptic connections within the spinal cord has been shown to be activity-dependent in rodents (Beggs et al 2002). This may mean that alterations in the pattern of sensory inputs, arising from sensory stimulation, tissue injury and pain during neonatal intensive care for example, will disrupt normal synaptic organization in the sensory system (Walker et al 2003). If so, abnormal or excessive activity related to skin inflammation or injury in the fetus or neonate may have the potential to cause long-term changes in sensory processing. This is supported by clinical studies suggesting that early pain related to surgical and procedural interventions during intensive care management of preterm neonates has long-term consequences for pain behaviour and perception in later life (Porter et al 1999).

Surprisingly there is no literature on the development of the projections from the dorsal column nuclei to the ventrolateral nucleus of the thalamus in man. The first thalamo-cortical afferents are observed at 5–7 weeks PCA (Kultas-Ilinsky et al 2004). As discussed previously, these afferents make temporary synapses with subplate neurons before invasion of the cortex occurs between 22 and 25 weeks PCA (Kostovic and Judas 2002). The mechanisms by which the thalamocortical connections in the developing cortex become topographically ordered are not completely understood. During the initial stage, in-growing thalamic axons are guided to their appropriate cortical targets by molecular cues intrinsic to the cortex. In the second phase, the topographical organization has been shown to be an activity-dependent process for several developing sensory systems, such as visual and somatosensory thalamocortical projections (for reviews see O'Leary et al 1995, Penn and Shatz 1999, Levitt 2003). If the source of activity is altered during this critical period then the normal patterns of connectivity are disrupted.

SOMATOSENSORY EVOKED POTENTIALS

An indication of the degree of maturation of somatosensory pathways can be obtained from somatosensory evoked potentials. Following electrical stimulation of the median the somatosensory pathways of a newborn can be assessed reliably over the Erb's point and over the spinal cord. For the first six months of postnatal age these subcortical responses are more constantly recordable than the cortical responses. The first cortical response to median nerve stimulation, termed N20 in mature adults, is called N1 in newborns. The early N1 deflection is measurable in most normal preterm infants from at least the seventh gestational month. However, although the overall waveform morphology of the N1 response is similar to that of the N20, the latencies of the responses are markedly longer and the responses smaller and wider in preterm babies than in adults. In longitudinal studies of preterm infants, the response latencies shorten and the responses become shorter in duration and more prominent with increasing age until adult-type responses are obtained between 2 and 3 years of age (Taylor et al 1996).

Corticospinal axonal projection and withdrawal

Studies within our laboratory of embryonic human brain development confirm the observations of Meyer and her colleagues that between 6 and 7 weeks PCA the cortical plate has not yet formed (Meyer et al 2000). It is surprising, therefore, that axons, which follow the course of the corticospinal tract, reach the medulla by 8 weeks PCA and are observed to decussate (Humphrey 1960, O'Rahily and Müller 1994) (Fig. 2.2). This must raise the question of whether these early axons arise in man from subplate neurons.

In adults, layer 5 of the neocortex is the exclusive source of cortical projection neurons to the spinal cord and cortical targets in the midbrain and hindbrain. In adulthood the distribution of layer 5 neurons projecting to each subcortical target is restricted to particular areas along the tangential extent of the neocortex. Corticotectal neurons which project to the superior colliculus are, for example, found primarily in the visual cortex, whereas corticospinal neurons are largely limited to the primary motor and somatosensory cortex. In rats, however, at birth, layer 5 neurons that project to the spinal cord or to the superior colliculus are present in a continuous distribution across the entire neocortex (Fig. 2.3). Using retrograde fluorescent tracers, it has been possible to demonstrate that the mature restricted distribution of layer 5 neurons is achieved not by cell death but by selective axonal elimination (Schreyer and Jones 1982, Stanfield et al 1982, Bates and Killackey 1984).

Subsequent studies using high resolution anterograde tracing with DiI have revealed that, during development, layer 5 neurons innervate their targets in the midbrain and hindbrain via collateral branches of corticospinal axons, and that, as a population, layer 5 neurons across the neocortex initially develop a similar set of collateral projections. Thus layer 5 projection neurons can best be regarded as a single class which initially share a developmental program directing them to project towards the caudal pole of the nervous system. To generate the mature pattern of layer 5 projections, functionally appropriate for each specialized area of the cortex, different combinations of branches are later selectively eliminated. Thus development of the mature patterning of cortical projections is a late event in corticogenesis (O'Leary and Koester 1993).

8

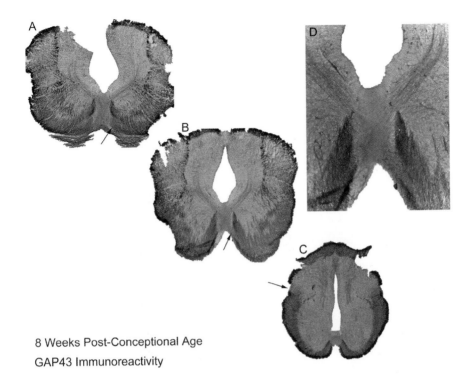

8 Weeks Post-Conceptional Age

GAP43 Immunoreactivity

Fig. 2.2 Horizontal sections from 8-week PCA fetus. These three sections from the caudal medulla (A, B) and rostral cervical spinal cord (C) from the same fetus demonstrate immunoperoxidase reactivity for GAP43 (a marker for growing axons) in nerve fibres following the course of the corticospinal tract. The arrows in A and B point to the location of the pyramids on the ventromedial surface of the medulla, which are very small at this stage of development. Small, GAP43 positive fibres can be seen leaving the pyramids and crossing over in a dorsolateral direction, indicating that axons have already entered the corticospinal decussation. This is shown more clearly in the higher-power figure (D, an enlargement of part of B). In the spinal cord, the dorsolateral funiculus (arrow) is small and contains some GAP43 immunoreactive fibres, which may be continuations of the axons observed at the decussation.

Recent studies provide new insights into the molecular events that underlie such axonal pruning (Ehlers 2003, Kantor and Kolodkin 2003). The mechanisms that control the final pattern of cortical projections, however, are not well understood, although the available evidence indicates a modulatory role for sensory input. For example, if somatosensory information is aberrantly routed to the visual cortex in developing rats prior to axonal withdrawal, layer 5 neurons in the visual cortex permanently retain their normally transient corticospinal axonal projections. Similarly, layer 5 neurons transplanted from visual cortex to motor cortex will permanently retain their projection to the spinal cord (Stanfield and O'Leary 1985, O'Leary and Stanfield 1989, O'Leary et al 1992).

In man there are no data to confirm or refute whether the initial axonal projection from layer 5 cortical neurons arises from the whole of the cortex. In the Macaque monkey a halving of the area of the cerebral cortex from which corticospinal axons originate has been

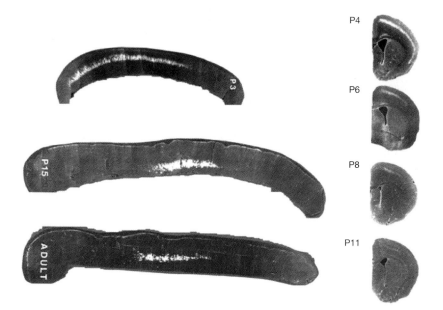

Fig. 2.3 On the left: sagittal sections through the cortex of a rat aged 3 postnatal days, 15 postnatal days and in adulthood, showing labelled cells following an injection of Fast Blue at the high cervical level (adapted from Schreyer and Jones 1982). On the right: coronal sections through the anterior parietal cortex in rats aged from 4 to 11 postnatal days (P4–P11), showing labelled cortical cells following injection of horseradish peroxidase into the high cervical spinal cord.

Source: Adapted from Bates and Killackey 1984, Schreyer and Jones 1988.

demonstrated during the first eight postnatal months, when brain volume overall increases by more than 30 per cent. These changes are associated with a threefold reduction in the number of retrogradely labelled cortical neurons, providing convincing evidence for an exuberant corticospinal projection and significant corticospinal axonal withdrawal in subhuman primates (Galea and Darian-Smith 1995).

Several studies in the rat indicate that a staggered outgrowth of corticospinal axons occurs, with many days elapsing between the appearance of the first projecting axons and the attainment of the peak number of corticospinal axons (Schreyer and Jones 1982, Gribnau et al 1986, Gorgels et al 1989, Gorgels 1990). Axonal collateral projection withdrawal also occurs over a protracted period and correlates with a dramatic reduction in corticospinal axonal numbers (Schreyer and Jones 1982, Gorgels et al 1989).

Staggered outgrowth of corticospinal axons also occurs in man. At 8 weeks PCA the pyramids are very small and they remain relatively small until there is a sudden and very large increase in size between 15 and 17 weeks PCA. There is a further large, but less rapid, increase in the size of the pyramid between 17 and 26 weeks, where it more than trebles in cross-sectional area (Humphrey 1960). Corticospinal axons reach as far as the lumbar enlargement by 18 weeks PCA (Humphrey 1960). By 40 weeks PCA corticospinal axons have begun to express neurofilaments and undergo myelination.

Corticospinal projections in several mammalian species develop transient ipsilateral projections early in development which are predominantly withdrawn by the time maturity is reached (Stanfield 1992). In the kitten, it has been demonstrated that unilateral inhibition of the motor cortex leads exuberant ipsilateral corticospinal projections from the uninhibited cortex to be maintained, at the expense of contralateral projections from the inhibited cortex, which become much reduced (Fig. 2.4) (Martin and Lee 1999, Martin et al 1999). The reduction in corticospinal projections from the inhibited cortex is due to interhemispheric competition between the corticospinal projections, and not due to activity blockade *per se*, since in a subsequent study bilateral inhibition of the motor cortices, which eliminated interhemispheric competition, led to qualitatively normal projections from both hemispheres (Martin and Lee 1999, Martin et al 1999).

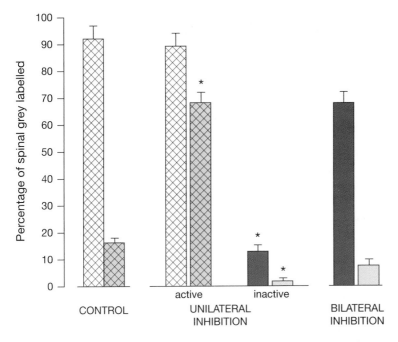

Fig. 2.4 The percentage of spinal grey matter labelled in the cervical spinal cord by anterograde transport of label placed on the forelimb area of the sensorimotor cortex in three groups of animals: four normal cats (CONTROL); four cats who had unilateral infusion of muscimol (UNILATERAL INHIBITION); and four cats who had bilateral muscimol infusions (BILATERAL INHIBITION). All infusions were made 3 mm below the pial surface at the centre of the forelimb area of the motor cortex. The infusions were continuous between postnatal weeks 3 and 7, which is the period of postnatal refinements of corticospinal terminations in cats. The left-hand hashed and solid bars represent cervical spinal cord contralateral to the cortex labelled, and the right-hand bars, the ipsilateral cervical spinal cord. Inactive (solid bars): data obtained from labelling projections from motor cortices infused with muscimol. Active (hashed bars): data obtained from labelling projections from normal motor cortices. Stars mark data significantly different from control values p<0.05.

Source: Data derived from Martin and Lee 1999, Martin et al 1999.

Focal transcranial magnetic stimulation (TMS) of the motor cortex in babies at the time of birth evokes responses in ipsilateral and contralateral muscles, demonstrating significant ipsilateral and contralateral corticospinal projections during development in man (Eyre et al 2001) (Fig. 2.5). In longitudinal and cross-sectional studies of normal babies and children, neurophysiological findings are consistent with the withdrawal of corticospinal axons over the first 24 postnatal months (Eyre et al 2001), as has been observed in sub-human primates (Galea and Darian-Smith 1995) (Fig. 2.6). Furthermore, rapid differential development of the ipsilateral and contralateral projections occurs over this time, so that responses at 2 years postnatal age in ipsilateral muscles are less frequent, significantly smaller, and have longer onset latencies and had higher thresholds than responses in contralateral muscles. The differential development of the ipsilateral responses is consistent with a greater withdrawal of ipsilateral corticomotoneuronal projections than contralateral, as has been observed during development of the corticospinal tract in animals. The small and late ipsilateral responses observed in older children and adults are consistent with the persistence of a small ipsilateral corticomotoneuronal projection, with slower conducting axons than contralateral projections (Eyre et al 2001, Eyre 2005).

Spinal innervation
Studies in animals reveal that early in development corticospinal axons initially occupy a larger terminal field within spinal grey matter and contact more spinal neurons than in the adult (Curfs et al 1994, Martin et al 1999). The elimination of supernumerary synapses and refinement of the area of termination during the process of axonal withdrawal occur in conjunction with the proliferation of synapses from the subset of axons that are maintained (Li and Martin 2001, 2002). In this way specificity in corticospinal connectivity is a dynamic process involving withdrawal of inappropriate connections and reinforcement and extension of appropriate connections, occurring at both the motor cortex and its sub-cortical projection sites including the spinal cord.

In man there is extensive innervation of spinal neurons prior to birth, including monosynaptic projections to alphamotoneurons of the ventral horn and inhibitory inter-neurons (Eyre et al 2000a, 2002, Eyre 2003a, 2003b) (Fig. 2.7). These observations in preterm and term babies should not be taken to mean that the corticospinal system is at that time capable of delivering control to the spinal cord for movement. It is proposed that the early corticospinal innervation, rather than furthering motor control *per se*, occurs to allow activity in the corticospinal system, together with sensory feedback, to shape development of the motor cortex and spinal motor centres (Eyre et al 2000a, 2001).

There is evidence from studies in the cat that the corticospinal system is incapable of exciting spinal motor circuits to a sufficient degree for controlling limb movements until their axon terminals are refined topographically. Given the importance of activity-dependent shaping of neuronal connectivity, such a mechanism would allow activity in the corticospinal system early in development to play a significant role in the development of circuit connectivity, without influencing movement (Meng and Martin 2003). There is indirect evidence to support the relevance of these observations in the cat to man. Generally in the first 12 to 24 months after birth, when axonal withdrawal and corticospinal connectivity refinement are likely to be still occurring (Eyre et al 2001), the thresholds for evoking muscle action potentials to TMS are high and the responses are inconsistent. This is followed by a drop in TMS threshold, the onset of consistent responses to TMS, and correlated improvement in hand skills, including the ability to perform relatively independent finger movements (Nezu et al 1997, Eyre et al 2000c).

Corticospinal activity during development is also involved in the shaping of spinal reflex development. Lesions in sensory motor cortex and/or infusion of muscimol over the motor cortex during development disturb the development of segmental afferent input in rats (Gibson et al 2000, Clowry et al 2004). Similar observations have been made in children who suffered lesions to the corticospinal system in the perinatal period (O'Sullivan et al 1998).

Activity-dependent development of the corticospinal tract

Substantial lesions of the sensorimotor cortex or corticospinal tract in subprimate mammals early in postnatal life lead to hypertrophy of the undamaged motor cortex and corticospinal projection (Hicks and D'Amato 1970, Huttenlocher and Raichelson 1989, Rouiller et al 1991, Jansen and Low 1996, Uematsu et al 1996). These changes are associated with maintenance of an increased ipsilateral corticospinal projection from the undamaged hemisphere. The cells of origin of the induced aberrant ipsilateral axons are more widely distributed than and distinct from the cells of origin of the crossed or contralateral corticospinal projection (Huttenlocher and Raichelson 1989, Reinoso and Castro 1989, Stanfield 1992, Jansen and Low 1996). There is no evidence for double labelling of corticospinal neurons in neonatally hemispherectomized animals that in adulthood had spinal cord injection of fluorescent tracers (Reinoso and Castro 1989). Thus induced ipsilaterally projecting corticospinal axons from the undamaged cortex do not arise as branches of the contralateral corticospinal projection, but arise from neurons which extend axons into the ipsilateral spinal cord during development, and whose axons would normally be withdrawn.

There are now repeated observations in man which demonstrate substantial plastic reorganization of the motor cortex and corticospinal projections following pre- or perinatal lesions to the corticospinal system (Benecke et al 1991, Carr et al 1993, Cao et al 1994, Lewine et al 1994, Maegaki et al 1995, Muller et al 1997, Nirkko et al 1997, Graveline et al 1998, Muller et al 1998, Hertz-Pannier 1999, Holloway et al 1999, Balbi et al 2000, Eyre et al 2000b, 2001, Thickbroom et al 2001). The findings of these studies are remarkably consistent with those made in animals following perinatal lesions to the corticospinal system.

HYPERTROPHY OF THE CONTRALESIONAL CORTICOSPINAL TRACT FOLLOWING UNILATERAL LESIONS

In children and adults who have suffered extensive damage to one motor cortex early in development, significant bilateral corticospinal innervation of spinal motoneuronal pools persists from the undamaged hemisphere. Thus focal TMS of the intact motor cortex evokes large responses in ipsilateral and contralateral muscles, which have similar latencies and thresholds (Fig. 2.8). These observations have been made following perinatal unilateral

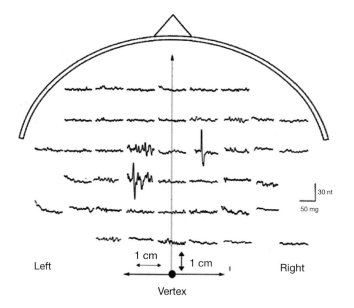

Left   1 cm   1 cm   Right

30 nt

50 mg

Vertex

Fig. 2.5 Mapping of the origin of responses evoked in right biceps brachii using TMS and a focal figure-of-eight coil. The coil was positioned using a latex 1 cm × 1 cm latex grid placed on the scalp. The individual was 5 weeks old. The filled circle marks the vertex. The traces are EMG recorded in right biceps brachii. TMS was applied at the beginning of each trace. Responses were obtained in right biceps brachii following stimulation of both the ipsilateral and contralateral cortex.

Fig. 2.6 A. Serial ipsilateral and contralateral responses recorded in the EMG of biceps following TMS of the left cortex in the same normal individual at increasing ages. The continuous line traces are from ipsilateral (left) biceps, and the dashed line traces are from contralateral (right) biceps. The stimulus artifact marks the application of TMS. The vertical line indicates the onset of the ipsilateral response when the individual was newborn. Thresholds for the responses are recorded on the right above the traces. Those in italics are for contralateral responses.

    B. Crosscorrelogram of multi-unit EMGs from contracting right and left biceps in the same newborn individual illustrated in **A,** demonstrating no evidence for common drive to the motoneuronal pools.

    C. The relative onset latencies for the ipsilateral and contralateral responses in the 18 neonates studied, calculated by subtracting the onset of the ipsilateral response from that of the contralateral. These data demonstrate the significantly shorter onset latency of ipsilateral responses in the newborn period.

    D–F. Longitudinal data from nine individuals, including the individual illustrated in **A,** studied at three-monthly intervals. Filled symbols and continuous lines represent data from ipsilateral responses, and open symbols and dashed lines from contralateral responses. The symbols represent the mean, and the vertical lines the 95 per cent confidence limits for mean. Threshold was measured as the percentage of maximum stimulator output. CMCD is the central conduction delay within the corticospinal tract. The amplitude ratio was calculated by dividing the peak to peak amplitude of the ipsilateral responses by that of the contralateral. The horizontal line in **F** indicates a ratio of one where responses are of equal size. These data demonstrate differential development of ipsilateral and contralateral responses evoked by TMS so that by 15 months ipsilateral responses have significantly higher thresholds, longer CMCDs and smaller amplitudes compared to contralateral responses.

Source: Adapted from Eyre et al 2001.

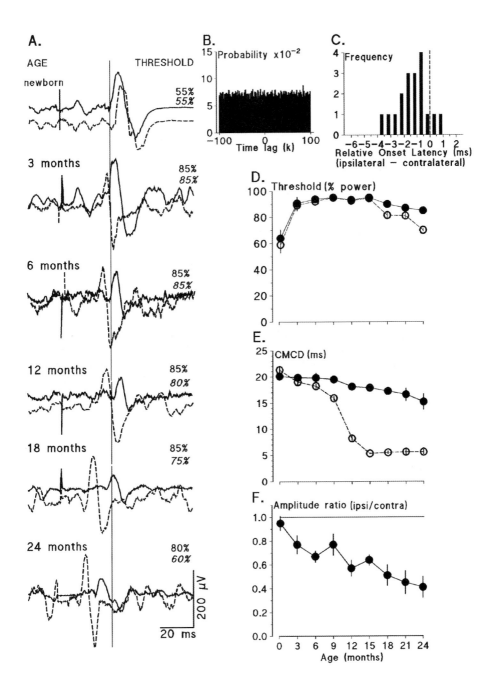

A.

AGE   THRESHOLD

newborn   55%
55%

3 months   85%
85%

6 months   85%
85%

12 months   85%
80%

18 months   85%
75%

24 months   80%
60%

200 μV

20 ms

B. Probability x10^{-2}

Time lag (k)

C. Frequency

Relative Onset Latency (ms)
(ipsilateral − contralateral)

D. Threshold (% power)

E. CMCD (ms)

F. Amplitude ratio (ipsi/contra)

Age (months)

15

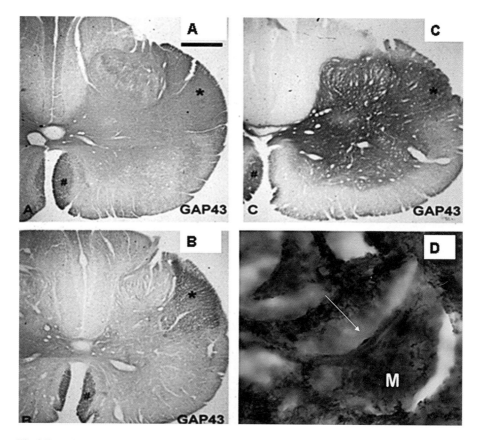

Fig. 2.7 Horizontal sections of human spinal cord C[5-6]. **A**, 24 weeks PCA. GAP43 immunoreactivity is widespread in white and grey matter. **B**, 27 weeks PCA. Corticospinal tracts are the only major axon tracts expressing GAP43 from which weaker immunoreactivity extends into the intermediate grey matter. **C**, 31 weeks PCA. Immunoreactivity is also now intense in the intermediate grey matter and present in motoneuronal pools and dorsal horn. **D**, 35 weeks PCA. Section counterstained with cresyl violet. M, Nissl stained motoneuronal cell body; solid arrow, GAP43 expressing varicose axons. Motoneuron cell bodies are closely apposed by GAP43 immunoreactive varicose axons. **A**, **B** and **C**, scale bar, 500μm. Stars mark the lateral, and hashes the anterior corticospinal tracts. **D**, scale bar, 20μm.

Source: Eyre et al 2000a.

brain damage arising from a variety of pathologies including infarction, dysplasia, and arteriovenous malformations (Benecke et al 1991, Maegaki et al 1995, Eyre et al 2000b, 2001). Short latency ipsilateral responses do not occur in normal individuals outside the perinatal period. Nor do they occur in individuals who acquired unilateral cortical lesions in adulthood, establishing that fast ipsilateral responses are not simply unmasked by unilateral lesions. Furthermore, the responses in contralateral muscles evoked by stimulation of the intact motor cortex, although within the normal range for age, are abnormally clustered towards short onset latencies and low thresholds (Eyre et al 2001).

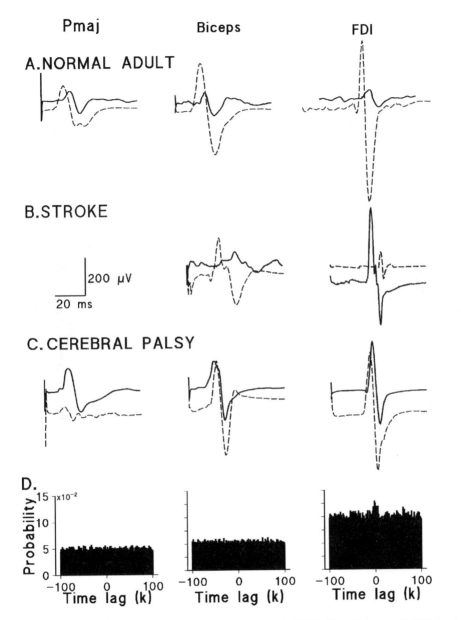

Fig. 2.8 Ipsilateral and contralateral responses recorded in the EMG of Pmaj, biceps and FDI following TMS of **A**, the left hemisphere in a normal adult, and the intact hemisphere in **B**, an individual with stroke, and **C**, an individual with spastic hemiplegic cerebral palsy. The continuous traces in **A**, **B** and **C** are from ipsilateral muscles, and the dashed traces are from contralateral muscles. TMS was delivered at the onset of each trace. **D.** Crosscorrelograms of multi-unit EMGs from contracting right and left Pmaj, biceps and FDI in the individual with spastic hemiplegic cerebral palsy and mirror movements whose responses are illustrated in **C** above. Graphs are plotted as a probability of an event from the right muscle correlating with an event in the left muscle at a time lag k.

Together these findings imply not only bilateral innervation of motoneuronal pools, but also an increase in the number of both fast conducting ipsilateral and contralateral corticospinal axons from the intact hemisphere following perinatal unilateral lesions of the corticospinal system. This conclusion is supported by direct measurement of corticospinal axonal number in the bulbar pyramid obtained at postmortem. These measurements demonstrate significant increases in the number of corticospinal axons, particularly larger-diameter axons, projecting from the intact hemisphere in adults with spastic hemiplegic cerebral palsy, in comparison to normal individuals and those with lesions acquired in adulthood (Verhaart 1950, Scales and Collins 1972).

Similarly, MRI studies of individuals with early unilateral brain damage demonstrate an increase in the size of the corticospinal projection from the undamaged hemisphere, accompanied by a shift of cortical sensorimotor functions to the intact hemisphere (Cao et al 1994, Lewine et al 1994, Maegaki et al 1995, Muller et al 1997, Nirkko et al 1997, Graveline et al 1998, Muller et al 1998, Hertz-Pannier 1999, Holloway et al 1999) (Fig. 2.9). Finally, short onset ipsilateral responses, observed bilaterally in individuals with Kallman's syndrome, are associated with significant bilateral hyperplasia of the corticospinal tract (Mayston et al 1997). Taken together these observations support persistence of ipsilateral and contralateral corticospinal projections from the intact hemisphere following unilateral brain damage early in development, which would normally have been withdrawn during subsequent development.

EVIDENCE FOR ACTIVITY-DEPENDENT COMPETITION BETWEEN THE
CORTICOSPINAL PROJECTIONS FROM EACH HEMISPHERE
Different patterns of corticospinal system development after unilateral and bilateral lesions to the corticospinal tract have been reported (Eyre et al 1989, 2000b, 2001). In individuals with spastic hemiplegic cerebral palsy, TMS of the damaged cortex either failed to evoke responses or evoked responses with abnormally high thresholds and prolonged onset latencies. In contrast, responses with relatively short onset latencies and low thresholds were evoked from the intact hemisphere. In individuals with spastic quadriparesis, responses from both hemispheres lay predominantly within the normal range. These observations are consistent with a significant reduction in the corticospinal projection from the damaged hemisphere and an increased projection from the intact hemisphere in individuals with unilateral lesions, whilst those with bilateral lesions maintain qualitatively normal projections from both hemispheres. Furthermore, these observations in man are similar to those obtained experimentally by Martin and his colleagues (Martin and Lee 1999, Martin et al 1999) when studying the kitten to demonstrate activity-dependent competition for synaptic space between the corticospinal projections from each hemisphere (Fig. 2.4).

IPSILESIONAL VERSUS CONTRALESIONAL REORGANIZATION
The exact factors that govern intrahemispheric versus interhemispheric reorganization after sensorimotor lesions during development are not understood. It is likely that reorganization is influenced by overall cortical development and specification at the time of the lesion, the fractional size of the lesion, the availability of sufficient and appropriate

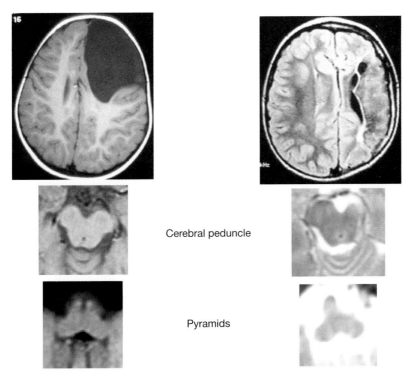

Cerebral peduncle

Pyramids

Fig. 2.9 MRI scans showing the cerebral cortex, cerebral peduncle and pyramids in the same individuals. Both suffered large perinatal infarcts of the right hemisphere and have left hemiparesis. *MRI scan on the left*: the individual had a persisting contralateral response following TMS of the infarcted hemisphere, although the site of origin was located more posteriorly and laterally than in the non-infarcted hemisphere. This individual did not have a fast ipsilateral response evoked following TMS of the undamaged hemisphere and shows no evidence of hypertrophy of the corticospinal projection from that hemisphere on the MRI scan. *MRI scan on the right*: individual with no response following TMS of the infarcted hemisphere and fast ipsilateral and contralateral responses evoked following TMS of the undamaged hemisphere. The MRI scan shows evidence of hypertrophy of the cerebral peduncle and pyramids from the undamaged hemisphere.

juxta-lesional cortex, the absence or presence of transient corticospinal projections (Martin and Lee 1999, Martin et al 1999, Eyre et al 2001), and the maturational status of the system as a whole at the time of the lesion (Eyre et al 2000a).

The temporal limit of plasticity of both the ipsi- and contralesional motor cortices and their corticospinal projections is at present unknown. The existence of critical periods for substantial experience-dependent plasticity has been clearly demonstrated for the visual, auditory and somatosensory systems and for language development in man.

By starting periods of monocular deprivation at progressively older ages, Hubel and Wiesel (1970) first documented that ocular dominance plasticity is confined to a critical period, which in the cat extends from 3 weeks to about 3 months of age. Deprivation-induced plasticity occurs rapidly at the height of the critical period. In the original studies by Hubel and Wiesel (1970) the monocular deprivation lasted for months. In later work, they found that robust effects were observed with as little as one week of deprivation. Subsequent studies by many other investigators showed that as little as eight hours of deprivation can produce synaptic depression in the visual cortex (Bear and Rittenhouse 1999). The neurophysiological consequences are maximal after 48 hours of monocular deprivation in animals at the height of the critical period. It is possible, therefore, that during critical periods, short periods of relative inactivity of motor cortex, induced by ischaemia, or over activity induced by seizures, may lead to permanent plastic changes in the development of the motor cortex and corticospinal projections.

REFERENCES

Anderson S, Kaznowski C, Horn C, Rubenstein J, McConnell S (2002) Distinct origins of neocortical projection neurons and interneurons in vivo. *Cereb Cortex* 12: 702–709.

Balbi P, Trojano L, Ragno M, Perretti A, Santoro L (2000) Patterns of motor control reorganization in a patient with mirror movements. *Clin Neurophysiol* 111: 318–325.

Bates C, Killackey H (1984) The emergence of a discretely distributed pattern of corticospinal projection neurons. *Dev Brain Res* 13: 265–273.

Bear M, Rittenhouse C (1999) Molecular basis for induction of ocular dominance plasticity. *J Neurobiol* 41: 83–91.

Beggs S, Torsney C, Drew L, Fitzgerald M (2002) The postnatal reorganization of primary afferent input and dorsal horn cell receptive fields in the rat spinal cord is an activity-dependent process. *Eur J Neurosci* 16: 1249–1258.

Benecke R, Meyer BU, Freund HJ (1991) Reorganisation of descending motor pathways in patients after hemispherectomy and severe hemispheric lesions demonstrated by magnetic brain stimulation. *Exp Brain Res* 32: 419–426.

Brodmann K (1909) *Vergleichende Lokalisationslehre der Grosshirnrinde in ihren Prinzipien dargestellt auf Grund des Zellenbaues*. Leipzig: Barth.

Cao Y, Vikingstad EM, Huttenlocher PR, Towle VL, Levin DN (1994) Functional magnetic resonance studies of the reorganisation of human sensorimotor area after unilateral brain injury in the perinatal period. *Proc Natl Acad Sci* 91: 9612–9616.

Carr L, Harrison L, Evans A, Stephens J (1993) Patterns of central motor reorganisation in hemiplegic cerebral palsy. *Brain* 166: 1223–1247.

Clowry G, Davies B, Upile N, Gibson C, Bradley P (2004) Spinal cord plasticity in response to unilateral inhibition of the rat motor cortex during development: changes to gene expression, muscle afferents and the ipsilateral corticospinal projection. *Eur J Neurosci* 20: 2555–2566.

Curfs MHJM, Gribnan AAM, Dederen PJWC (1994) Selective elimination of transient corticospinal projections in the rat cervical spinal grey matter. *Brain Res Dev Brain Res* 78: 182–190.

De Carlos J, O'Leary D (1992) Growth and targeting of subplate axons and establishment of major cortical pathways. *J Neurosci* 12: 1192–1211.

Ehlers M (2003) Deconstructing the axon: Wallerian degeneration and the ubiquintin-proteasome system. *Trend Neurosci* 27: 1–60.

Eyre J (2003a) Developmental plasticity of the corticospinal system. In: Boniface S, Ziemann U, editors. *Plasticity of the Nervous System*. Cambridge: Cambridge University Press, pp. 62–91.

Eyre JA (2003b) Development and plasticity of the corticospinal system in man. *Neural Plast* 10: 93–106.

Eyre J (2004) Developmental plasticity of the corticospinal system. In: Boniface S, Ziemann U, editors. *Plasticity of the Human Brain*. Cambridge: Cambridge University Press.

Eyre JA (2005) Developmental aspects of corticospinal projections. In: Eisen A, editor. *Motor Neuron Diseases Handbook of Clinical Neurophysiology*. Amsterdam: Elsevier.

Eyre J, Gibson M, Koh T, Miller S (1989) Corticospinal transmission excited by electromagnetic stimulation of the brain is impaired in children with spastic hemiparesis but not those with quadriparesis. *J Physiol* (Lond) 414: 9.

Eyre J, Miller S, Clowry G, Conway E, Watts C (2000a) Functional corticospinal projections are established prenatally in the human foetus permitting involvement in the development of spinal motor centres. *Brain* 123: 51–64.

Eyre J, Taylor J, Villagra F, Miller S (2000b) Exuberant ipsilateral corticospinal projections are present in the human newborn and withdrawn during development probably involving an activity-dependent process. *Dev Med Child Neurol* 82: 12.

Eyre JA, Miller S, Clowry GJ, Conway EA, Watts C (2000c) Functional corticospinal projections are established prenatally in the human foetus permitting involvement in the development of spinal motor centres. *Brain* 123: 51–64.

Eyre J, Taylor J, Villagra F, Smith M, Miller S (2001) Evidence of activity-dependent withdrawal of corticospinal projections during human development. *Neurology* 57: 1543–1554.

Eyre JA, Miller S, Clowry GJ (2002) The development of the corticospinal tract in humans. In: Pascual-Leone A, Davey G, Rothwell J, Wasserman EM, editors. *Handbook of Transcranial Magnetic Stimulation*. London: Arnold, pp. 235–249.

Galea MP, Darian-Smith I (1995) Postnatal maturation of the direct corticospinal projections in the macaque monkey. *Cereb Cortex* 5: 518–540.

Ghosh A, Shatz C (1992) Involvement of subplate neurons in the formation of ocular dominance columns. *Science* 255: 1441–1443.

Gibson CL, Arnott GA, Clowry GC (2000) Plasticity in the rat spinal cord seen in response to lesions to the motor cortex during development but not to lesions in maturity. *Exp Neurol* 166: 422–434.

Gorgels T (1990) A quantitative analysis of axon outgrowth, axon loss and myelination in the rat pyramidal tract. *Dev Brain Res* 54: 51–61.

Gorgels T, De Kort E, Van Aanholt H, Nieuwenhuys R (1989) A quantitative analysis of the development of the pyramidal tract in the cervical spinal cord in the rat. *Anat Embryol* 179: 377–385.

Graveline C, Mikulis D, Crawley A, Hwang P (1998) Regionalized sensorimotor plasticity after hemispherectomy fMRI evaluation. *Ped Neurol* 19: 337–342.

Gribnau A, de Kort E, Dederen P, Nieuwenhuys R (1986) On the development of the pyramidal tract in the rat. II. An anterograde tracer study of the outgrowth of the corticospinal fibers. *Anat Embryol* (Berl): 175: 101–110.

Hertz-Pannier L (1999) Plasticité au cours de la maturation cérébrale: bases physogiques et étude par IRM fontionelle. *J Neuroradiol* 26: IS66–IS74.

Hicks S, D'Amato C (1970) Motor-sensory and visual behaviour after hemispherectomy in newborn and mature rats. *Exp Neurol* 29: 416–438.

Holloway V, Chong W, Connelly A, Harkness W, Gadian D (1999) Somatomotor fMRI and the presurgical evaluation of a case of focal epilepsy. *Clin Radiol* 54: 301–303.

Hubel D, Wiesel T (1970) Laminar and columnar distribution of geniculocortical fibres in the Macaque monkey. *J Comp Neurol* 146: 421–450.

Humphrey T (1960) The development of the pyramidal tracts in human fetuses, correlated with cortical differentiation. In: Tower DB, Schade JB, editors. *Structure and Function of the Cortex. Proceedings of the Second International Meeting of Neurobiologists*. Amsterdam: Elsevier, pp. 93–103.

Hüppi PS, Warfield S, Kikinis R, Barnes PD, Zientara GP, Jolesz FA, Tsuji MK, Volpe JJ (1998) Quantitative magnetic resonance imaging of brain development in premature and mature newborns. *Ann Neurol* 43: 224–235.

Huttenlocher PR, Raichelson RM (1989) Effects of neonatal hemispherectomy on location and number of corticospinal neurons in the rat. *Dev Brain Res* 47: 59–69.

Inder T, Huppi S, Zientara G, Maier S, Jolesz F, di Salvo D, Robertson R, Barnes P, Volpe J (1999) Early detection of periventricular leukomalacia by diffusion-weighted magnetic resonance imaging techniques. *J Pediatr* 134: 631–634.

Jansen EM, Low WC (1996) Quantitative analysis of contralateral hemisphere hypertrophy and sensorimotor performance in adult rats following unilateral neonatal ischemic-hypoxic brain injury. *Brain Res* 708: 93–99.

Kanold P (2004) Transient microcircuits formed by subplate neurons and their role in functional development of thalamocortical connections. *Neuroreport* 15: 2149–2153.

Kantor D, Kolodkin A (2003) Curbing the excesses of youth: molecular insights into axonal pruning. *Neuron* 38: 849–852.

Koester S, O'Leary D (1992) Functional classes of cortical projection neurons develop dendritic distinctions by class-specific sculpting of an early common pattern. *J Neurosci* 12: 1382–1392.

Konstantinidou AD, Silos-Santiago I, Flaris N, Snider WD (1995) Development of primary afferent projection in the human spinal cord. *J Comp Neurol* 354: 1–12.

Kostovic I, Judas M (2002) Correlation between the sequential ingrowth of afferents and transient patterns of cortical lamination in preterm infants. *Anat Rec* 267: 1–6.

Kostovic I, Rakic P (1990) Developmental history of the transient subplate zone in the visual and somatosensory cortex of the macaque monkey and human brain. *J Comp Neurol* 297: 441–470.

Kultas-Ilinsky K, Fallet C, Verney C (2004) Development of the human motor-related thalamic nuclei during the first half of gestation, with special emphasis on GABAergic circuits. *J Comp Neurol* 476: 267–289.

Levitt P (2003) Structural and functional maturation of the developing primate brain. *J Pediatr* 143 (4 Suppl): S35–S45.

Lewine JD, Astur RS, Davis LE, Knight JE, Maclin EL, Orrison WW (1994) Cortical organization in adulthood is modified by neonatal infarct: a case study. *Radiology* 190: 93–96.

Li Q, Martin J (2001) Postnatal development of corticospinal axon terminal morphology in the cat. *J Comp Neurol* 435: 127–141.

Li Q, Martin J (2002) Postnatal development of connectional specificity of corticospinal terminals in the cat. *J Comp Neurol* 447: 57–71.

McConnell S (1988) Development and decision-making in the mammalian cerebral cortex. *Brain Res* 472: 1–23.

McConnell S (1995) Constructing the cerebral cortex: neurogenesis and fate determination. *Neuron* 15: 761–768.

Maegaki Y, Yamamoto T, Takeshita K (1995) Plasticity of central motor and sensory pathways in a case of unilateral extensive cortical dysplasia. Investigation of magnetic resonance imaging, transcranial magnetic stimulation and short latency somatosensory evoked potentials. *Neurology* 45: 2255–2261.

Marin-Padilla M (1971) Early prenatal ontogenesis of the cerebral cortex (neocortex) of the cat (Felis domestica). A Golgi study. I. The primordial neocortical organization. *Z Anat Entwicklungsgesch* 134: 117–145.

Marin-Padilla M (1972) Prenatal ontogenetic history of the principal neurons of the neocortex of the cat (Felis domestica). A Golgi study. II. Developmental differences and their significances. *Z Anat Entwicklungsgesch* 136: 125–142.

Martin JH, Lee SJ (1999) Activity-dependent competition between developing corticospinal terminations. *Neuroreport* 10: 2277–2282.

Martin JH, Kably B, Hacking A (1999) Activity-dependent development of cortical axon terminations in the spinal cord and brain stem. *Exp Brain Res* 125: 184–199.

Mayston M, Harrison L, Quinton R, Stephens J, Krams M, Bouloux P (1997) Mirror movements in X-linked Kallmann's syndrome. I. A neurophysiological study. *Brain* 120: 1199–1216.

Meng Z, Martin J (2003) Postnatal development of corticospinal postsynaptic action. *J Neurophysiol* 90: 683–692.

Meyer G, Schaaps J, Moreau L, Goffinet A (2000) Embryonic and early fetal development of the human neocortex. *J Neurosci* 20: 1858–1868.

Mrzljak L, Uylings H, Kostovic I, Van Eden C (1988) Prenatal development of neurons in the human prefrontal cortex: I. A qualitative Golgi study. *J Comp Neurol* 271: 355–386.

Mrzljak L, Uylings H, Kostovic I, van Eden C (1992) Prenatal development of neurons in the human prefrontal cortex. *J Comp Neurol* 22: 485–496.

Muller RA, Rothermel RD, Behen ME, Muzik O, Chakraborty PK, Chugani HT (1997) Plasticity of motor organization in children and adults. *Neuroreport* 8: 3103–3108.

Muller RA, Watson CE, Muzik O, Chakraborty PK, Chugani HT (1998) Motor organization after early middle cerebral artery stroke: a PET study. *Pediatr Neurol* 19: 294–298.

Nezu A, Kimura S, Uehara S, Kobayashi T, Tanaka M, Saito K (1997) Maturity of corticospinal pathway and problem of clinical application. *Brain Dev* 19: 176–180.

Nirkko AC, Rosler KM, Ozdoba C, Heid O, Schroth G, Hess CW (1997) Human cortical plasticity. Functional recovery with mirror movements. *Neurology* 48: 1090–1093.

Okado N (1981) Onset of synapse formation in the human spinal cord. *J Comp Neurol* 201: 211–219.

O'Leary D, Koester S (1993) Development of projection neuron types, axon pathways, and patterned connections of the mammalian cortex. *Neuron* 10: 991–1006.

O'Leary D, Nakagawa Y (2002) Patterning centers, regulatory genes and extrinsic mechanisms controlling arealization of the neocortex. *Curr Opin Neurobiol* 12: 14–25.

O'Leary D, Stanfield B (1989) Selective elimination of axons extended by developing cortical neurons is dependent on regional locale: experiments utilizing fetal cortical transplants. *J Neurosci* 9: 2230–2246.

O'Leary D, Schlaggar B, Stanfield B (1992) The specification of sensory cortex: lessons from cortical transplantation. *Exp Neurol* 115: 121–126.

O'Leary D, Borngasser D, Fox K, Schlaggar B (1995) Plasticity in the development of neocortical areas. *Ciba Found Symp* 193: 214–230.

O'Rahily R, Müller F (1994) *The Human Embryonic Brain: An Atlas of Developmental Stages*. New York: Wiley-Liss.

O'Sullivan MC, Miller S, Ramesh V, Conway E, Gilfillan K, McDonough S, et al (1998) Abnormal development of biceps brachii phasic stretch reflex and persistence of short latency heteronymous excitatory responses to triceps brachii in spastic cerebral palsy. *Brain* 121: 2381–2395.

Penn AA, Shatz CJ (1999) Brain waves and brain wiring: the role of endogenous and sensory-driven neural activity in development. *Pediatr Res* 45: 447–458.

Porter F, Grunau R, Anand K (1999) Long-term effects of pain in infants. *J Dev Behav Pediatr* 20: 253–261.

Rakic P (1972) Mode of cell migration to the superficial layers of fetal monkey neocortex. *J Comp Neurol* 145: 61–84.

Rakic P (1974) Neurons in rhesus monkey visual cortex: systematic relation between time of origin and eventual disposition. *Science* 183: 425–427.

Rauschecker J, Korte M (1993) Auditory compensation for early blindness in cat cerebral cortex. *J Neurosci* 13: 4538–4548.

Reinoso BS, Castro AJ (1989) A study of corticospinal remodelling using retrograde fluorescent tracers in rats. *Exp Brain Res* 74: 387–394.

Rickmann M, Wolff J (1981) Differentiation of 'preplate' neurons in the pallium of the rat. *Bibl Anat* 19: 142–146.

Rouiller EM, Liang P, Moret V, Wiesendanger M (1991) Trajectory of redirected corticospinal axons after unilateral lesion of the sensorimotor cortex in neonatal rat; a phaseolus vulgaris-leucoagglutinin (PHA-L) tracing study. *Exp Neurol* 114: 53–65.

Scales DA, Collins GH (1972) Cerebral degeneration with hypertrophy of the contralateral pyramid. *Arch Neurol* 26: 186–190.

Schreyer D, Jones E (1982) Growth and target finding by axons of the corticospinal tract in prenatal and postnatal rats. *Neuroscience* 7: 1837–1853.

Schreyer D, Jones E (1988) Topographical sequence of outgrowth of corticospinal axons in the rat: a study using retrograde axonal labeling with Fast blue. *Dev Brain Res* 38: 89–101.

Shatz C, Ghosh A, McConnell S, Allendoerfer K, Friauf E, Antonini A (1990) Pioneer neurons and target selection in cerebral cortical development. *Cold Spring Habour Symp Quant Biol* 55: 469–480.

Stanfield BB (1992) The development of the corticospinal projection. *Prog Neurobiol* 38: 169–202.

Stanfield BB, O'Leary DD (1985) The transient corticospinal projection from the occipital cortex during postnatal development of the rat. *J Comp Neurol* 238: 236–248.

Stanfield BB, O'Leary DDM, Fricks C (1982) Selective collateral elimination in early postnatal development restricts cortical distribution of rat pyramidal tract neurones. *Nature* 298: 371–373.

Taylor M, Boor R, Ekert P (1996) Preterm maturation of the somatosensory evoked potential. *Electroencephalogr Clin Neurophysiol* 100: 448–452.

Thickbroom G, Byrnes M, Archer S, Nagarajan L, Mastaglia F (2001) Differences in sensory and motor cortical organization following brain injury early in life. *Ann Neurol* 49: 320–327.

Uematsu J, Ono K, Yamano T, Shimanda M (1996) Development of corticospinal tract fibres and their plasticity. II Neonatal unilateral cortical damage and subsequent development of the corticospinal tract in mice. *Brain Dev* 18: 173–178.

Verhaart JWC (1950) Hypertrophy of the pes pedunculi and pyramid as a result of degeneration of the contralateral corticofugal fibre tracts. *J Comp Neurol* 92: 1–15.

Walker S, Meredith-Middleton J, Cooke-Yarborough C, Fitzgerald M (2003) Neonatal inflammation and primary afferent terminal plasticity in the rat dorsal horn. *Pain* 105: 185–195.

Wiesel T, Hubel D (1965) Comparison of the effects of unilateral and bilateral eye closure on cortical unit responses in kittens. *J Neurophysiol* 28: 1029–1040.

Zecevic N, Milosevic A, Rakic S, Marin-Padilla M (1999) Early development and composition of the human primordial plexiform layer: an immunohistochemical study. *J Comp Neurol* 412: 241–254.

Zhou C, Qiu Y, Pereira FA, Crair MC, Tsai SY, Tsai MJ (1999) The nuclear orphan receptor COUP-TFI is required for differentiation of subplate neurons and guidance of thalamocortical axons. *Neuron* 24: 847–859.

3
NEUROLOGICAL ASSESSMENT IN NORMAL YOUNG INFANTS

Eugenio Mercuri, Leena Haataja and Lilly Dubowitz

Since the pioneering work of Saint-Anne Dargassies, who developed an examination based on the evaluation of active and passive tone, there have been a number of methods used for assessing the neurological and neurobehavioural status of the infant after the neonatal period (Andre-Thomas et al 1960, Milani-Comparetti and Gidoni 1967, Touwen 1976, Saint-Anne Dargassies 1977, Baird and Gordon 1983, Ellison et al 1983, Palmer et al 1984, Campbell and Wilheim 1985, Gorga et al 1985, Amiel-Tison and Grenier 1986, Amiel-Tison and Stewart 1989, Nickel et al 1989, Hempel 1993, Kuenzle et al 1994). However, despite the large number of tests available, the search has continued for a neurological examination which could be easily and reliably used in routine clinical settings and which would combine neurological findings with behaviour characteristics and motor milestones (Vohr 1999).

In 1981 we published a method for the neurological assessment of the newborn infant based on a proforma with definitions for performing the test and diagrams to aid recording (Dubowitz and Dubowitz 1981). As this method proved user-friendly in both clinical and research settings, and could be performed and recorded even by relatively inexperienced staff, we aimed to develop a neurological examination, based on the same principles, for use after the neonatal period in infants up to 24 months of age.

Development of the Hammersmith Infant Neurological Examination

The Hammersmith Infant Neurological Examination has now been used in our clinical practice for a number of years and has undergone several modifications. The examination originally included several items evaluating posture, and active and passive tone, but we subsequently also included the assessment of other aspects of neurological status such as cranial nerve function, movements, reflexes and protective reactions. In our latest version (Haataja et al 1999) we also included some items, adapted from the Bayley scales (Bayley 1993), assessing behavioural state, as this may affect the result of the examination. The number and nature of the additional items had to be limited to items which are easily performed and interpreted in clinical settings.

We also included a list of items which reflect the development of gross and fine motor function. The ability to acquire motor milestones is an important part of the neurological development of infants, and their absence is an important sign of abnormal neurological maturation. These developmental items were placed in a separate section of the proforma.

The final version of the proforma consists of 37 items divided into three sections. The first section includes 26 neurological items, the second includes eight items assessing the development of motor function, and the third evaluates behavioural state with three items.

Validation of the examination

The examination was initially designed as a clinical tool to be used as a follow-up assessment for infants above 6 months of age. When we developed this method we felt that the proforma should be structured in a way that could allow users to identify abnormal neurological signs, or at least to detect signs that would require further assessment.

In order to standardize the examination, we assessed a cohort of 135 low-risk term infants at 12 and 18 months, who had been recruited at birth, had normal neonatal neurological investigation and normal cranial ultrasound, and had no known perinatal risk factors, and thus were regarded as the optimal study population (Dubowitz et al 1998, Mercuri et al 1998, Dubowitz et al 1999). All the examinations were performed between 11 and 19.5 months of age (92 infants at the mean age of 12.2 months and 43 infants at the mean age of 18.2 months), and the results were analysed calculating the frequency distribution of the findings observed in each item (Haataja et al 1999).

The first section with 26 neurological items was then redesigned on the basis of the findings of this study. Column 1 represents those most frequently seen in the normal population (75 per cent or more), while those in column 2 are seen less frequently (in 25 per cent or less but in more than 10 per cent), and the findings in columns 3 and 4 are those seen in 10 per cent or less. An isolated finding outside column 1 or 2 does not always indicate a neurological abnormality, but rather that the finding observed is not that commonly observed in a low-risk population and therefore should be reassessed. The risk of neurological abnormalities, however, increases in parallel to the increasing number of findings in column 3 and 4.

Our results recorded at 12 and 18 months showed no age-dependency in the items included in the main section (section 1) (Haataja et al 1999). We subsequently decided to validate the examination in infants younger than 10 months, aiming to establish to what extent the items are age-dependent. We therefore applied the infant neurological examination to a cohort of 74 healthy term infants assessed between 12 and 32 weeks (Haataja et al 2003). The examination was not performed in infants below 12 weeks, as many items, such as posture in sitting and head control, depend on maturity, and are not suitable for younger infants.

We found that while all the infants examined between 28 and 32 weeks showed similar findings to those assessed between 11 and 19 months, infants examined before 6 months showed some differences, mainly related to immature axial tone and incomplete development of saving reactions (Haataja et al 2003).

Timing and sequence of the examination

The examination has to be performed while the infant is awake and vigilant. The posture and tone items should optimally be tested with the infant lying on a mat. The examiner is allowed to use toys to try to engage the child's confidence and cooperation. With the

25

exception of cranial nerve assessment, the examination should be performed with the child undressed, with only a nappy on. The examiner is encouraged to record the items in sequence, in order to avoid failing to record any of the items. However, the flow of the examination has to be adapted to the clinical situation. If the child dislikes being handled, making particular items difficult to assess, it is worth retrying after a short break.

Performing and scoring the examination

The response to any item is indicated by circling the particular item. If a response does not fall clearly into one of the options offered, but falls between two options, then mark across the vertical line dividing the two. In case of asymmetry, mark the observation separately for the left and right side (in many boxes left (L) and right (R) are readily marked). An additional column on the right-hand side of the proforma makes it possible to draw attention to asymmetry of response. In particular items there are two drawings in the same box. In this case mark the one closest to what is seen. In case of deviation from given responses, draw the deviation on the figures. The summary space on the front page of the proforma is reserved for any specific comments on the examination or the infant's somatic status (e.g. respiratory infection, medication, etc.). In the following section we define the items in detail and illustrate the individual neurological criteria.

Section 1: Neurological examination

ASSESSMENT OF CRANIAL NERVE FUNCTION

Examination of the infant's cranial nerve function begins by observing spontaneous *facial appearance* during the assessment. Facial expressions are observed for integrity or asymmetry (cranial nerve 7). *Eye movements and visual responsivity* (cranial nerves 2, 3, 4 and 6) should be formally assessed by getting the infant to follow a target (e.g. a red ball) in a circular manner. The *auditory response* (cranial nerve 8) should be tested by producing a sound (e.g. a rattle) out of the baby's sight, and observing the reaction. Despite positive reactions, we strongly recommend a formal hearing test for all infants. Parents are asked in detail about possible problems with *sucking and swallowing* during daily feeds, as well as the presence of excessive dribbling (cranial nerves 5, 7, 9, 10 and 12). The items assessed in the cranial nerve subsection do not change with age.

In a complete neurological assessment, the pupillary light reflex, corneal reflex, gag reflex and funduscopic examination should also be performed.

ASSESSMENT OF POSTURE

The posture items 'in sitting' are meant to be assessed while the infant sits with a slight support at the hips or on their own.

The *head posture* in sitting is judged by the overall performance of the infant during the whole assessment.

Age-dependent changes: The findings in this item change with age. In our cohort, by 16 weeks of age more than 90 per cent of the infants were able to keep the head upright and the chin in the midline related to the chest (column 1).

TABLE 3.1
Assessment of cranial nerve function

	Column 1 (score 3)	Column 2 (score 2)	Column 3 (score 1)	Column 4 (score 0)
Facial appearance (at rest and when crying or stimulated)	smiles or reacts to stimuli by closing eyes and grimacing		closes eyes but not tightly, poor facial expression	expressionless, does not react to stimuli
Eye appearance	normal conjugated eye movements		Intermittent deviation of eyes or abnormal movements	Continuous deviation of eyes or abnormal movements
Auditory response test the response to rattle or bell	reacts to stimuli on both sides		doubtful reaction to stimuli or asymmetrical	does not react to stimuli
Visual response test the ability to follow a red ball or moving object	follows the object for a complete arc		follows the object for an incomplete arc *or* asymmetry	does not follow the object
Sucking/ swallowing watch the infant suck on breast or bottle	good suck and swallowing		poor suck and/or swallowing	no sucking reflex, no swallowing

Head posture

	1	2	3		4	
In sitting	straight; in midline		slightly to side *or* backward *or* forward		markedly to side *or* backward *or* forward	

Trunk posture

	1	2	3	4
In sitting (hold at hips if unstable)	straight		slightly curved or bent to side	very rounded, rocketing back, or bent sideways

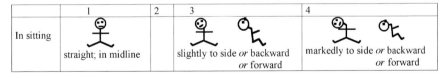

The *trunk posture* in sitting has to be judged for its possible roundness and asymmetry or midline deviation.

Age-dependent changes: The findings in this item change with age. In our cohort all the infants scored in columns 1 (87 per cent) or 2 (13 per cent) by 28 weeks of age.

27

Arm posture

	1	2	3	4
At rest	in neutral position, central straight *or* slightly bent		*slight* internal rotation *or* external rotation	*marked* internal rotation *or* external rotation *or* dystonic posture hemiplegic posture

The *arm posture* refers to the observed spontaneous posture of the infant's arms.

Hand posture

	1	2	3	4
	hands open		*intermittent* adducted thumb *or* fisting	*persistent* adducted thumb *or* fisting

The *hand posture* refers to the observed most prevalent spontaneous hand position during the assessment.

Age-dependent changes: The findings in the items assessing arm and hand posture do not change with age. More than 90 per cent of infants in our cohort had findings in column 1 irrespective of their age.

Leg posture

	1	2	3	4
In sitting		able to sit with straight back and legs straight or knees slightly flexed (long sitting)	able to sit with straight back but knees flexed at 15–20 degrees	unable to sit straight unless knees markedly flexed
In supine and in standing	legs in neutral position, straight *or* slightly bent	*slight* external rotation	*marked* internal rotation *or* external rotation at hips	fixed extension or flexion *or* contractures at hips and knees

The *leg posture* is assessed in long sitting, i.e. with the infant sitting on a flat surface with legs out straight in front of him/her. The ability to keep legs out straight without, or with, flexed knees is observed, recording the angle of the flexed knees as well as the straightness of the back.

Age-dependent changes: The findings in this item change with age. In our cohort more than 90 per cent of infants had findings in columns 1 or 2 by the age of 28 weeks.

Foot posture

	1	2	3	4
In supine and in standing	central in neutral position toes straight midway between flexion and extension	*slight* internal rotation *or* external rotation	*intermittent* tendency to stand on tiptoes *or* toes up *or* curling under	*marked* internal rotation *or* external rotation at the ankle *persistent* tendency to stand on tiptoes *or* toes up or curling under

In the *foot posture* some rotation of the forefoot is frequently observed (column 2), but generally this comes from the hip, and is not genuinely present at the ankle. The persistent tendency to have toes up or curled under the forefoot or to stand on tiptoes (column 4) is abnormal at any age.

Foot posture is tested both in supine and in standing posture. The infant is held in the standing position (usually by 5 to 6 months of age the baby fully supports his weight) or stands unassisted.

Age-dependent changes: In our cohort more than 90 per cent of infants had findings in column 1 irrespective of their age.

ASSESSMENT OF MOVEMENTS

Movements

	1	2	3	4
Quantity watch infant lying in supine	normal		excessive *or* sluggish	minimal *or* none
Quality	free, alternating, smooth		jerky, slight tremor	• cramped & synchronous • extensor spasms • athetoid • ataxic • very tremulous • myoclonic spasm • dystonic movement

These items are based on the examiner's observations of the infant's spontaneous voluntary motor activity during the course of the assessment. For the judgement to be reliable, the infant should be observed not only in the supine position but also when performing voluntary tasks. The examiner has to score separately the quantity and quality of movements, since, for example, the quantity can be within normal limits but the quality abnormal. In

29

our cohort the majority of infants scored in column 1 in both items irrespective of age at testing.

ASSESSMENT OF MUSCLE TONE

This section of the examination should be performed with the child lying on a mat.

Scarf sign

	1	2	3	4
Take the infant's hand and pull the arm across the chest until there is resistance. Note the position of the elbow	Range: R L R L		R L	R L or R L

The *scarf sign* assesses the tone of the shoulder girdle. The arm is pulled across the chest gently but firmly until there is resistance. The child's head is kept in the midline and the position of the elbow is recorded. Note if the elbow comes as far as the outer border of the chest (column 3), to the middle of the ipsilateral side of the chest, to the midline, or crosses the midline to the middle of the contralateral side (mark as appropriate in column 1).

Age-dependent changes: The findings in this item do not change with age. In our cohort more than 90 per cent of the infants tested from the age of 12 weeks onwards scored in column 1.

Passive shoulder elevation

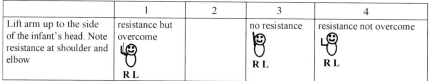

	1	2	3	4
Lift arm up to the side of the infant's head. Note resistance at shoulder and elbow	resistance but overcome R L		no resistance R L	resistance not overcome R L

Passive shoulder elevation is performed by holding the arm at the wrist and lifting it up to the side of the head. Record the resistance felt at shoulder and elbow. If some resistance is met which can easily be overcome, score in column 1. If there is almost no resistance to this manoeuvre and the arm goes straight up, score in column 3. If the resistance cannot be overcome, score in column 4. It is a good idea to repeat the shoulder elevation two or three times to feel for possible asymmetry.

Age-dependent changes: The findings in this item show little change with age. In our cohort the findings in column 2 were relatively common between 12 and 16 weeks of age, but thereafter the majority of findings were in column 1.

Forearm supination and pronation are scored by the resistance felt while rotating the forearm. The upper arm should be steadied.

Forearm pronation/supination

	1	2	3	4
Steady upper arm while pronating and supinating forearm, note resistance	full pronation and supination, no resistance		full pronation and supination but resistance to be overcome	full pronation and supination not possible, marked resistance

Age-dependent changes: The findings in this item show little change with age. In our cohort the findings in column 3 were relatively common between 12 and 16 weeks of age, but thereafter the majority of findings were in column 1.

Hip adduction

	1	2	3	4
With the infant's legs extended, open them as far as possible The angle formed by the legs is noted	**Range: 150°–80°** R L R L	150°–160° R L	>170° R L	<80° R L

Hip adduction assessment requires the child to be lying horizontal, ideally with a loosened nappy. The legs must be kept straight and in the midline, and then gently abducted as far as possible. The angle formed by the legs is scored. This manoeuvre tests adductor tightness.

Age-dependent changes: The findings in this item show little change with age. In our cohort tested from 12 weeks onwards the majority of findings were in column 1.

Popliteal angle

	1	2	3	4
Legs are flexed at the hip simultaneously on to the abdomen, then extended at the knee until there is resistance Note angle between lower and upper leg	**Range: 150°–110°** R L R L	150°–160° R L	~90° or >170° R L R L	<80° R L

Popliteal angle is scored with the child in the supine position, preferably without a nappy. The hips are flexed simultaneously so that the anterior aspect of the thighs is lying on the abdomen, making sure, at the same time, to keep the child's bottom touching the bed (if the bottom is allowed to lift up, the measured popliteal angle will be bigger). The lower legs are extended at the knees as far as possible and the angle between the lower and upper leg is recorded. This manoeuvre especially tests the hamstring tightness.

Age-dependent changes: The findings in this item change with age; the finding in column 3 (~90°) is relatively frequent until 24 weeks of age, but afterwards more than 90 per cent of the infants in our cohort scored in column 1.

Ankle dorsiflexion

	1	2	3	4
With knee extended, dorsiflex ankle. Note the angle between foot and leg	**Range: 30°–85°** ↘ ↘ R L R L	20°–30° ↘ R L	<20°or 90° ↘ ⌐ R L R L	>90° ⌐ R L

Ankle dorsiflexion has to be scored with the leg straight at the knee and hip. The knee is held down by the examiner placing their hand on top of it; at the same time their other hand is placed flat on the sole of the foot and the ankle is dorsiflexed maximally. The angle between the foot and leg is scored. It is a good idea to repeat the dorsiflexion if the child pushes intentionally against in order to feel for possible asymmetry.

Age-dependent changes: The findings in this item do not change with age. In our cohort more than 90 per cent of the infants tested from the age of 12 weeks onwards scored in column 1.

Pull to sit

	1	2	3	4
Pull infant to sit by wrists				

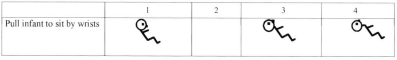

Pull to sit (a traction manoeuvre) is performed by holding the child by the wrists and pulling them gently towards the sitting position. The position of the head (take the ear as a reference) in relation to the shoulder and body is observed while pulling up.

Age-dependent changes: The findings in this item show little change with age after 16 weeks. In our cohort the findings in column 3 were relatively common between 12 and 16 weeks of age, but thereafter the majority of findings were in column 1.

Ventral suspension

	1	2	3	4
Hold infant in ventral suspension; note position of back, limbs and head				

Ventral suspension is performed by holding the infant around the abdomen and lifting him up horizontally. The flexion of limbs and the position of the back (straight/rounded) and head are observed.

Age-dependent changes: The findings in this item do not change with age after 12 weeks. In our cohort more than 90 per cent of the infants scored in column1.

This section does not include a complete list of all testable reflexes and reactions at infant age. Less experienced examiners often find these items difficult to perform and interpret; the infant's state can influence the responses and thus the inter-observer reliability may remain unacceptably low. The items selected for inclusion in our examination have been chosen based on our clinical experience of how best to avoid the above problems, while still keeping certain items with clinical value in differentiating deviant development.

Tendon reflexes

	1	2	3	4
	easily elicitable biceps knee ankle	mildly brisk biceps knee ankle	brisk biceps knee ankle	clonus or absent biceps knee ankle

To elicit the deep *tendon reflexes* the examiner has to be careful to catch the extremity at rest. It is preferable to use the reflex hammer for testing, but if the infant is apprehensive it may be better to tap sharply with the fingers when the child relaxes. The tendon reflexes are scored for their elicitability, and it is important to note any asymmetry.

Age-dependent changes: The findings in this item do not change with age.

Arm protection

	1	2	3	4
Pull the infant by one arm from the supine position and note the reaction of the opposite side	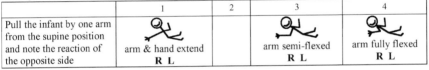arm & hand extend **R L**		arm semi-flexed **R L**	arm fully flexed **R L**

Arm protection precedes the postural reflex of lateral propping. To perform the test the infant lies supine and the flat of the examiner's hand is placed on one hip. With the other hand, the child is pulled up by his contralateral wrist, and it should be observed whether he puts his free arm down on the mat/examination bed to support himself. The test is repeated the other way around to test the other side.

Age-dependent changes: The findings in this item change with age. Although this reaction can be observed even under 1 month of age, it is only consistent from the age of 3–4 months onwards.

Even though it is not scored in this examination, we also recommend that the examiner tests the lateral saving reaction (protective extension) from the age of 5 months onwards. The lateral saving reaction occurs when the infant is falling to one side or other in the sitting position and extends the arm laterally to catch himself. Persistent asymmetry of the reactions (both arm protection and lateral saving reflex) can be early signs of hemiparesis.

Kicking in vertical suspension is performed by holding the child vertically just under the armpits, with his back to the examiner so that he can see the carer, and see whether he kicks his legs equally and well. Sometimes one has to get someone to tickle his feet to encourage a response. At later ages (>18 months) infants may not kick much. The purpose

Kicking in vertical suspension

	1	2	3	4
Hold infant under axilla, make sure legs do not touch any surface	kicks symmetrically		kicks one leg more or poor kicking	no kicking even if stimulated or scissoring

is mainly to look for subtle differences: whether the kicking is asymmetrical (column 3) or totally absent (column 4).

Age-dependent changes: The findings in this item do not change with age, and more than 90 per cent of the infants in our cohort had findings in column 1. The finding in column 4 is abnormal at any age.

Lateral tilting

	1	2	3	4
With infant held vertically, tilt quickly to horizontal Note spine, limbs and head (describe side up)	R L	R L	R L	R L

Lateral tilting is performed by holding the child just above the hips (not high under the armpits), with his back towards the examiner so that the infant is facing the carer. While tilting the infant from vertical to horizontal, the response of the upper side trunk muscles and head and limb positions are observed. If the infant does not have muscle strength and tone to produce antigravity movement, he flops when tilted (column 4).

Age-dependent changes: The findings in this item change with age. In our cohort more than 90 per cent of infants scored in columns 1 or 2 after 28 weeks of age. Note the particularly large normal variation in this item; 16 per cent of low-risk infants scored in column 2 at the mean age of 12 months (Haataja et al 1999).

Forward parachute reflex

	1	2	3	4
With infant held vertically, suddenly tilt forwards Note reaction of the arms	symmetrical, positive		partial/asymmetrical reaction	no reaction

The *forward parachute reflex* is one of the postural reflexes, which is stimulated by holding the infant just above the waist and tilting him forward towards a mat.

Age-dependent changes: The findings in this item change with age. The reaction is age-dependent, and starts appearing from 5–6 months onwards, and is usually repeatedly positive by 9 months in a normal child. The examiner should also observe for symmetry of the extending hands.

ASYMMETRIES

Mild asymmetrical findings (maximum of one column difference), especially in tone and reflexes/reactions items, are quite common as transient aberrant signs in infancy. However, marked asymmetry even in one examination and sustained asymmetry of any degree in the follow-up assessments should be reassessed.

Section 2: Developmental milestones

Head control	unable to maintain head upright (normal <3 m)	wobbles (normal at 4 m)	all the time maintained upright (normal at 5 m)			
Sitting	cannot sit	with support at hips (normal at 4 m)	props (normal at 6 m)	stable sit (normal at 7–8 m)	pivots (rotates) (normal at 9 m)	Observed: Reported (age):
Voluntary grasp	no grasp	uses whole hand	index finger and thumb but immature grasp	pincer grasp		Observed: Reported (age):
Ability to kick (in supine)	no kicking	kicks horizontally, legs do not lift	upward (vertically) (normal at 3 m)	touches leg (normal at 4–5 m)	touches toes (normal at 5–6 m)	Observed: Reported (age):
Rolling	no rolling	rolling to side (normal at 4 m)	prone to supine	supine to prone		Observed: Reported (age):
Crawling	does not lift head	on elbow (normal at 3 m)	on outstretched hand (normal at 4 m)	crawling flat on abdomen (normal at 8 m)	crawling on hands and knees (normal at 10 m)	Observed: Reported (age):
Standing	does not support weight	supports weight (normal at 4 m)	stands with support (normal at 7 m)	stands unaided (normal at 12 m)		Observed: Reported (age):
Walking		bouncing (normal at 6 m)	cruising (walks holding on) (normal at 12 m)	walking independently (normal at 15 m)		Observed: Reported (age):

This section includes eight items which document developmental progress. These items are not scored but they can act as an *aide-mémoire* for clinical work. They also give valuable information about the infant's motor progress in follow-up. The items may be recorded in two ways: as reported by the caretaker, and as observed by the examiner. The strips were

35

designed according to the gradient of normal maturation. The normative values in these strips are adapted from Illingworth's work (Illingworth 1991). As these items are age-dependent and we only have the frequency distribution for infants at 12 and 18 months of age, it was not possible to score these findings using the same method as for the items in section 1.

Section 3: Behaviour

State of consciousness	unrousable	drowsy	sleepy but wakes easily	awake but no interest	loses interest	maintains interest
Emotional state	irritable, not consolable	irritable, mother can console	irritable when approached	neither happy nor unhappy	happy, smiling	
Social orientation	avoiding, withdrawn	hesitant	accepts approach	friendly		

This section includes three items evaluating behavioural state, adapted from the Bayley scales (Bayley 1993). These are graded into 4, 5 and 6 columns respectively and scored according to the number of the column circled.

Optimality scores

When we validated the examination in a cohort of low-risk full-term infants tested at 12 and 18 months, we also devised an optimality score mainly for research purposes. The optimality score is based on the distribution frequency of the findings observed in full-term infants examined at 12 and 18 months. The scoring system has been devised so that for each item a score of 3 is given to the finding in column 1, a score of 2 to column 2, a score of 1 to column 3, and a score of 0 to column 4. If the finding falls between two columns, it is given the appropriate half-score between the columns (e.g. an item falling between score 1 and 2 is scored 1.5). In the case of asymmetry the left and right side are scored separately, and the mean of the separate scores is taken as the score of this particular item.

The examination is constructed to give subscores of all the tested subsections (cranial nerves, posture, movements, tone, reflexes and reactions), and the global optimality score is achieved by adding up all the scores from individual items. Thus the global score can vary from a minimum of 0 to a maximum of 78. Based on the calculated frequency distribution of the global scores at 12 and 18 months, the optimality was set at or above the 10th percentile, and suboptimality below the 10th percentile. Accordingly, a global score equal to or above 73 was regarded as optimal at 12 months, and a global score equal to or above 74 at 18 months (Haataja et al 1999).

We have subsequently examined 74 infants aged between 3 and 8 months in order to establish whether the optimality scoring system could be applied to younger infants. Our results suggest that the optimality scoring system developed for infants at 12 and 18 months should not be applied in infants younger than 6 months, as many items show age-dependent changes, and that it should also be used with caution in infants aged between 6 and 9 months, as a few items will still have a wider variability (Haataja et al 2003).

REFERENCES

Amiel-Tison C, Grenier A (1986) *Neurological Assessment During the First Years of Life.* New York: Oxford University Press.

Amiel-Tison C, Stewart A (1989) Follow up studies during the first five years of life: a pervasive assessment of neurological function. *Arch Dis Child* 64: 496–502.

Andre-Thomas A, Chesni Y, Saint-Anne Dargassies S (1960) *The Neurological Examination of the Infant.* Clinics in Developmental Medicine 1. London: Heinemann.

Baird HW, Gordon EC (1983) *Neurological Evaluation of Infants and Children.* Clinics in Developmental Medicine 84/85. London: Heinemann.

Bayley N (1993) *Bayley Scales of Infant Development, 2nd edn.* San Antonio: The Psychological Corporation (BSID-II).

Campbell SK, Wilheim IJ (1985) Development from birth to 3 years of age of 15 children at high risk for central nervous system dysfunction. *Phys Ther* 65: 463–469.

Dubowitz L, Dubowitz V (1981) *The Neurological Assessment of the Preterm and Full Term Infant.* Clinics in Developmental Medicine 79. London: Heinemann.

Dubowitz L, Mercuri E, Dubowitz V (1998) An optimality score for the neurologic examination of the term newborn. *J Pediatr* 133: 406–416.

Dubowitz L, Dubowitz V, Mercuri E (1999) *The Neurological Assessment of the Preterm and Full Term Newborn Infant, 2nd edn.* Clinics in Developmental Medicine 148. London: Mac Keith Press.

Ellison PH, Browning CA, Larson B, Denny J (1983) Development of a scoring system for the Milani-Comparetti and Gidoni method of assessing neurologic abnormality in infancy. *Phys Ther* 63: 1414–1423.

Gorga D, Stern FM, Ross G (1985) Trends in neuromotor behavior of preterm and fullterm infants in the first year of life: a preliminary report. *Dev Med Child Neurol* 27: 756–766.

Haataja L, Mercuri E, Regev R, Cowan F, Rutherford M, Dubowitz V, Dubowitz L (1999) Optimality score for the neurologic examination of the infant at 12 and 18 months of age. *J Pediatr* 135: 153–161.

Haataja L, Cowan F, Mercuri E, Bassi L, Guzzetta A, Dubowitz L (2003) Application of a scorable neurologic examination in healthy term infants aged 3 to 8 months. *J Pediatr* 143: 546. (Letter.)

Hempel MS (1993) The neurological examination for toddler-age. Thesis, University of Groningen, Holland.

Illingworth RS (1991) *The Normal Child, 10th edn.* Edinburgh: Churchill Livingstone.

Kuenzle C, Baenziger O, Martin E, Thun-Hohenstein L, Steinlin M, Good M, et al (1994) Prognostic value of early MR imaging in term infants with severe perinatal asphyxia. *Neuropediatrics* 4: 191–200.

Mercuri E, Dubowitz L, Paterson-Brown S, Cowan F (1998) Incidence of cranial ultrasound abnormalities in apparently well neonates on a postnatal ward: correlation with antenatal and perinatal factors and neurological status. *Arch Dis Child Fetal Neonatal Ed* 79: F185–F189.

Milani-Comparetti A, Gidoni EA (1967) Routine developmental examination in normal and retarded children. *Dev Med Child Neurol* 9: 631–638.

Nickel RE, Renken CA, Gallenstein JS (1989) The Infant Motor Screen. *Dev Med Child Neurol* 31: 35–42.

Palmer FB, Shapiro BK, Wachtel RC, Ross A, Accardo PJ (1984) Primitive Reflex Profile: a quantitation of primitive reflexes in infancy. *Dev Med Child Neurol* 24: 375–383.

Saint-Anne Dargassies S (1977) *Neurological Development in the Full-term and Premature Neonate.* Amsterdam: Elsevier.

Touwen B (1976) *Neurological Development in Infancy.* Clinics in Developmental Medicine 58. London: Heinemann.

Vohr BR (1999) The quest for the ideal neurologic assessment for infants and young children. *J Pediatr* 135: 140–142. (Editorial.)

4
CLASSICAL NEUROLOGICAL EXAMINATION IN YOUNG INFANTS WITH NEONATAL BRAIN LESIONS

Eugenio Mercuri, Leena Haataja, Daniela Ricci, Frances Cowan and Lilly Dubowitz

The Hammersmith Infant Neurological Examination has been used for over 20 years as a clinical tool in the follow-up of newborns at risk of neurological sequelae, such as preterm infants and full-term infants with neonatal encephalopathy or with other congenital or acquired brain lesions (Dubowitz et al 1998). The sequential use of the examination, which is easy to perform and facilitates reliable recording of the findings, has allowed the natural evolution of neurological signs to be better understood both in infants with normal neurological development and in those with neurological abnormalities. Using the clinical examination in combination with brain imaging and neurophysiological techniques we have also been able to identify specific clinical patterns associated with different types of brain lesions (Mercuri et al 1999a, Haataja et al 2001, Frisone et al 2002). This has proved to be particularly useful not only in following the evolution of abnormal neurological signs associated with specific lesions, but also in documenting when abnormal signs are no longer seen or when abnormal neurological signs appear in infants with brain lesions in whom cerebral palsy or other neurological abnormalities may become obvious after a clinically silent interval (Bouza et al 1994).

The examination was originally developed with the primary aim that inspection of the proforma would help to identify deviant signs in the clinic, but subsequently we devised a scoring system with ranges for optimal scores and different levels of suboptimality mainly for use in a research setting (Haataja et al 1999). The introduction of a quantitative scoring system has allowed a better correlation between the severity of neurological findings and neuroimaging, and has also provided interesting data on the prognostic value of the examination. Our main experience has been in full-term infants with focal infarction and neonatal encephalopathy, and in preterm infants with and without brain lesions.

Hypoxic-ischaemic encephalopathy
Perinatal hypoxic-ischaemic events are the major cause of morbidity in term infants with neonatal encephalopathy (Cowan et al 2003, Pierrat et al 2005). Our experience is that most of these infants have no evidence of antenatal lesions on brain MRI, but do have a significant increase in perinatal risks compared to controls, suggesting a perinatal hypoxic-ischaemic event. These infants have often been labelled as suffering from hypoxic-ischaemic encephalopathy (HIE) (Sarnat and Sarnat 1976). Our definition of HIE is that of neurological abnormalities in the first 48 hours after evidence of fetal distress, i.e. meconium-stained

liquor and/or cardiotocographic abnormalities, and low Apgar scores (below 4 at 1 minute and below 7 at 5 minutes) (Mercuri et al 2002) and low cord pH (below 7.1).

Several studies have shown that the presence and the severity of neonatal neurological abnormalities in these infants are related to the pattern of lesions on brain MRI (Rutherford et al 1996, Mercuri et al 1999a), but less has been reported about the evolution of clinical signs in the first year. In our experience, infants who had neonatal HIE but who had a normal brain MRI or mild white matter changes may have minor neurological abnormalities in the first two weeks after birth but they have normal examinations when examined after the third week and throughout the first two years (Dubowitz et al 1998, Mercuri et al 1999a). These infants all have a normal outcome. At the other end of the spectrum, infants with severe basal ganglia lesions, with or without associated white matter lesions, show abnormal axial and limb tone, reduced visual alertness and poor sucking in the first weeks after birth and these abnormalities persist when examined at 5–7 weeks, 6 and 12 months (Fig. 4.1) (Dubowitz et al 1998, Ricci et al 2006).

The group of infants with less severe basal ganglia or with diffuse white matter changes, in contrast, show a different evolution of neurological signs (Fig. 4.2). Although these infants also show reduced axial and limb tone, reduced visual alertness and often poor sucking in the first weeks after birth, the examination performed at 5–7 weeks shows a marked improvement of limb tone, vision and sucking. While sucking and vision, however, remain normal or with minimal abnormalities at 6 and 12 months, limb tone, which appears to be normal at 5–7 weeks, is often found to be increased between 3 and 6 months. These findings suggest that the apparent improvement noted at 5–7 weeks is only a transient phase at the time when the tone changes from hypotonia to hypertonia.

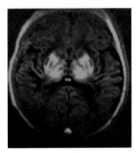

Axial tone				Limb tone				Movements				Sucking				Vision			
1-2 w	5-7 w	6 m	12 m	1-2 w	5-7 w	6 m	12 m	1-2 w	5-7 w	6 m	12 m	1-2 w	5-7 w	6 m	12 m	1-2 w	5-7 w	6 m	12 m
▼	▼	▼	▼	▼	▲	▲	▲	●	●	●	●	●	●	●	●	●	●	●	●

Fig. 4.1 Sequential examinations at 1–2 weeks, 5–7 weeks, 6 months and 12 months in a child with severe basal ganglia lesions. Note that axial tone, movements, sucking and vision remain persistently abnormal throughout all the examinations. Limb tone also remains abnormal but changes from hypotonia in the first two weeks to increased tone from 5 weeks onwards. (○ = normal, ● = abnormal, ▼ = decreased, ▲ = increased)

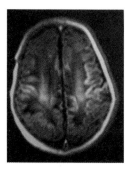

Axial tone				Limb tone				Movements				Sucking				Vision			
1-2 w	5-7 w	6 m	12 m	1-2 w	5-7 w	6 m	12 m	1-2 w	5-7 w	6 m	12 m	1-2 w	5-7 w	6 m	12 m	1-2 w	5-7 w	6 m	12 m
▼	○	▼	▼	▼	○	▲	▲	●	○	●	●	●	○	○	○	●	○	○	○

Fig. 4.2 Sequential examinations at 1–2 weeks, 5–7 weeks, 6 months and 12 months in a child with severe white matter lesions. Note that axial tone, movements, sucking and vision are all abnormal on the examination performed at 1–2 weeks, but limb tone, sucking and vision appear to normalize at 5–7 weeks. At 6 months, however, while sucking and vision are still normal, limb tone is increased. (○ = normal, ● = abnormal, ▼ = decreased, ▲ = increased)

These findings highlight the importance of performing sequential neurological examinations in order to follow the evolution of clinical signs, and suggest that caution should be exercised in counselling parents when assessing infants with such lesions at 5–7 weeks of age, when the neurological examination may only show a slightly reduced axial tone and mild abnormalities in movements.

OPTIMALITY SCORES IN INFANTS WITH HIE

We have applied the optimality scoring system to the examinations performed between 9 and 14 months in a cohort of 53 term infants with hypoxic-ischaemic encephalopathy (HIE) (Haataja et al 2001). (For details of the scoring system see Chapter 3, p. 36.)

Thirty-one out of the 53 infants examined had an optimal total score (73 or above), and 22 had a suboptimal score (under 73). The distribution of scores was related to the pattern of lesions on neonatal MRI. The scores were always optimal in the infants with normal or minor neonatal MRI findings, but the scores decreased with increasing severity of basal ganglia involvement. The lowest scores were found in the infants with the most severe basal ganglia and white matter lesions, while infants with diffuse white matter lesions but normal basal ganglia had intermediate scores. Table 4.1 shows the range and median of the optimality scores in the various imaging subgroups.

The use of the optimality score also provided useful prognostic information on the severity of the functional outcome. In our study, global scores between 67 and 78 were always found in infants who achieved independent ambulation by 2 years, while scores between 40 and 67 predicted restricted mobility. None of the infants with scores under 40 were able to sit unsupported at 2 or 4 years.

TABLE 4.1
Range and median scores of the neurological examination and neonatal MRI findings

MRI finding	Median score	Range of the scores
Normal (n=16)	78	74.5–78
Moderate WM (n=6)	77.5	75–78
Minimal BG (n=10)	77.5	70–78
Moderate BG (n=5)	57	40.5–76
Moderate WM and BG (n=3)	47.5	26–69
Severe WM (n=4)	59	45.5–70
Severe WM haemorrhages (n=2)	52	39–65
Severe BG and diffuse WM (n=5)	25	15.5–34.5
Severe BG/subcortical WM (n=2)	14.5	10.5–18.5

BG = basal ganglia; WM = white matter

Cerebral infarction

Neonatal cerebral infarction or stroke can be defined as a sudden severe ischaemic insult usually to grey and white matter caused by embolic, thrombotic or ischaemic events. In the last two decades, as a result of the wider availability of brain imaging in neonates, cerebral infarction has been shown to be more common than previously estimated (Mercuri et al 1999b). The population-based data from Estan and Hope (1997) give an incidence of 1 in 4000 term infants, but this was based on ultrasound and CT assessment of the lesions in a group of infants requiring admission to a neonatal intensive care unit and is almost certainly an underestimate of the incidence. De Vries's data suggest that focal lesions of this nature occur in 1 per cent of the preterm population (de Vries et al 1997). Lesions in the territory of the middle cerebral artery are the most common type of infarction in full-term infants and, as observed in adult stroke, the left side is three to four times more often affected than the right.

Hemiplegia is the typical motor sequela in infants with focal infarction. The incidence of hemiplegia reported in various studies, however, is very variable, ranging from 8 to 100 per cent of the cases, the difference probably reflecting the population studied – from our experience only infants with infarction affecting cerebral hemispheric tissue as well as the basal ganglia and the posterior limb of the internal capsule will develop hemiplegia (Mercuri et al 1999b, 2004, Boardman et al 2005). Unfortunately most studies do not relate the occurrence of hemiplegia to a detailed description of the tissue involved. In our studies, which are not population-based and obtained from term infants mainly presenting with seizures, between 20 and 30 per cent of infants with infarction develop hemiplegia.

Previous studies have reported that infants with so-called congenital hemiplegia may have a clinically silent interval, up to 9–12 months, when clinical signs of hemiplegia are not evident (Bouza et al 1994). Serial neurological examinations in infants with neonatal cerebral infarction have allowed the accurate timing of any clinical signs of hemiplegia, providing information on which are the first definitive signs and in what order they appear

(Bouza et al 1994, Dubowitz et al 1998). These data are related to lesions occurring in the perinatal period in symptomatic infants.

The initial neonatal examination in infants with cerebral infarction can be quite variable, ranging from normal to the presence of marked asymmetry in tone and movement (Mercuri et al 1999b). In most cases the initial finding is generalized hypotonia, but, as the majority of these infants have convulsions and are on anticonvulsant drugs, the significance of this finding is uncertain. A proportion of these infants show some asymmetry of limb tone generally within a few weeks, often with relative hypotonia rather than hypertonia contralateral to the lesion. This initial asymmetry is often not seen at 2–3 months and these early asymmetries are not always associated with later hemiplegia.

The timing of the appearance of the first clinical signs of hemiplegia is variable and reflects to some extent the severity of hemiplegia: in general, the worse the hemiplegia, the earlier the clinical signs appear and the more severe they are.

The first signs, however, can be very subtle and should be carefully looked for. Asymmetry of spontaneous movements can already be identified between 9 and 16 weeks (Guzzetta et al 2003). Other common early abnormal signs observed after 12 weeks are asymmetry of kicking when the infant is held in vertical suspension (Bouza et al 1994), with a relative paucity of kicking on the affected side (Fig. 4.3a). There may also be asymmetry of the popliteal angles (Fig. 4.3b), but the affected side is not always the tighter. Other signs subsequently seen are asymmetries in passive tone, such as in the angle of the hip adductor, on shoulder abduction, and in active truncal tone on lateral tilting (Fig. 4.4). After four months, the arm protective reaction, seen when a child is pulled up from supine by one arm, is also often asymmetrical (Fig. 4.5) in infants who will develop hemiplegia (Bouza et al 1994).

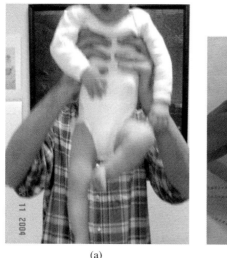
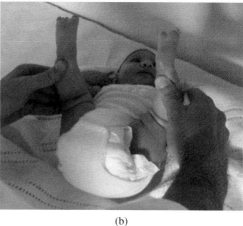

(a)   (b)

Fig. 4.3 (a) Asymmetry of kicking. (b) Asymmetry of popliteal angle.

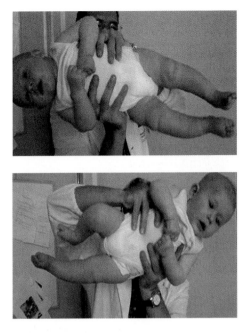

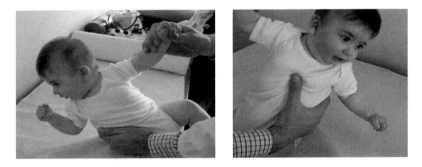

Fig. 4.4 Asymmetrical lateral tilting.

Fig. 4.5 Asymmetrical arm protective reaction.

Other asymmetries of tone and movements, such as in pronation/supination of the forearm and ankle dorsiflexion, also become more obvious between 9 and 12 months.

After 9 months asymmetries in function also become more obvious. A strong hand preference is generally present in all children with hemiplegia by 12 months (Fig. 4.6) but can already be found from 4 months onwards in children who will develop severe hemiplegia. Children with hemiplegia have a tendency to reach over using the non-affected hand even if objects are presented on the side of the affected hand. Dystonic posturing of the hand and hand fisting are also typical findings from 5–6 months onwards, but only in children who will develop severe hemiplegia.

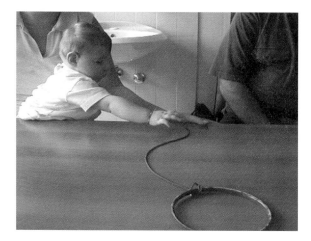

Fig. 4.6 Child with left hemiplegia reaching over using the non-affected hand.

Asymmetrical gait, with hyperextension of the knee, and, when present, a tendency to walk on tiptoes, and inverted foot also become obvious after 12 months.

OPTIMALITY SCORES IN INFANTS WITH CEREBRAL INFARCTION
Serial neurological examinations are a valuable tool for detecting and following systematically the evolution of the asymmetries and other neurological signs in a child with hemiplegia. The application of the optimality scoring system to these infants, as we have currently evaluated it, is, however, limited compared to other groups such as infants with HIE where lesions tend to be bilateral and symmetrical. Even when some abnormalities are present, these are mainly asymmetries of tone and posture. At present, when a child has different scores between the sides for limb tone or posture for a particular item, the score for that item is the average of the individual scores for each side.

While this will reduce the total score, it is rarely very low and is indeed often close to optimal, either because the normal scores from the non-hemiplegic side compensate for the abnormal side or because both sides, while different, may be within the optimal range for that item. In this group of infants the number and persistence of the asymmetries should be noted separately. In infants with HIE the optimality scores have proven to be a reliable prognostic indicator of the ability to walk unaided at 2 years. The relatively good scores in children with hemiplegia reflect the fact that almost all are independently mobile by 2 years of age, and the scores are only slightly lower in those in whom the walking ability is significantly delayed or those with severe hemiplegia (unpublished data).

Preterm infants
The infant examination has been regularly used for over 20 years in the follow-up of preterm infants, and in particular in those with severe brain lesions such as cystic periventricular leukomalacia (cPVL), intraventricular haemorrhage (IVH) and haemorrhagic parenchymal

infarction (HPI). In preterm infants with predominantly unilateral lesions, such as HPI, serial neurological examinations help to detect and follow systematically the evolution of possible asymmetries and other neurological signs, which, as previously reported in term infants with cerebral infarction, may only become obvious some months after they have reached term age equivalent (de Vries et al 1990).

In infants with more diffuse lesions sequential examination will help to follow the maturation of tone and other neurological signs over time. Most of the cerebral lesions sustained by preterm infants occur many weeks before they reach term age, and the neonatal neurological examination at term age may already provide useful information on the pattern and severity of neurological abnormalities which are variable in different patterns of lesions. We have previously reported, for example, that by term age infants with severe cPVL present with increased extensor tone in the legs and increased flexor tone in the arms, predominant extensor tone of the trunk and head, abnormal finger posture, poor visual attention (depending on the site of the cPVL) and irritability. These signs, already present at term age, can also be observed in the follow-up examinations (Fig. 4.7a–c) and, when present, are always associated with the most severe outcome (de Vries et al 1990). In contrast, infants with large IVH will generally show normal or slightly decreased axial and limb tone, better visual attention, though it may be delayed in some infants, and less irritability.

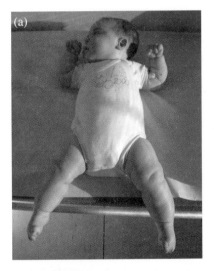

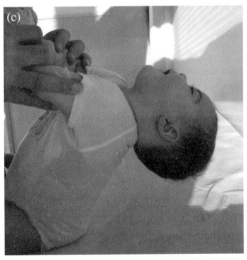

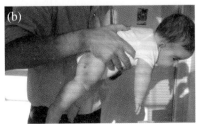

Fig. 4.7 Note the increased extensor tone in the legs with increased flexor tone in the arms (a), and the predominant extensor axial tone (b and c).

The optimality scoring system has been applied to a cohort of 74 preterm infants whose gestational age ranged between 24 and 30.5 weeks (Frisone et al 2002). The infants were examined between 9 and 18 months chronological age (6–15 months corrected). These findings have been subsequently confirmed in a larger cohort of infants with the same range of gestational age (Mercuri et al 2003).

The main interest was not only to establish the possible prognostic value of the optimality scores in predicting motor outcome but also to establish whether the range of scores in low-risk preterm infants was different from those found in low-risk full-term infants.

In preterm infants with severe brain lesions the range of optimality scores reflects the variability in motor outcome better than cranial ultrasound findings. Major abnormalities, such as cPVL (grades 2 and 3) (de Vries et al 1992) and IVH, can be associated with both optimal and suboptimal scores and with variable outcome. Children who do not achieve the ability to sit unsupported or walk at 2 years generally have optimality scores below 52, while infants who are able to sit but not to walk at 2 years have scores between 52 and 64. The sensitivity of an optimality score above 64, obtained between 9 and 15 months chronological age, to predict walking at 2 years is 98 per cent and the specificity is 85 per cent.

In preterm infants with normal scans or with only minor lesions and normal motor outcome the range of scores was wider than that found in low-risk term infants. One-third of infants with normal motor outcome at 2 years had suboptimal scores, though above 64. In these infants the lower scores were mainly found in maturational items such as axial tone and saving reactions (Table 4.2).

The results showed that this standardized scorable neurological examination, which can be performed in very preterm infants as early as 9 months chronological age, predicts gross motor outcome at 2 years of age. The scores showed no significant association with the degree of prematurity or the age at assessment. These findings are extremely useful in very preterm infants who are at high risk of severe neurological and developmental disabilities and in whom the early prediction of motor function can be difficult. Although

TABLE 4.2
List of items which more frequently had suboptimal scores in the infants
with a suboptimal global score and normal motor outcome

Items	Suboptimal scores
Lateral tilting	75%
Passive shoulder abduction	60%
Trunk posture	40%
Legs posture	35%
Forward parachute	33%
Arm protection	25%
Popliteal angle	25%
Ankle dorsiflexion	23%

high-quality early and sequential ultrasound examinations (de Vries et al 2004) are a very good predictor of cerebral palsy in the preterm infant, as is MRI at term age equivalent in preterm infants with HPI (de Vries et al 2004), such information is frequently not available in the routine clinical situation, particularly away from tertiary medical centres. Parents are naturally anxious to be reassured that their very vulnerable preterm infants, who are often somewhat delayed in their gross motor skills, are likely to attain independent walking. By using this simple but standardized neurological examination and scoring system in the clinic, robust and reliable reassurance can be given without recourse to more technical, time-consuming and expensive investigations.

Other applications

In the last few years the protocol has also found wide application in many different environments, and not only in research settings, combining clinical data with highly sophisticated instrumental techniques, but also in small units in developing countries. We have constructed a simple neurological examination especially for rural settings – the Shoklo Neurological Test, which is aimed at screening and following up the short- and long-term adverse effects of serious infections, drugs and toxins in children aged from 9 to 36 months (Haataja et al 2002).

The examination includes some items assessing hand coordination and eight items assessing tone and behaviour from the Hammersmith Infant Neurological Examination. We selected only items that could be reliably performed even by less experienced health workers, e.g. paramedical staff. The test was validated in a cohort of low-risk term infants in London, and shown to correlate favourably with the Griffiths Developmental Scales. In order to evaluate the Shoklo Neurological Test in less optimal conditions, it was applied to a cohort of 128 infants from a Karen refugee camp. After appropriate training, the paramedical staff performed well in quality control situations, showing inter-tester agreement of 95 per cent. This test can be used in resource-poor settings for clinical and research purposes (Haataja et al 2002).

REFERENCES

Boardman JP, Ganesan V, Rutherford MA, Saunders DE, Mercuri E, Cowan F (2005) Magnetic resonance image correlates of hemiparesis after neonatal and childhood middle cerebral artery stroke. *Pediatrics* 115: 321–326.
Bouza H, Rutherford M, Acolet D, Pennock JM, Dubowitz LM (1994) Evolution of early hemiplegic signs in full-term infants with unilateral brain lesions in the neonatal period: a prospective study. *Neuropediatrics* 25: 201–207.
Cowan F, Rutherford M, Groenendaal F, Eken P, Mercuri E, Bydder GM, Meiners LC, Dubowitz LM, de Vries LS (2003) Origin and timing of brain lesions in term infants with neonatal encephalopathy. *Lancet* 361: 736–742.
de Vries LS, Pierrat V, Minami T, Smet M, Casaer P (1990) The role of short latency somatosensory evoked responses in infants with rapidly progressive ventricular dilatation. *Neuropediatrics* 21: 136–139.
de Vries LS, Eken P, Dubowitz L (1992) The spectrum of leukomalacia using cranial ultrasound. *Behav Brain Res* 49: 1–6.
de Vries L, Groenendal F, Eken P, van Haastert IC, Rademakers KJ, Meiners LC (1997) Infarcts in the vascular distribution of the middle cerebral artery in preterm and fullterm infants. *Neuropediatrics* 28: 88–96.

de Vries LS, Van Haastert IL, Rademaker KJ, Koopman C, Groenendaal F (2004) Ultrasound abnormalities preceding cerebral palsy in high-risk preterm infants. *J Pediatr* 144: 815–820.

Dubowitz L, Dubowitz V, Mercuri E (1998) *The Neurological Assessment of the Preterm and Full-term Newborn Infant, 2nd edn.* Clinics in Developmental Medicine 148. Cambridge: Mac Keith Press.

Estan J, Hope P (1997) Unilateral neonatal cerebral infarction in full term infants. *Arch Dis Child Fetal Neonatal Ed* 76: F88–F93.

Frisone MF, Mercuri E, Laroche S, Foglia C, Maalouf EF, Haataja L, Cowan F, Dubowitz L (2002) Prognostic value of the neurologic optimality score at 9 and 18 months in preterm infants born before 31 weeks' gestation. *J Pediatr* 140: 57–60.

Guzzetta A, Mercuri E, Rapisardi G, Ferrari F, Roversi MF, Cowan F, Rutherford M, Paolicelli PB, Einspieler C, Boldrini A, Dubowitz L, Prechtl HF, Cioni G (2003) General movements detect early signs of hemiplegia in term infants with neonatal cerebral infarction. *Neuropediatrics* 34: 61–66.

Haataja L, Mercuri E, Regev R, Cowan F, Rutherford M, Dubowitz V, Dubowitz L (1999) Optimality score for the neurologic examination of the infant at 12 and 18 months of age. *J Pediatr* 135: 153–161.

Haataja L, Mercuri E, Guzzetta A, Rutherford M, Counsell S, Frisone MF, Cioni G, Cowan F, Dubowitz L (2001) Neurologic examination in infants with hypoxic-ischemic encephalopathy at age 9 to 14 months: use of optimality scores and correlation with magnetic resonance imaging findings. *J Pediatr* 138: 332–337.

Haataja L, McGready R, Arunjerdja R, Simpson JA, Mercuri E, Nosten F, Dubowitz L (2002) A new approach for neurological evaluation of infants in resource-poor settings. *Ann Trop Paediatr* 22: 355–368.

Mercuri E, Guzzetta A, Haataja L, Cowan F, Rutherford M, Counsell S, Papadimitriou M, Cioni G, Dubowitz L (1999a) Neonatal neurological examination in infants with hypoxic ischaemic encephalopathy: correlation with MRI findings. *Neuropediatrics* 30: 83–89.

Mercuri E, Rutherford M, Cowan F, Pennock J, Counsell S, Papadimitriou M, Azzopardi D, Bydder G, Dubowitz L (1999b) Early prognostic indicators of outcome in infants with neonatal cerebral infarction: a clinical, electroencephalogram, and magnetic resonance imaging study. *Pediatrics* 103: 39–46.

Mercuri E, Rutherford M, Barnett A, Foglia C, Haataja L, Counsell S, Cowan F, Dubowitz L (2002) MRI lesions and infants with neonatal encephalopathy. Is the Apgar score predictive? *Neuropediatrics* 33: 150–156.

Mercuri E, Guzzetta A, Laroche S, Ricci D, vanHaastert I, Simpson A, Luciano R, Bleakley C, Frisone MF, Haataja L, Tortorolo G, Guzzetta F, de Vries L, Cowan F, Dubowitz L (2003) Neurologic examination of preterm infants at term age: comparison with term infants. *J Pediatr* 142: 647–655.

Mercuri E, Barnett A, Rutherford M, Guzzetta A, Haataja L, Cioni G, Cowan F, Dubowitz L (2004) Neonatal cerebral infarction and neuromotor outcome at school age. *Pediatrics* 113: 95–100.

Pierrat V, Haouari N, Liska A, Thomas D, Subtil D, Truffert P, Groupe d'Etudes en Epidemiologie Perinatale (2005) Prevalence, causes, and outcome at 2 years of age of newborn encephalopathy: population based study. *Arch Dis Child Fetal Neonatal Ed* 90: F257–F261.

Ricci D, Guzzetta A, Cowan F, Haataja L, Rutherford M, Dubowitz L, Mercuri E (2006) Sequential neurological examinations in infants with neonatal encephalopathy and low Apgar scores: relationship with brain MRI. *Neuropediatrics* 37: 148–153.

Rutherford M, Pennock J, Schwieso J, Cowan F, Dubowitz L (1996) Hypoxic-ischaemic encephalopathy: early and late magnetic resonance imaging findings in relation to outcome. *Arch Dis Child Fetal Neonatal Ed* 75: F145–F151.

Sarnat HB, Sarnat MS (1976) Neonatal encephalopathy following fetal distress. A clinical and electroencephalographic study. *Arch Neurol* 33: 696–705.

5
OTHER APPROACHES TO NEUROLOGICAL ASSESSMENT

Giovanni Cioni, Christa Einspieler and Paola Paolicelli

Introduction

In recent years clinicians interested in the neurological assessment of newborns and young infants have paid increasing attention to newer approaches to the assessment of the nervous system. These approaches are mainly based on the knowledge that from the first weeks of gestation the human nervous system is capable of many complex and rapidly changing functions. Convergent findings of different disciplines (psychology, neuroscience, paediatrics) have contributed to overcome the traditional image of the 'incompetent' and immature newborn.

It is now accepted that the young nervous system (of a fetus, a newborn or a young infant) is not a simple collection of reflexes, but a complex organism producing a great deal of endogenously generated behaviours, able to use them for his adaptive needs, in interaction with his environment.

Many attempts have been made to integrate these findings and to introduce new items, exploring more complex motor, perceptual, cognitive and communicative functions, into the neurological assessment of newborns and young infants. However, the practical contribution of these attempts, in relation to clinical practice, is in many cases still not fully established.

To be really useful, new methods of neurological assessment have to fulfil a series of basic requirements, clearly indicated by Prechtl (1990). They have to include items strictly related to the age-specific repertoire of the CNS, which changes very rapidly during the pre- and early postnatal periods. New functions emerge, others undergo a regression. The concept of ontogenetic adaptation of the organism to the age-specific requirements of the environment (Oppenheimer 1981) may account for rapid transformations of neural functions.

However, not all the age-specific functions of the infant's repertoire are suitable for clinical assessment. Diagnostic tools need to be non-invasive, and non-time-consuming. Both conditions are needed to allow repeated longitudinal observations, particularly of fragile individuals such as preterm infants. Moreover, the reliability and prognostic value of these methods have to be carefully tested. New methods of functional evaluation of newborns and infants which fulfil these conditions may help in understanding the possible consequences of brain lesions, detected by brain imaging techniques.

So far the most valuable contribution to establishing new approaches to clinical evaluation of fetal, neonatal and infant movements emerges from the work of Prechtl and his co-workers, which will be described in the following pages.

Assessment of general movements

GOALS AND OBJECTIVES OF GM OBSERVATION

To functionally assess the young nervous system, the quality of a certain type of pattern of spontaneous movements, the so-called general movements (GMs), can be observed and assessed, because it has been demonstrated that these movements in particular are an excellent marker for early brain impairment and dysfunction (Prechtl 1990). The young human nervous system generates endogenously (i.e. without being constantly triggered by specific sensory input) a variety of motor patterns such as startles, GMs, isolated limb movements, twitches, stretches, yawning, and breathing movements. They emerge as early as 9 to 12 weeks postmenstrual age (de Vries et al 1982) and continue after birth without changing their form, irrespective of when birth occurs (Prechtl 2001a).

Of the many distinct movement patterns appearing during the course of development from fetus to young infant, the one most effective for the functional assessment of the young nervous system is GMs. They are complex, occur frequently, and last long enough to be observed properly (Prechtl 2001b). GMs involve the whole body in a variable sequence of arm, leg, neck and trunk movements. They wax and wane in intensity, force and speed, and they have a gradual beginning and end. Rotations along the axis of the limbs and slight changes in the direction of movements make them fluent and elegant and create the impression of complexity and variability (Prechtl 1990). While before term we call these movements fetal or preterm GMs (Einspieler et al 2004), at term age until about 6 to 9 weeks post-term age they are called writhing movements (Hopkins and Prechtl 1984; Fig. 5.1).

Even if age-related minor differences exist, GMs have, by and large, a similar appearance from early fetal life until the end of the second month post-term. At 6 to 9 weeks post-term age, GMs with a writhing character gradually disappear while fidgety GMs gradually emerge (Hopkins and Prechtl 1984, Prechtl et al 1997a; Fig. 5.1). Fidgety movements are present up to the end of the first half-year of life, at which point intentional and antigravity movements start to dominate.

Preterm GMs

No difference can be observed between fetal and preterm GMs, indicating that neither the increase of the force of gravity after birth nor maturation has an influence on the appearance of GMs. The GMs of a preterm infant may occasionally have large amplitudes and are often of fast speed (Cioni and Prechtl 1990, Prechtl et al 1997b, Einspieler et al 2004).

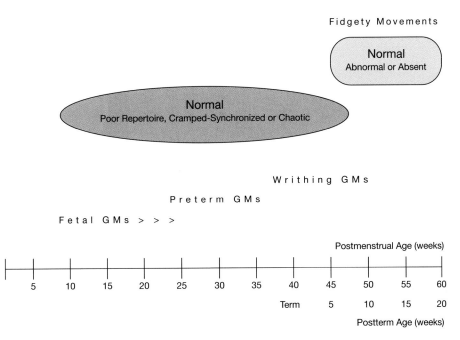

Fig. 5.1 Developmental course of normal and abnormal general movements.

Writing movements

At term age and during the first two months post-term, GMs are commonly referred to as writhing movements. They are characterized by small to moderate amplitude and by slow to moderate speed. Typically, they are ellipsoid in form, which creates the impression of a writhing quality (Hopkins and Prechtl 1984, Cioni et al 1989, Prechtl et al 1997b, Einspieler et al 2004). EMG recordings reveal that the burst duration is significantly longer during preterm GMs than during writhing GMs. However, burst amplitude values and tonic background data do not change from preterm GMs to writhing GMs (Hadders-Algra and Prechtl 1992).

At 6 to 9 weeks post-term age, writhing movements gradually disappear while fidgety GMs gradually emerge (Hopkins and Prechtl 1984, Cioni and Prechtl 1990, Hadders-Algra and Prechtl 1992, Prechtl et al 1997a, 1997b; Fig. 5.1).

Fidgety movements

Fidgety movements are small movements of moderate speed and variable acceleration of neck, trunk and limbs, in all directions, continual in the awake infant, except during fussing and crying (Prechtl et al 1997a, 1997b, Einspieler et al 2004). EMG recordings (Hadders-Algra et al 1992) and 3-D-motion analyses (Coluccini et al 2002) reveal that movement velocity and amplitude as well as tonic background activity decrease during the transformation from writhing to fidgety movements.

Various other movements may occur together with fidgety movements, such as wiggling-oscillating and saccadic arm movements, swipes, mutual manipulation of fingers, manipulation (fiddling) of clothing, reaching and touching, legs lifting with or without hand–knee contact, trunk rotation, and axial rolling (Hopkins and Prechtl 1984, Einspieler et al 2004).

As GMs include activity of all segments from cervical to lumbar spinal cord, it is likely that the generating neuronal structure is located supraspinally (Prechtl 1997). As they emerge at 9 to 10 weeks postmenstrual age, it is unlikely that higher structures than the brainstem are involved. It can also be assumed that GMs of writhing quality and those of fidgety quality are generated by different central pattern generators. Their temporal overlap at the transformation from one type into the other (Fig. 5.1) makes this most plausible (Prechtl 1997, 2001b). That writhing movements do not disappear during sleep even at 6 months is indicative of the prolonged preservation of their central pattern generator during the fidgety movement period and thereafter (Einspieler et al 1994).

GENERAL MOVEMENTS CHANGE THEIR QUALITY IF THE NERVOUS SYSTEM IS IMPAIRED

GMs in low-risk and high-risk or brain-damaged infants are not different with respect to the rate of their occurrence, i.e. their quantity (Prechtl and Nolte 1984, Ferrari et al 1990). The quality of GMs is probably modulated by corticospinal or reticulospinal pathways, and hence can be affected by impairments of these structures. Disruption of the corticospinal projections by periventricular lesions of the corona radiata or internal capsule due to haemorrhages or hypoxic-ischaemic lesions leads to abnormal GMs (Prechtl 1997). Preterm and writhing GMs lose their complex and variable character and have a poor repertoire, or are cramped-synchronized, or chaotic. Fidgety movements can be either abnormal or absent (Fig. 5.1). All normal and abnormal GM patterns are illustrated by a video (Prechtl et al 1997b) and a CD-ROM (Einspieler et al 2004).

Poor repertoire GMs

The sequence of the successive movement components is monotonous and movements of the different body parts do not occur in the complex way seen in normal GMs (Ferrari et al 1990, Prechtl et al 1997b). Poor repertoire GMs are frequent in infants with brain ultrasound abnormalities and can be followed by normal, abnormal or an absence of fidgety movements. Hence, the predictive value of poor repertoire GMs is low (Prechtl et al 1997a, Einspieler et al 2004, Nakajima et al 2005).

Cramped-synchronized GMs

GMs appear rigid and lack the normal smooth and fluent character; all limb and trunk muscles contract and relax almost simultaneously (Ferrari et al 1990, Prechtl et al 1997b). If this abnormal pattern is observed consistently over a number of weeks it is of high predictive value for the development of spastic cerebral palsy (Ferrari et al 2002).

Chaotic GMs
Movements of all limbs are of large amplitude and occur in a chaotic order without any fluency or smoothness. They consistently appear to be abrupt (Bos et al 1997a, Ferrari et al 1997). Chaotic GMs are rare; infants with chaotic GMs often develop cramped-synchronized GMs a few weeks later (Einspieler et al 2004).

Abnormal fidgety movements
These look like normal fidgety movements but their amplitude, speed and jerkiness are exaggerated (Prechtl et al 1997a, 1997b). Abnormal fidgety movements are rare and their predictive value is low (Einspieler et al 2004).

Absence of fidgety movements
If fidgety movements are never observed from 9 to 20 weeks post-term we call this abnormality 'absence of fidgety movements'. Other movements can, however, be commonly observed (Prechtl et al 1997a, 1997b). The absence of fidgety movements is highly predictive for later neurological impairments, particularly for cerebral palsy (Prechtl et al 1997a, Cioni et al 2000, Einspieler et al 2002, Guzzetta et al 2003).

THE ASSESSMENT PROCEDURE
In order to provide a reliable assessment of GMs the recording procedure has to be standardized (Einspieler et al 1997, 2004). The comfortably dressed infant, preferably with bare arms and legs, is videoed in supine position. The duration of the recording depends on the age of the infant. In order to collect about three GMs for reliable assessment we usually record preterm infants for 30 to 60 minutes, independent of whether the infant is asleep or awake. The observer does not need to be present during the recording, and the whole recording does not need to be assessed. Afterwards, the recording is re-viewed and about three GM sequences are copied onto an assessment tape. From term age onwards, 5 to 10 minutes of optimal recording are usually sufficient. The sequential recordings taken at different ages should be stored on the assessment tape for the documentation of the individual developmental course (Einspieler et al 1997, 2004). Recordings of a fussing or crying infant cannot be analysed.

The assessment is based on global visual Gestalt perception, which is a powerful but vulnerable instrument in the analysis of complex phenomena (Lorenz 1971). Hence, attention to details must be avoided by all means.

Studies in preterm infants during individualized developmental care (Constantinou et al 1999, Baldi 2002) or in 3-month-old infants during visual, acoustic, proprioceptive or social stimulation (Dibiasi and Einspieler 2002, 2004) indicated that GMs were hardly influenced by environmental stimulation. For the assessment of GMs, however, environmental stimulation may interfere with the observer's Gestalt perception: for example, the presence of caregivers, siblings or twins on the video, or mirror images of the infant, or a bed crowded with toys, or an irritating coloured blanket should be avoided (Einspieler et al 2004).

The experienced observer does not need more than one to three minutes to judge a GM recording. However, a snapshot assessment of a single recording is less accurate than an individual developmental trajectory (Prechtl 1990, Einspieler and Prechtl 2005) which preferably documents two to three recordings of the preterm period (with three GM sequences in each), one recording at term or early post-term age or both, and at least one recording between 9 and 15 weeks post-term (Einspieler et al 2004). An individual developmental trajectory indicates the consistency or inconsistency of normal or abnormal findings. The prediction of the individual neurological development is based on such a trajectory.

The observer should never assess for longer periods than about 45 minutes without taking a break, as tiredness interferes with visual Gestalt perception (Einspieler et al 1997). If many recordings of abnormal GMs are seen in a series it is advisable for the observer to watch a criterion standard normal recording from time to time. This is necessary for re-calibrating the Gestalt perception.

TRAINING AND INTER-RATER RELIABILITY

Updated information about this approach can be found in *Prechtl's Method on the Qualitative Assessment of General Movements in Preterm, Term and Young Infants* (Einspieler et al 2004). Standardized basic and advanced training courses, lasting four days, are provided by the GM Trust group (www.general-movements-trust.info). A basic training course enables professionals in the field of infant and child neurology to apply Prechtl's GM assessment accurately. Evaluation of almost 9000 assessments performed by some 800 observers demonstrated that 83 per cent of the assessments were correct, i.e. in agreement with the criterion standard. In addition, discrimination between normal and abnormal GMs was in agreement with the criterion standard in 92 per cent (Valentin et al 2005).

Eleven studies on 358 infants assessed by 90 observers revealed an inter-rater agreement of between 89 and 93 per cent (for a review see Einspieler et al 2004). The average kappa (Cohen 1969) in another four studies on 108 infants assessed by 11 observers was 0.88 (van Kranen-Mastenbroek et al 1992, Bos et al 1997b, 1998, Cioni et al 2000). Analysis of 20 GM recordings repeated after a time interval of two years obtained a 100 per cent test–retest reliability for global judgement, and an 85 per cent reliability for detailed analysis (Einspieler 1994).

SEMI-QUANTITATIVE ASSESSMENT AND MOTOR OPTIMALITY SCORES

A semi-quantitative assessment of GM quality can be achieved by applying Prechtl's optimality concept (Prechtl 1980). A score for optimal or non-optimal performance is given to every movement criterion, such as amplitude, speed, movement character, sequence, range in space, onset and cessation of GMs: the higher the sum of the optimality scores, the more optimal the quality of the GMs.

Two different optimality scoring lists have been reported: the first for preterm and term age (Ferrari et al 1990); and the second (shown in Fig. 5.2) covering the motor behaviour of 3- to 5-month-old infants (Bos et al 2003).

With this semi-quantitative and detailed approach the power of the global Gestalt perception is lost. However, it is helpful to semi-quantitatively describe any change in the quality of GMs, assessing either improvement or worsening.

Assessment of Motor Repertoire - 3 to 5 Months
Christa Einspieler and Arie Bos, the GM Trust 2001

Name: ....

born: .... Postmenstrual Age: .... Birth weight: ....

Recording Date: .... Postterm Age: ....

Number of movement patterns observed: ⊔⊔ normal (N) ⊔⊔ abnormal (A)

N A	fidgety movements	N	hand-face contact	N A	legs lift, flexion at knees
N A	swiping movements	N	hand-mouth contact	N A	legs lift extension at knees
N A	wiggling-oscillating movem.	N	hand-hand contact	N	hand-knee contact
N A	saccadic arm movements	N	hand-hand manipulation	N A	arching
N A	kicking	N A	fiddling / clothes, blanket	N A	trunk rotation
N A	excitement bursts	N	reaching	N	axial rolling
A	'cha-cha-cha movements'	N A	foot-foot contact	N A	visual scanning
N A	smiles	N	foot-foot manipulation	N	hand regard
N A	mouth movements	N A	segmental movements arms	N	head anteflexion
N A	tongue movements	N A	segmental movements legs	A	arm movements in circles
N A	head rotation	A	segm: discrepancy arm-leg	A	almost no leg movements

Number of postural patterns observed: ⊔⊔ normal (N) ⊔⊔ abnormal (A)

N A	head in midline (20 °)	N	variable finger postures	A	hyperextension of the neck
N A	symmetrical	A	predominant fisting	A	hyperextension of trunk
N A	spontaneous ATNR absent or	A	finger spreading	A	extended arms/ on / above
	could be overcome	A	few finger postures		surface are predominant
A	body and limbs 'flat' on	A	synchronised opening and	A	extended legs / on / above
	surface		closing of the fingers		surface are predominant

Movement character (global score):

N	smooth and fluent	A	stiff	A	predominantly slow speed
A	jerky	A	cramped	A	predominantly fast speed
A	monotonous	A	synchronous	A	predomin. large amplitude
A	tremulous	A	cramped-synchronised	A	predomin. small amplitude

Motor Optimality List:

1.	Fidgety Movements	normal	☐	12
		abnormal	☐	4
	± + ++ P D	absent	☐	1
2.	Repertoire of	age-adequate	☐	4
	co-existent other movements	reduced	☐	2
		absent	☐	1
3.	Quality of other movements	N > A	☐	4
		N = A	☐	2
		N < A	☐	1
4.	Posture	N > A	☐	4
		N = A	☐	2
		N < A	☐	1
5.	Movement character	smooth and fluent	☐	4
		abnormal, not cramped-synchr.	☐	2
		cramped-synchronised	☐	1

Motor Optimality Score:
Maximum: 28; Minimum: 5

Fig. 5.2 Proforma for the assessment of spontaneous motor repertoire of 3- to 5-month-old infants.

Moreover, a GM optimality score can be used for statistical calculations and comparisons with other measurements. For example, Einspieler (1994) has reported a high correlation between the GM optimality score and the pO_2-values obtained during night polysomnographies in 3- to 20-week-old infants, indicating that drops in pO_2 resulted in a less optimal GM performance.

MAIN APPLICATIONS IN THE FOLLOW-UP OF HIGH-RISK INFANTS
The methodological breakthrough of Prechtl's GM assessment lies in the fact that it predicts severe neurological deficits at a much earlier age than was previously possible (Prechtl et al 1997a). In addition, it accurately identifies those infants with normal GMs despite being at-risk due to their history, who will have a normal neurological outcome (Prechtl 2001b).

Early specific markers for spastic cerebral palsy
The first longitudinal study on the predictive value of the various abnormal GM patterns revealed cramped-synchronized GMs as highly predictive for spastic cerebral palsy (Ferrari et al 1990). The largest longitudinal study of 130 infants, consisting of the whole spectrum from normal to abnormal brain ultrasound findings due to hypoxic-ischaemic lesions or haemorrhages, confirmed the significance of cramped-synchronized GMs. All infants who at repeated assessments consistently showed cramped-synchronized GMs later developed spastic cerebral palsy (Prechtl et al 1997a). The earlier consistent cramped-synchronized GMs occurred, the worse the later motor impairment (Ferrari et al 2002).

There is yet another early marker for later development of cerebral palsy. Almost all infants who never had fidgety movements developed cerebral palsy. An absence of fidgety movements can be preceded by cramped-synchronized GMs or, exceptionally, by poor repertoire GMs. The validity of fidgety movements as a marker is clearly demonstrated if we look at an individual developmental trajectory consisting of transient cramped-synchronized GMs. Transient cramped-synchronized GMs were associated with cerebral palsy if fidgety movements were absent. If transient cramped-synchronized GMs were followed by normal fidgety movements, the neurological outcome was normal (Ferrari et al 2002).

Thus, specific early signs of later spastic cerebral palsy are consistent cramped-synchronized GMs and/or absence of fidgety movements. Both abnormal qualities of GMs can be seen at an age at which, on a standard neurological examination, no evidence of cerebral palsy is yet present, namely as early as from fetal life onwards (Prechtl and Einspieler 1997) or from preterm or term birth until the third month post-term (Prechtl et al 1997a).

Early signs of hemiplegia
The observation of abnormal movements from birth onwards refuted the hypothesis of a silent period of later hemiplegia. Two studies have shown that infants with subsequent hemiplegia had 'absence of fidgety movements' following bilateral cramped-synchronized or poor repertoire GMs (Cioni et al 2000, Guzzetta et al 2003). The first asymmetrical sign,

independent of the head position, was segmental movements, which were reduced or absent contralateral to the side of the lesion. Segmental movements are distinct movements of hand and feet, fingers and toes, occurring either isolated or as part of GMs. In the latter case they are not part of limb flexion or extension (Cioni et al 1997a, van der Heide et al 1999). This asymmetry occurred in preterm born infants from the third month post-term age onwards (Cioni et al 2000). In term born infants with neonatal infarction the asymmetry of segmental movements was present from the second month (Guzzetta et al 2003).

The prediction of dyskinetic cerebral palsy
Until the second month post-term, the infant who will later develop dyskinetic cerebral palsy displays a poor repertoire of GMs, 'arm movements in circles' and finger spreading. Characteristically, these abnormal arm and finger movements remain until at least 5 months post-term. The abnormal unilateral or bilateral 'arm movements in circles' are monotonous, slow forward rotations from the shoulder. In particular, the monotony in speed and amplitude is the most characteristic quality of 'arm movements in circles'. Usually these abnormal arm movements are accompanied by finger spreading (Einspieler et al 2002).

From 3 months onwards, a lack of movements towards the midline, particularly foot–foot contact, is an additional specific sign of later dyskinetic cerebral palsy. In addition, the majority of cases display neither hand–hand contact nor hand–mouth contact (Einspieler et al 2002).

Common to both spastic and dyskinetic cases is the absence of fidgety movements and the absence of antigravity movements, i.e. legs lifting, during the third to fifth month (Einspieler et al 2002). The absence of fidgety movements is of particular interest. Prechtl (1997) suggested a specific central pattern generator for fidgety movements, located, most likely, in the brainstem. The absence of fidgety movements in both forms of cerebral palsy, caused by different brain lesions, indicates that intact corticospinal fibres as well as the output from the basal ganglia and cerebellum are necessary to generate normal fidgety movements (Einspieler et al 2002).

GMs and mild neurological impairments
Abnormal fidgety movements are less predictive for neurological outcome than absence of fidgety movements (Prechtl et al 1997a), but they have been discussed in the context of the development of mild neurological impairments (Bos et al 1999, 2002, Einspieler et al 2004).

Hadders-Algra and co-workers described how 'mildly abnormal GMs' in infants aged 3 to 4 months (the period of fidgety movements) were predictive for the development of minor neurological deficits (MND), attention deficit hyperactivity disorder, and boisterous, disobedient behaviour of 4- to 9-year-old children (Hadders-Algra and Groothuis 1999, Hadders-Algra et al 2004). According to Hadders-Algra, 'mildly abnormal GMs' lack fluency but still show some complexity and variation (Hadders-Algra et al 1997, Hadders-Algra 2004). However, the classification 'mildly abnormal GMs' does not exist in Prechtl's GM assessment. Results from Bruggink et al (2006) indicate that the quality of the early motor repertoire, in particular an abnormal quality of FMs and an abnormal quality of the concurrent motor repertoire at 11–16 weeks post-term, is associated with the development of complex MND at 7 to 11 years of age.

The longest-lasting follow-up study to date (12 to 15 years) demonstrated that the GM quality was not predictive for MND at puberty age (Einspieler et al 2006). However, children with a history of abnormal fidgety movements had fine manipulative disabilities at prepuberty age.

Predictive values

Several papers have indicated that the sensitivity of this method for predicting severe neurological impairment is about 94 per cent (Ferrari et al 1990, Prechtl et al 1993, Cioni et al 1997b, 1997c, Prechtl et al 1997a, Ferrari et al 2002). The specificity of the same studies was lower during the preterm and writhing movement period (46 to 93 per cent) due to a considerable number of infants with poor repertoire GMs who normalized at the fidgety movement period and who had a normal outcome. With increasing age, specificity increased, revealing values between 82 and 100 per cent during the third month, when normal fidgety movements predict a normal neurological outcome (Einspieler and Prechtl 2005). Normal GMs at all ages (likelihood ratio LR- = 0.04, 95 per cent confidence interval: 0.005 to 0.27) as well as cramped-synchronized GMs (LR+ = 45, 95 per cent confidence interval: 6.4 to 321) and the absence of fidgety movements (LR >51) have excellent likelihood ratios (Einspieler et al 2004).

GMs and pervasive disorders

More recently, standardized measures of early spontaneous movements, including GM assessment, have been applied to other severe developmental disorders, such as Rett syndrome (Einspieler et al 2005) and autism spectrum disorders (ASD) (Phagava et al 2005). Apparently normal early development was one of the initial criteria for these disorders, but several investigators considered them to be developmental disorders manifesting very soon after birth. The results provided by standardized observations of spontaneous movement patterns seem to indicate that both Rett syndrome and ASD are manifest within the first months of life. Although not necessarily specific, the signs observed are of value in alerting clinicians to the possibility of the diagnosis at an early stage when intervention is likely to be most effective.

On-line vs off-line assessment of GMs

In all the studies described above, the standardized technique of assessing GMs has been applied, based on the observation of video-recordings with specific methodological features (Einspieler et al 2005). The use of a precise method of video observation has proven useful for the overall reliability of the examination. Undisturbed by other environmental impressions, the observer can assess the video-recording on the basis of his or her visual *gestalt* perception of the movement quality, with the additional advantage of repeated playback, even at different speeds. The full application of the standard methodology, however, is not always easy to accomplish routinely in clinical settings, as it requires the use of video equipment and additional dedicated time, which are not always available, especially outside the context of specifically designed follow-up programs. Moreover, the standard method has the disadvantage of not allowing the observer to give an immediate clinical response to the family, particularly in case of doubtful results. For these reasons, in many clinical contexts the assessment of GMs is also performed with the unaided eye, and the judgement is based on the direct observation of infant behaviour.

Only one study so far has investigated the reliability of this modified version of the method in a large number of preterm, term and young infants at neurological risk (Guzzetta et al 2007). While being video-recorded, each infant's spontaneous motor activity was directly observed and assessed by means of a written proforma. A blind evaluation of the video was subsequently performed by a different evaluator. The correlation coefficient between the two techniques was 0.42 at writhing age, and 0.79 at fidgety age. Both methods showed a very high sensitivity for the neurological outcome, as no false negatives were observed. The direct assessment showed a lower specificity, particularly during the writhing period. These results support the use of the direct assessment of GMs when the full application of the standard video observation cannot be routinely applied, restricting the use of video-recordings to the abnormal or doubtful cases. This may facilitate the integration of the assessment of spontaneous movements into more general protocols of neurological examination (Dubowitz et al 1999) and into clinical follow-up programs.

OTHER METHODS OF GENERAL MOVEMENT ASSESSMENT
Other authors have confirmed the importance of the assessment of spontaneous movements for early diagnosis, but using criteria for normality and abnormality of movements different from Prechtl's method.

Touwen (1990) did not describe specific movement patterns but classified the qualitative characteristics of movements according to three paired categories: *patterned* (movement patterns are consistently composite and recognizable) versus *unpatterned* (no consistent pattern can be recognized, movements are defined as 'chaotic' or 'erratic'); *smooth* (movements are continuous and fluent with gradual acceleration and deceleration) versus *jerky* (movements are abrupt with sudden acceleration and deceleration); *variable* (movements change in speed, amplitude and direction with various patterns and postures) versus *stereotyped* (movements are invariant in type, speed, direction and amplitude).

Van Kranen-Mastenbroek et al (1992, 1994) suggested five different categories of general movements, ranging from normal GMs (Type I) to different kinds of abnormalities (Types II, III, IV, V). The main difference compared to Prechtl's method lies in the attention to many details (onset of movements, variability in amplitude, overall amplitude, speed of arms compared to legs, etc.), while a global Gestalt judgement is only used as the last item of the examination.

Hadders-Algra et al (1997, 2004) introduced new terminology and enlarged the categorization of the existing types of GM abnormalities. In particular, normal GMs are defined according to Prechtl's definition (Prechtl 1990, Prechtl et al 1997a), while abnormal GMs are distinguished according to an interpretative instead of descriptive criterion, as 'mildly' and 'definitely' abnormal. Data related to the predictive values of these different categories have been reported in this chapter.

Kakebeeke et al (1997, 1998) used a 10-point scale based on the assessment of fluency, spatio-temporal variability and sequencing of GMs, by assessing separately arms and legs. No data on the predictive value of this scale are available.

An item scoring the quality of spontaneous movements is also included in the neurological assessment of newborns and young infants by Dubowitz et al (1999; and Chapter 4), but a specific study of the value of this item has not been provided. The validity of this integrated approach, which does not use video-recording, is indirectly supported by the results of on-line GM assessment (see previous section).

The 'complementary' neuromotor examination

The so-called 'complementary' neuromotor examination of the newborn and the young infant is a clinical technique suggested by Grenier in the 1980s to enlarge, and make more comprehensive, the traditional neurological assessment during the first years of life (Amiel-Tison and Grenier 1985, Grenier et al 1985).

According to Grenier, the classical neurological examination, mainly based on sub-cortical responses (i.e. reflexes, passive muscle tone, etc.), does not permit the observation of motor activities likely to be mediated by higher centres, otherwise hidden by primitive and obligatory neurological reactions (i.e. Moro reflex, asymmetrical tonic neck responses, etc.). These reactions, typical of the first months of life, are related to the position of the head and have a strong influence on upper and lower limb posture and movements.

Grenier named the repertoire of movements elicited by means of specific facilitations, mainly postural, that can be obtained by supporting the head, '*motricité libérée*'. Movements patterns characteristic of '*motricité libérée*' could anticipate the motor behaviour of older infants, and they may be relevant in predicting normal neurological and cognitive development. According to Grenier, the patterns of '*motricité libérée*' are never observed in infants with brain dysfunction, and they are useful in predicting, at a very early age, an unfavourable neurological outcome (cerebral palsy).

The complementary neuromotor examination is carried out in the presence of the parents, who are directly involved in the stimulation of their infant in order to increase his attention; at the same time they also have the opportunity to verify the infant's hidden capacities and integrity of the nervous system.

The examination is characterized by three different progressive phases: '*deparassitage*' (liberation), 'liberated state' and 'guided motricity'.

Manual support and proprioceptive stimulation are given to the neck and the spine while the infant is kept alert and attentive to the examiner. Muscle tone and primary reflexes are modified: head control, relaxation of upper limbs, decrement of obligatory movements and primary reflexes are gradually observed ('*deparassitage*').

The new behavioural state of sensorial ability and interaction, called the 'liberated state', is different from any of the five classical states described by Prechtl (1974), being characterized by active participation of the infant and by the expression of hidden motor abilities (e.g. a 17-day-old infant reaching and grasping an object). During the 'liberated state', with the help and 'guide' of the examiner, the infant can also perform dynamic tests, such as lateral support on right and left arm, and lateral abduction of the hip.

This approach is still in use in some French units, both in full-term and in preterm infants (Grenier et al 1995, Hernandorena et al 1995). However, the technique is time-consuming, not applicable in very immature infants, and no clear evidence is available, so far, on its value in clinical follow-up.

Behavioural assessment scales

The Neonatal Behavioural Assessment Scale (NBAS) is a technique developed by Brazelton (1973) for examining the behaviour of term infants during the first couple of months of age. Its conceptual basis is founded on the assumption that the newborn has active and specific responses to environmental stimulations, rather than passive behaviour. NBAS involves the exploration of spontaneous neonatal behaviour and the ability to modify the infant's behavioural functioning by means of facilitations by the examiner: this establishes an interactive relationship with the infant, based on his individual characteristics.

There are two key principles which lie behind this method: first, the 'best performance' concept, from the infant's point of view; and, second, the flexibility of the examiner in modifying and adapting the examination to the specific and individual characteristics of the infant, in order to obtain optimal behavioural responses.

According to this approach the behaviour of the newborn and young infant is organized into four functional systems (autonomic nervous system regulation, motor activity organization, behavioural state organization, social abilities): each system interacts with the others, and is influenced by the environment.

The stability of the autonomic nervous system is expressed by the presence or absence of tremors or startles or changing of skin colour; motor organization is represented by evaluation of muscle tone, reflexes and motor activity; the organization of behavioural states includes lability of states, irritability, peak of excitement, consolability and self-quieting activity; and the quality of attention and interaction consists of levels of alertness and the ability to focus attention on the source of stimulation or on a visual/auditory stimulus.

The NBAS includes 28 behavioural items and 18 neurological items related to reflexes (see Fig. 5.3). The upper age limit for its use is indicated at around 2 months (corrected, if preterm infants are considered).

The application of the NBAS is related to the dynamic content of the interaction between the infant and his/her caregivers. The interactive characteristics of the scale make it quite different from other methods of examination; in particular the 'objectivity' of the examiner is replaced by a flexible approach more similar to a parental style. In addition, the parents, who are present during the observation of the infant's responses, are able to gain a better understanding of his capacities.

The NBAS has a preferential order of evaluation, but the order can be flexible and adapted to the infant's response to the examination; for this reason the experience of the examiner is very important. The scale represents not only a research instrument – in recent years it has developed a wider application in the clinical field.

It has to be underlined that the scale allows evaluation of behavioural organization, whereas it was not designed for neurological diagnosis; in this respect, the presence of a neurological section, related to muscle tone and reflexes, might be confusing.

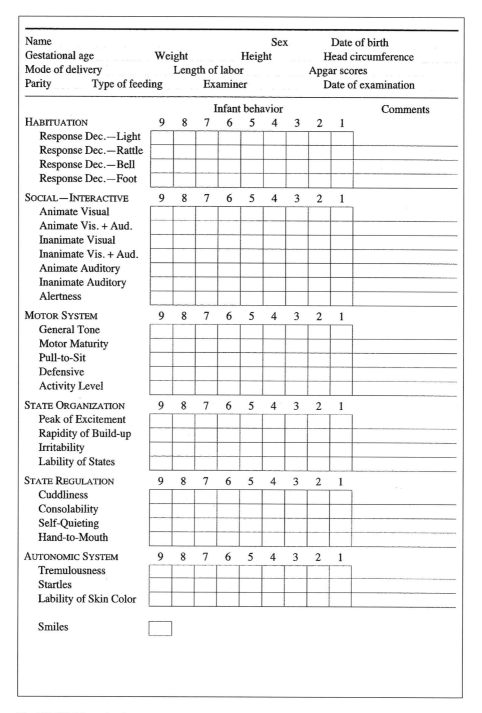

	Infant behavior									Comments
HABITUATION	9	8	7	6	5	4	3	2	1	
Response Dec.—Light										
Response Dec.—Rattle										
Response Dec.—Bell										
Response Dec.—Foot										
SOCIAL—INTERACTIVE	9	8	7	6	5	4	3	2	1	
Animate Visual										
Animate Vis. + Aud.										
Inanimate Visual										
Inanimate Vis. + Aud.										
Animate Auditory										
Inanimate Auditory										
Alertness										
MOTOR SYSTEM	9	8	7	6	5	4	3	2	1	
General Tone										
Motor Maturity										
Pull-to-Sit										
Defensive										
Activity Level										
STATE ORGANIZATION	9	8	7	6	5	4	3	2	1	
Peak of Excitement										
Rapidity of Build-up										
Irritability										
Lability of States										
STATE REGULATION	9	8	7	6	5	4	3	2	1	
Cuddliness										
Consolability										
Self-Quieting										
Hand-to-Mouth										
AUTONOMIC SYSTEM	9	8	7	6	5	4	3	2	1	
Tremulousness										
Startles										
Lability of Skin Color										
Smiles										

Name   Sex   Date of birth
Gestational age   Weight   Height   Head circumference
Mode of delivery   Length of labor   Apgar scores
Parity   Type of feeding   Examiner   Date of examination

Fig. 5.3 NBAS scoring form.

SUPPLEMENTARY ITEMS	Infant behavior									Comments
	9	8	7	6	5	4	3	2	1	
Quality of Alertness										
Cost of Attention										
Examiner Facilitation										
General Irritability										
Robustness/Endurance										
State Regulation										
E's Emotional Resp.										

REFLEXES	0	1	2	3	Asym	Comments
Plantar Grasp						
Babinski						
Ankle Clonus						
Rooting						
Sucking						
Glabella						
Passive Resist.—Legs						
Passive Resist.—Arms						
Palmar Grasp						
Placing						
Standing						
Walking						
Crawling						
Incurvation						
Tonic Dev. Head/Eyes						
Nystagmus						
TNR						
Moro						

SUMMARY: INFANT

Strengths   Concerns

SUMMARY: PARENT(S)

Strengths   Concerns

RECOMMENDATIONS FOR CAREGIVING:

Fig. 5.3 *continued*

In the literature, there is a recent proposal for a new evaluation instrument, the Neonatal Intensive Care Network Neurobehavioural Scale (Lester et al 2004), in order to offer a more complete behavioural and neurological examination in preterm as well as in full-term infants.

On the basis of Brazelton's assessment of term infants, Als et al (1982) standardized a behavioural scale for preterm infants, the Assessment of Preterm Infant Behaviour (APIB), an interesting clinical instrument which aims to evaluate the global maturational level of the preterm infant, to identify the aspects at risk of developmental problems, and to plan a better individualized intervention in the neonatal intensive care unit (NICU), and afterwards.

Behavioural evaluation using the APIB has been validated for clinical research. The difference in maturity between newborns at term and preterm infants without brain lesions is reported (Huppi et al 1996, Mouradian et al 2000), and this immaturity, persisting until 40 weeks postconceptional age, seems to be associated with a delay in structural maturation observed on MRI (Huppi et al 1996).

The availability of a profile of behavioural functioning of the newborn is an important starting point for early intervention. In the context of the interaction between the functional subsystems and the environment, early intervention has to be individualized, that is, based on the infant's behavioural responses, in association with adjustments in the environment of the NICU (lights and sound level, frequency of noxious interventions, etc.), specific motor facilitation (posture in flexion, not during feeding time), and assistance with the transition from waking to sleeping (individualized developmental care).

Recent studies report significant results from early intervention programmes in high- and in low-risk preterm infants (Parker et al 1992, Buchler et al 1995, Als et al 1996, Huppi et al 1996, Stevens et al 1996) and also better performance on behavioural, electrophysiological and brain structural measures demonstrated on MRI (Als 2004). A recent Cochrane review (Symington and Pinelli 2006) suggests that these interventions may have some benefit for the outcomes of preterm infants; however, there continues to be conflicting evidence from the many studies. According to this review, before a clear direction for practice can be supported, evidence demonstrating more consistent effects of developmental care interventions on short- and long-term clinical outcomes is needed. Moreover, the economic impact of the implementation and maintenance of developmental care practices should be considered by individual institutions.

Among the limitations of these behavioural scales, in the context of assessment, we have to underline that adaptations for ages beyond the first two months are not available. Moreover, for the same test a high intraindividual day-to-day variability in the responses has been shown (Sameroff 1978). In addition, these techniques are time-consuming and not easily applicable in a clinical setting. However, as indicated above, they can have applications in interventions concerning early stimulation of neurologically impaired infants, and in studies on the effect of environmental risk factors on infants' development.

Conclusions

Recent findings have contributed to a new approach to the neurological assessment of newborn and young infants. Assessment of the quality of execution of movement patterns and of general movements in particular, as well as the other methods described in this chapter, or others that could not be reported here – such as the Test of Infant Motor Performance proposed by Campbell (2001) and described in Chapter 13 (see pages 230–32) – provide an important contribution to the early diagnosis, prognosis and treatment of high-risk infants. However, these methods should always complement, and not replace, traditional neurological examination techniques. They have different properties and diagnostic tasks. Moreover, traditional neurological assessment provides a more comprehensive picture of the various neural subsystems, some of which cannot be tested by GM observation and other approaches.

REFERENCES

Albers S, Jorch G (1994) Prognostic significance of spontaneous motility in very immature preterm infants under intensive care treatment. *Biol Neonat* 66: 182–187.

Als H (2004) Early experience alters brain function and structure. *Pediatrics* 113: 846–857.

Als H, Lester BM, Tronick EZ, Brazelton TB (1982) Toward a research instrument for the assessment of preterm infants' behavior (APIB). In: Fitzgerald H, Lester M, Yooman MW, editors. *Theory and Research in Behavioral Pediatrics*. New York: Plenum Press, pp 35–132.

Als H, Duffy FH, Mc Annulty GB (1996) Effectiveness of individualized neurodevelopmental care in the newborn intensive care unit (NICU). *Acta Paediatr* 416: 21–30.

Amiel-Tison C, Grenier A (1985) *La Surveillance Neurologique au Cours de la Première Année de la Vie*. Paris: Masson.

Baldi I (2002) The preterm infant with prolonged periventricular hyperechogenicity: prognostic role of neurological assessment and the effects of neonatal care. (In Italian.) MD thesis, University of Pisa.

Bos AF, van Loon AJ, Hadders-Algra M, Martijn A, Okken A, Prechtl HFR (1997a) Spontaneous motility in preterm, small for gestational age infants. II. Qualitative aspects. *Early Hum Dev* 50: 131–147.

Bos AF, van Asperen RM, de Leeuw DM, Prechtl HFR (1997b) The influence of septicaemia on spontaneous motility in preterm infants. *Early Hum Dev* 50: 61–70.

Bos AF, Martijn A, van Asperen RM, Hadders-Algra M, Okken A, Prechtl HFR (1998) Qualitative assessment of general movements in high risk preterm infants with chronic lung disease requiring dexamethasone therapy. *J Pediatr* 132: 300–306.

Bos AF, Einspieler C, Prechtl HFR, Touwen B, Okken-Beukens M, Stremmelar F (1999) The quality of spontaneous motor activity in preterm infants as early predictive signs for minor neurological abnormalities at two years. Newsletter. *Neonat Neurol* 8: 4–5.

Bos AF, Einspieler C, Prechtl HFR (2002) Motor repertoire at early age for prediction of neurological deficits at 2 y. *Pediatr Res* 52: 796. (Abstract.)

Bourgeois JP (2001) Synaptogenesis in the neocortex of the newborn: the ultimate frontier for individuation. In: Lagercrantz H, Hanson M, Evrard P, Rodeck C, editors. *The Newborn Brain. Neuroscience and Clinical Applications*. Cambridge: Cambridge University Press, pp 91–113.

Brazelton TB (1973). *Neonatal Behavioral Assessment Scale*. Clinics in Developmental Medicine 50. Philadelphia: JB Lippincott.

Bruggink JLM, Einspieler C, Butcher PR, Stremmelaar EF, Bos AF (2006) Can mild neurological abnormalities at 7 to 11 years be predicted from the motor repertoire at early age in preterm infants? *PAS* 3570: 310. (Abstract.)

Buchler DM, Als H, Duffy FH, MC Annulty GB, Liederman J (1995) Effectiveness of individualized developmental care for low risk preterm infants: behavioral and electrophysiologic evidence. *Pediatrics* 96: 923–932.

Campbell SK (2001) *The Test of Infant Motor Performance. Test User's Manual Version 1.4*. Chicago: Infant Motor Performance Scales, LLC.

Cioni G, Castellacci AM (1990) Development of fetal and neonatal motor activity: implications for neurology. In: Block H, Bertenthal BI, editors. *Sensory-motor Organizations and Development in Infancy and Early Childhood.* Amsterdam: Kluwer Academic Publishers, pp 135–144.

Cioni G, Prechtl HFR (1990) Preterm and early postterm motor behaviour in low-risk premature infants. *Early Hum Dev* 23: 159–193.

Cioni G, Ferrari F, Prechtl HFR (1989) Posture and spontaneous motility in fullterm infants. *Early Hum Dev* 7: 247–262.

Cioni G, Paolicelli PB, Rapisardi G, Castellacci AM, Ferrari A (1997a) Early natural history of spastic diplegia and tetraplegia. *Eur J Pediatr Neurol* 1: 33. (Abstract.)

Cioni G, Ferrari F, Einspieler C, Paolicelli PB, Barbani MT, Prechtl HFR (1997b) Comparison between observation of spontaneous movements and neurological examination in preterm infants. *J Pediatr* 130: 704–711.

Cioni G, Prechtl HFR, Ferrari F, Paolicelli PB, Einspieler C, Roversi MF (1997c) Which better predicts later outcome in fullterm infants: quality of general movements or neurological examination? *Early Hum Dev* 50: 71–85.

Cioni G, Bos AF, Einspieler C, Ferrari F, Martijn A, Paolicelli PB, Rapisardi G, Roversi MF, Prechtl HFR (2000) Early neurological signs in preterm infants with unilateral intraparenchymal echodensity. *Neuropediatrics* 31: 240–251.

Cohen J (1960) A coefficient of agreement for nominal scales. *Ed Psychol Meas* 20: 37–46.

Coluccini M, Maini S, Sabatini A, Prechtl HFR, Cioni G (2002) Kinematic analysis of general movements in early infancy. *Dev Med Child Neurol* 44: 14. (Abstract.)

Constantinou JC, Adamson-Macedo EN, Stevenson DK, Mirmiran M, Fleisher BE (1999) Effects of skin-to-skin holding on general movements of preterm infants. *Clin Pediatr* 38: 467–471.

Culp RE, Culp AM, Harmon RJ (1989) A tool for educating parents about their premature infants. *Birth* 16: 23–26.

de Vries JIP, Visser GHA, Prechtl HFR (1982) The emergence of fetal behaviour. I. Qualitative aspects. *Early Hum Dev* 7: 301–322.

Dibiasi J, Einspieler C (2002) Can spontaneous movements be modulated by visual and acoustic stimulation in 3-month-old infants? *Early Hum Dev* 68: 27–37.

Dibiasi J, Einspieler C (2004) Load perturbation does not influence spontaneous movements in 3-month-old infants. *Early Hum Dev* 77: 37–46.

Dubowitz LMS, Dubowitz V, Mercuri E (1999) *The Neurological Assessment of the Preterm and Full-Term Newborn Infant, 2nd edn.* Clinics in Developmental Medicine 148. Cambridge: Cambridge University Press.

Einspieler C (1994) Abnormal spontaneous movements in infants with repeated sleep apnoeas. *Early Hum Dev* 36: 31–48.

Einspieler C, Prechtl HFR (2005) Prechtl's assessment of general movements: a diagnostic tool for the functional assessment of the young nervous system. *Ment Retard Dev Disabil Res* 11: 61–7. (Review.)

Einspieler C, Prechtl HFR, van Eykern L, de Roos B (1994) Observation of movements during sleep in ALTE and apnoeic infants. *Early Hum Dev* 40: 39–50.

Einspieler C, Prechtl HFR, Ferrari F, Cioni G, Bos AF (1997) The qualitative assessment of general movements in preterm, term and young infants – review of the methodology. *Early Hum Dev* 50: 47–60.

Einspieler C, Cioni G, Paolicelli PB, Bos AF, Dressler A, Ferrari F, Roversi MF, Prechtl HFR (2002) The early markers for later dyskinetic cerebral palsy are different from those for spastic cerebral palsy. *Neuropediatrics* 33: 73–78.

Einspieler C, Prechtl HFR, Bos AF, Ferrari F, Cioni G (2004) *Prechtl's Method on the Qualitative Assessment of General Movements in Preterm, Term and Young Infants.* Clinics in Developmental Medicine 167. London: Mac Keith Press.

Einspieler C, Kerr AM, Prechtl HF (2005) Is the early development of girls with Rett disorder really normal? *Pediatr Res* 57: 696–700.

Einspieler C, Marschik PB, Milioti S, Nakajima Y, Bos AF, Prechtl HF (2006) Are abnormal fidgety movements an early marker for complex minor neurological dysfunction at puberty? *Early Hum Dev*, in press.

Ferrari F, Gioni C, Prechtl HFR (1990) Qualitative changes of general movements in preterm infants with brain lesions. *Early Hum Dev* 23: 193–233.

Ferrari F, Prechtl HFR, Cioni G, Roversi MF, Einspieler C, Gallo C, Paolicelli PB, Cavazzutti GB (1997) Behavioural states, posture and spontaneous movements in infants affected by brain malformation. *Early Hum Dev* 50: 87–113.

Ferrari F, Cioni G, Einspieler C, Roversi MF, Bos AF, Paolocelli PB, Ranzi A, Prechtl HFR (2002) Cramped synchronised general movements in preterm infants as an early marker for cerebral palsy. *Arch Pediatr Adolesc Med* 156: 460–467.

Geerdink JJ, Hopkins B (1993) Qualitative changes in general movements and their prognostic values in preterm infants. *Eur J Paediatr* 152: 362–367.

Grenier A, Hernandorena X, Sainz M, Contaires B, Carré M, Bouchet E (1995) Examen neuromoteur complémentaire de nourrissons à risque de sequelles. Pourquoi? Comment? *Arch Pédiatr* 2: 1007–1012.

Guzzetta A, Mercuri E, Rapisardi G, Ferrari F, Roversi F, Cowan F, Rutherford M, Paolicelli PB, Einspieler C, Boldrini A, Dubowitz L, Prechtl HFR, Cioni G (2003) General movements detect early signs of hemiplegia in term infants with neonatal cerebral infarction. *Neuropediatrics* 34: 61–66.

Guzzetta A, Belmonti V, Battini R, Boldrini A, Paolicelli PB, Cioni G (2007) Does the assessment of general movements without video observation reliably predict neurological outcome? *Eur J Pediatr Neurol* (in press).

Hadders-Algra M (2004) General movements: a window for early identification of children at high risk for developmental disorders. *J Pediatr* 145: S12–S18.

Hadders-Algra M, Groothuis AM (1999) Quality of general movements in infancy is related to neurological dysfunction, ADHD, and aggressive behaviour. *Dev Med Child Neurol* 41: 381–391.

Hadders-Algra M, Prechtl HFR (1992) Developmental course of general movements in early infancy I: Descriptive analysis of change in form. *Early Hum Dev* 28: 201–213.

Hadders-Algra M, Van Eykern LA, Klip-Van den Nieuwendijk AW, Prechtl HF (1992) Developmental course of general movements in early infancy. II. EMG correlates. *Early Hum Dev* 28: 231–251.

Hadders-Algra M, Klip-van den Nieuwendijk AW, Martijn A, van Eykern LA (1997) Assessment of general movements: towards a better understanding of a sensitive method to evaluate brain function in young infants. *Dev Med Child Neurol* 39: 88–98.

Hadders-Algra M, Mavinkurve-Groothuis AMC, Groen SE, Stremmelaar EF, Martijn A, Butcher PR (2004) Quality of general movements and the development of minor neurological dysfunction at toddler and school age. *Clin Rehabil* 18: 287–299.

Hernandorena X, Contaires B, Carré M, Sainz M, Bouchet E, Grenier A (1995) Surveillance neurologique des nouveau-nés à risque d'infirmité motrice cérébrale. *Arch Pédiatr* 2: 941–947.

Hopkins B, Prechtl HFR (1984) A qualitative approach to the development of movements during early infancy. In: Prechtl HFR, editor. *Continuity of Neural Functions from Prenatal to Postnatal Life.* Clinics in Developmental Medicine 94. Oxford: Blackwell, pp 179–197.

Huppi PS, Schuknecht B, Boesch C, Bossi E, Fselblinger J, Fusch C, Herschkowitz N (1996) Structural and neurobehavioral delay in postnatal brain development of preterm infants. *Pediatr Res* 39: 895–901.

Kakebeeke TH, von Siebenthal K, Largo RH (1997) Differences in movement quality at term among preterm and term infants. *Biol Neonat* 71: 367–378.

Kakebeeke TH, von Siebenthal K, Largo RH (1998) Movement quality in preterm infants prior to term. *Biol Neonat* 73: 145–154.

Lester BM, Tronick EZ, Brazelton TB (2004) The Neonatal Intensive Care Network Neurobehavioral Scale procedures. *Pediatrics* 113: 641–667.

Lorenz K (1971) Gestalt perception as a source of scientific knowledge. (English translation of a German paper of 1959.) In: Lorenz K, editor. *Studies in Animal and Human Behaviour*, Vol. II. London: Methuen, pp 281–322.

Mouradian LE, Als H, Coster WJ (2000) Neurobehavioral functioning of healthy preterm infants of varying gestational ages. *J Dev Behav Pediatr* 21: 408–416.

Nakajima Y, Einspieler C, Marschik PB, Bos AF (2005) Does a detailed assessment of poor repertoire general movements help to identify those infants who will develop normally? *Early Hum Dev* 82: 53–59.

Parker SI, Zahr LK, Cole JG, Brecht ML (1992) Outcome after developmental intervention in the neonatal intensive care unit for mothers of preterm infants with low socioeconomic status. *J Pediatr* 120: 780–785.

Phagava H, Muratori F, Maestro S, Guzzetta A, Cioni G (2005) Retrospective analysis of general movements in infants with autism spectrum disorder: a pilot study. *Eur J Neurol* 12(Suppl 2): 239–240.

Prechtl HFR (1974) The behavioural state of the newborn (a review). Duivenvoorde Lecture. *Brain Res* 76: 185–212.

Prechtl HFR (1980) The optimality concept. *Early Hum Dev* 4: 201–205.

Prechtl HFR (1990) Qualitative changes of spontaneous movements in fetus and preterm infants are a marker of neurological dysfunction. *Early Hum Dev* 23: 151–158.

Prechtl HFR (1997) State of the art of a new functional assessment of the young nervous system. An early predictor of cerebral palsy. *Early Hum Dev* 50: 1–11.

Prechtl HFR (2001a) Prenatal and early postnatal development of human motor behaviour. In: Kalverboer AF, Gramsbergen A, editors. *Handbook of Brain and Behaviour in Human Development.* Amsterdam: Kluwer, pp 415–427.

Prechtl HFR (2001b) General movement assessment as a method of developmental neurology: new paradigms and their consequences. The 1999 Ronnie MacKeith Lecture. *Dev Med Child Neurol* 43: 836–842.

Prechtl HFR, Einspieler C (1997) Is neurological assessment of the fetus possible? *Eur J Obstetr Gynecol Repr Biol* 75: 81–84.

Prechtl HFR, Nolte R (1984) Motor behaviour of preterm infants. In: Prechtl HFR, editor. *Continuity of Neural Functions from Prenatal to Postnatal Life.* Clinics in Developmental Medicine 94. Oxford: Blackwell, pp 79–92.

Prechtl HFR, Ferrari F, Cioni G (1993) Predictive value of general movements in asphyxiated fullterm infants. *Early Hum Dev* 35: 91–120.

Prechtl HFR, Einspieler C, Cioni G, Bos AF, Ferrari F, Sontheimer D (1997a) An early marker for neurological deficits after perinatal brain lesions. *Lancet* 349: 1361–1363.

Prechtl HFR, Bos AF, Cioni G, Einspieler C, Ferrari F (1997b) *Spontaneous Motor Activity as a Diagnostic Tool.* Demonstration Video. London, Graz: The GM Trust (www.general-movements-trust.info).

Sameroff, AJ (1978): Summary and conclusion: the future of newborn assessment. In: Sameroff AJ, editor. *Organization and Stability of Newborn Behaviour Assessment Scale. Monographs of the Society for Research in Child Development* 177(43): 102–123.

Seme-Ciglenečki P (2003) Predictive value of assessment of general movements for neurological development of high-risk preterm infants: comparative study. *Croat Med J* 44: 721–727.

Stevens B, Johnston C, Petryshen H, Taddio A (1996). Premature infant pain profile: development and initial validation. *Clin J Pain* 12: 13–22.

Symington A, Pinelli J (2006): Developmental care for promoting development and preventing morbidity in preterm infants. *Cochrane Database Syst Rev* 19: CD001814.

Touwen BCL (1990) Variability and stereotypy of spontaneous motility as a predictor of neurological development of preterm infants. *Dev Med Child Neurol* 32: 501–509.

Valentin T, Uhl K, Einspieler C (2005) The effectiveness of training in Prechtl's method on the qualitative assessment of general movements. *Early Hum Dev* 81: 623–627.

van der Heide JC, Paolicelli PB, Boldrini A, Cioni G (1999) Kinematic and qualitative analysis of lower-extremity movements in preterm infants with brain lesions. *Phys Ther* 79: 546–557.

van Kranen-Mastenbroek V, van Oostenbrugge R, Palmans L, Stevens A, Kingma H, Blanco C, Hasaart T, Vles J (1992) Inter- and intra-observer agreement in the assessment of the quality of spontaneous movements in the newborn. *Brain Dev* 14: 289–293.

van Kranen-Mastenbroek V, Kingma H, Caberg H, Ghys A, Blanco C, Hasaart T, Vles J (1994) Quality of spontaneous general movements in full-term small for gestational age and appropriate for gestational age newborn infants. *Neuropediatrics* 25: 145–153.

6
MAGNETIC RESONANCE IMAGING OF THE INFANT BRAIN

Mary Rutherford, Eugenio Mercuri and Frances Cowan

Introduction

Magnetic resonance (MR) imaging has a vital role to play in paediatric neurology. In most cases the examination provides the most valuable information if performed within the neonatal period. However, this relies on the neonate presenting with distinguishing signs or symptoms, and on the availability of MR imaging within the hospital. Unfortunately MR imaging of the sick neonate is not easy, and experience – both in the practicalities of performing a successful examination and in the interpretation of the results – is limited to relatively few centres. Centres performing serial examinations, however, can provide invaluable information which helps in the interpretation of scans performed in later infancy in other units.

In this chapter we will propose a few recommendations related to practical issues, such as sedation or safety procedures, suggesting the most appropriate sequences and timing to use in the first years of life. We will also describe how MR imaging can be used to follow the physiological maturation of the developing brain and the evolution of the patterns of lesions most frequently observed in the neonatal period.

Practical issues

SEDATION

Successful imaging of the neonate or young child requires careful preparation of the infant and close cooperation between radiologist, radiographer, neonatologists and paediatricians. To this end neonates may be successfully imaged during natural sleep, following a feed or under light sedation with, for instance, chloral hydrate. We use a dose of between 25 and 50 mg/kg orally, via nasogastric tube or rectally (Cowan 1998). Severely encephalopathic neonates may not require sedation or may already be sedated by anticonvulsant medication. All neonates, sedated or not, should be monitored during scanning with MR-compatible pulse oximetry and ECG. A qualified paediatrician should be in attendance throughout. Older children can be successfully sedated with chloral hydrate for the purposes of MR imaging. We use a higher dose of between 75 and 100 mg/kg for children over the age of 6 months (Cowan 1998). It should not be necessary to use a general anaesthetic below the age of 2 years, but these children usually require the maximum dose of chloral hydrate. They also require monitoring throughout the scan and afterwards until they have woken.

All neonates and children require a careful metal check prior to an MR scan. Excessive noise, particularly with fast sequences such as diffusion-weighted or perfusion-weighted imaging, may wake a sleeping infant or even harm the developing auditory system, and ear protection should be used. We use mouldable dental putty as individualized earplugs, and neonatal earmuffs (Natus MiniMuffs; www.natus.com). Infants may move even when asleep, but moulded airbags or foam placed snugly around the infant's head will keep this to a minimum. Swaddling the infants will keep them warm and also reduce movements. For older children, headphones and adult-style earplugs can be used. Foam around the head will also reduce motion (Pennock 2002).

HARDWARE AND SOFTWARE ADAPTATIONS

Image quality is governed by the signal to noise ratio. To this end the head coil used should fit as snugly as possible around the head. In the absence of a dedicated neonatal or infant head coil, an adult knee coil – available with most commercial scanners – will accommodate the head of an infant up to approximately 2 months of age.

Most MR sequences designed for imaging the adult brain will need to be adapted to obtain high quality images of the immature brain (under 2 years), with its higher water content. The exact imaging parameters depend on the specific system and magnet strength being used.

T1 and T2 refer to the MR parameters known as longitudinal and transverse relaxation times respectively. These times vary with different tissue types. Images that are T1- or T2-weighted provide complementary information about normal anatomy and about pathology. Diffusion-weighted imaging measures the amount of random water motion or diffusivity within the brain. This diffusivity, measured as an apparent diffusion co-efficient (ADC), is reduced in areas of acute infarction (see Fig. 6.5). This is partly explained by a decrease in freely moving extracellular water and an increase in relatively restricted intracellular water, seen as cytotoxic oedema. Once cells have undergone necrosis and the infarction is established, usually during the second week after injury, diffusivity pseudonormalizes.

FLAIR imaging is essentially T2-weighted but the signal intensity from cerebrospinal fluid is nulled. This makes it easier to distinguish high signal intensity glial tissue, particularly when it is in a periventricular area.

We would routinely perform the following sequences:

- T1-weighted sequence acquired in the transverse plane. This is ideal for assessing the basal ganglia and thalami and provides the best views of the posterior limb of the internal capsule. (Fig. 6.1)
- T2-weighted sequence acquired in the transverse plane. This is better than T1-weighted imaging for early ischaemia and provides excellent grey/white matter contrast in the very immature brain (Fig. 6.1)
- T1-weighted sequence acquired in the sagittal plane (Fig. 6.2). A volume acquisition is ideal as it provides thin slices and can be reformatted into any plane. It can be used

for absolute quantification of brain structures (Fig. 6.3). T2-weighted sequences can also be reformatted (Fig. 6.4).

- Diffusion-weighted imaging, which is ideal for early (<1 week) identification of ischaemic tissue (Fig. 6.5).

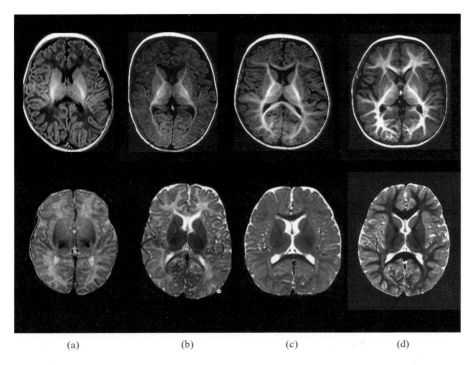

(a)   (b)   (c)   (d)

Fig. 6.1 Normal appearances of the brain at term on T1-weighted images (top row) and T2-weighted images (bottom row) at term (a), 3 months (b), 1 year (c) and 2 years (d).

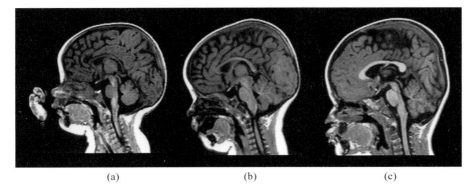

(a)   (b)   (c)

Fig. 6.2 T1-weighted images in sagittal plane. The appearances of the corpus callosum (a) at term, (b) at 3 months, with some high signal intensity consistent with myelin, and (c) at 1 year when it is fully myelinated.

71

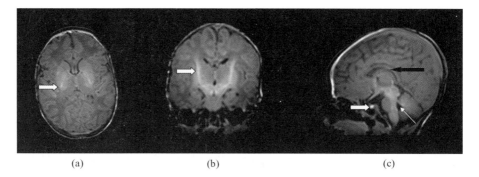

(a)   (b)   (c)

Fig. 6.3 T1-weighted volume acquisition which may be reformatted into any plane. (a) and (b) Note the myelination in the posterior limb of the internal capsule (arrows). (c) In the sagittal plane the corpus callosum can be clearly seen (black arrow) along its entire length. The pituitary may be seen as high signal intensity within the pituitary fossa (thick white arrow). The vermis of the cerebellum can be assessed and the fourth ventricle clearly seen (thin black arrow).

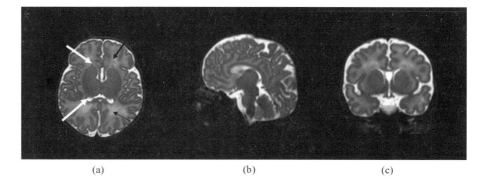

(a)   (b)   (c)

Fig. 6.4 T2-weighted images of a neonatal brain. Multislice acquisition producing a 'pseudo' volume with isotropic images suitable for reformatting into any plane. There is a residual low signal intensity germinal matrix in the temporal horn and over the head of the caudate nucleus (arrows). There are obvious caps anterior to the anterior horns (black arrow) which have a low signal intensity component consistent with migrating cells. Arrowheads are seen posteriorly in the periventricular white matter (black short arrow).

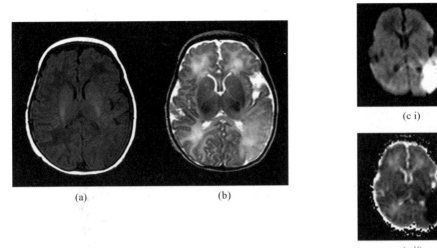

Fig. 6.5 Diffusion-weighted imaging. A 5-day-old neonate with a perinatally acquired left-sided middle cerebral artery infarct. (a) T1-weighted images show relatively subtle loss of grey white matter differentiation within the left posterior parietal lobe. (b) T2-weighted images show more obvious loss of grey white matter differentiation. (ci) The diffusion-weighted image shows high signal intensity and the ADC trace map. (cii) This shows corresponding low signal intensity consistent with restricted diffusion.

Normal appearances of the developing brain from term to 2 years

CORTEX

The brain of the term infant appears mature in terms of its cortical folding. By 38 weeks all the sulci are formed, though they become deeper over the following few weeks (Figs 6.1, 6.5) and the Sylvian fissure may close further. The cortical folding at term age of infants born very preterm appears similar to that of term born infants but it is not as mature and complex (Ajayi-Obe et al 2000).

Normal cortex is of high signal intensity on T1-weighted images and low signal intensity on T2-weighted images. The highest signal contrast is seen around the Rolandic or central sulcus (Fig. 6.6), a region where the adjacent white matter is rapidly myelinating at this age. This cortical high signal decreases over the next two months on T1-weighted images, and over six months on T2-weighted images, depending to some extent on the particular sequences used. This change may be due to a reduction in cellularity and an increasing number of synapses. At the same time white matter is myelinating and changing its signal intensity in the reverse direction to the cortex. Thus, in the first months after the neonatal period, MR images go through a phase of relative isointensity compared to earlier and later images. The phenomenon also applies to injured tissue and may make interpretation of normality and damage difficult in the early months after the neonatal period.

At term, the germinal matrix which gives rise to the cortex has largely involuted compared to the preterm brain (Fig. 6.7), but occasionally remnants of it are seen in the

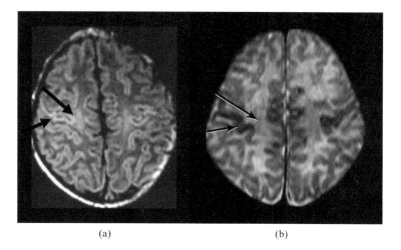

(a)   (b)

Fig. 6.6 Normal appearance of the centrum semiovale showing a well-folded cortex. (a) T1-weighted sequence. There is high signal intensity around the central sulcus (bottom arrow) and high signal in the white matter consistent with myelination (top arrow). (b) T2-weighted sequence. There is low signal intensity around the central sulcus (bottom arrow) and more diffuse low signal in the white matter consistent with myelination (bottom arrow).

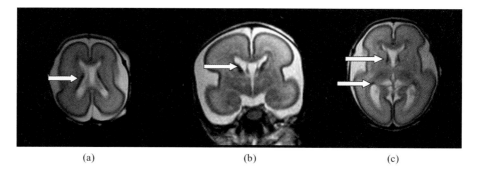

(a)   (b)   (c)

Fig. 6.7 Fast spin echo sequence of a preterm brain at 25 weeks' gestation. The low signal intensity germinal matrix can be clearly seen over the caudate nucleus in the transverse plane (a), over the head of the caudate nucleus in the coronal plane (b), and in the transverse plane (c), and in the roof of the temporal horn (c) (lower arrow). Bands of alternating signal intensity, consistent with migrating cells, are seen around the ventricles.

caudothalamic notch and posterior to the thalami at their junction with the optic radiation and in the anterior periventricular white matter. These are best seen on fast spin echo (FSE) T2-weighted sequences (Fig. 6.4).

CENTRAL GREY MATTER

The basal ganglia and thalami are relatively large in the term infant. The head of caudate nucleus, the lentiform nucleus (globus pallidus and putamen) and thalami are clearly

74

separated by the internal capsule. The globus pallidus and the ventrolateral nucleus of the thalamus (VLNT) and to a lesser extent the posterior putamen are of high signal on T1-weighted images (Fig. 6.1). This high signal in the globus pallidus and putamen becomes less obvious over the next few weeks but it may make interpretation of abnormal signal in kernicterus difficult near to term. The VLNT remains differentiated from the surrounding tissue for several months.

Iron deposition, which reduces the signal intensity in the globus pallidus, substantia nigra and red nucleus (and later the dentate nucleus) on T2-weighted images, should not be seen before 9 years of age. Vascular spaces are often seen in the lower basal ganglia near the anterior commissure and should not be confused with abnormal spaces seen in, for example, Leigh's disease.

MESENCEPHALON AND BRAINSTEM
The pyramidal tracts in the mesencephalon and brainstem are beginning to myelinate in their most lateral portions at term. From birth to 3 months, tracts and nuclei in the brainstem become increasingly obvious, particularly on T1-weighted images.

WHITE MATTER
White matter is relatively immature and largely unmyelinated at term age. Myelination, which has been confined to the brainstem, globus pallidus and VLNT up to term, shows an enormous spurt in the white matter from about 38 weeks' gestation onwards. This continues over the first year, to a lesser extent in year two and, to a small degree, into adolescence.

At term age myelin is seen on MR images in the brainstem, the posterior limb of the internal capsule (PLIC) and the central white matter of the centrum semiovale (Figs 6.1, 6.3). Myelin appears earlier and proceeds faster on T1-weighted images than it does on conventional T2-weighted FSE images. Myelin is seen as high signal on T1-weighted images in the posterior third to half of the internal capsule at term, and the absence of this normal appearance from 37 weeks onwards has great significance for future neurodevelopment and is a very important marker to note on scans. On T2-weighted images only a small region in the most posterior portion of the PLIC appears myelinated; it has a characteristic globular appearance (Figs 6.1, 6.4). On FSE images the region of short T2 is longer and may be as extensive as the high signal on the T1-weighted images. In preterm infants at term the PLIC appears to myelinate slightly earlier than in infants born near term, though the quality of the myelin may not be optimal.

At term age the bulk of the cerebral hemispheres is still composed of unmyelinated white matter which is generally of intermediate to low signal on T1-weighted, and of high signal on T2-weighted, images (Fig. 6.1). It should not be of uniform signal intensity but change slightly the more peripheral it is and become closer to that of cortex, though it should always remain clearly demarcated from cortex. Around the anterior horns of the ventricles there are small 'caps' of low signal intensity on T2-weighted images, which are migrating cells originating in the germinal matrix (Fig. 6.4). Adjacent, but more peripheral, is an arrow-shaped region ('arrowhead') of higher signal on T2-weighted images and low signal on T1-weighted images. This tissue is relatively cell poor on histology. Similar areas are also seen superior to the body and posterior to the occipital horns of the ventricles. These features are much more prominent earlier in gestation and should not normally be very obvious at term age or beyond (Fig. 6.7).

The changes in myelination of the white matter over the first year are dramatic. White matter provides the bulk of the brain volume and is the major contributor to brain growth over the first two years. Before term, myelin is best seen on FSE T2-weighted images. After term, for about eight to ten months, myelin is better seen on T1-weighted sequences. After that time the major changes on T1-weighted images have occurred and further maturation and detail are again better seen on T2-weighted images (Fig. 6.1).

As a general rule, myelination occurs in a caudal to cephalic direction and in the hemispheres is seen first parietally then occipitally, frontally and temporally. Primary tracts myelinate before those in the association areas of the hemispheres. In the brainstem

TABLE 6.1
Timing of myelination in the major regions of the brain

Region	Age of myelination on T1-weighted images	Age of myelination on T2-weighted images
Posterior brainstem	Complete at term	Complete at term
Anterior brainstem	Beginning at term	4 months
Posterior limb of the internal capsule	One-third myelinated at term; complete by 1 month	Small posterior region myelinated at term; complete by 6 months
Anterior limb of the internal capsule	Beginning at 2 months and complete by 3 months	Beginning at 6 months and complete by 8 months
Central centrum semiovale	Beginning at term, reaching motor cortex by 3 months	1–2 months, reaching cortex by 3–4 months
Optic radiations	1 month	2–4 months
Splenium of the corpus callosum	3 months	6 months
Genu of the corpus callosum	5 months	8 months
Hippocampus	Term to 1 month	??
Cerebellar peduncles	Term	2 months
Cerebellar hemispheres	Term (central); 4 months (peripheral)	8–18 months
Occipital white matter	2–3 months, reaching cortex by 6–7 months	4–7 months, continuing subcortically from 9 to 12 months
Frontal white matter	5–6 months	11–14 months, continuing subcortically to 18 months
Temporal white matter	Beginning around 7–8 months, more peripherally by 1 year	16–18 months, continuing subcortically to 24 months
Subcortical white matter and U fibres	24 months	–

myelination occurs dorsally before ventrally, and in sensory before motor tracts. Details of sites and timing of myelination are given in Table 6.1. In summary, on T1-weighted images the internal capsule is myelinated to the genu by 1 month and in its entirety by 3 months (Fig. 6.1). The next regions to myelinate are the central semiovale, the optic radiations and the corpus callosum (Fig. 6.2). On T2-weighted images the changes are slower and more prolonged, and hence subtle changes and delays in myelination in the second year are better demonstrated with T2-weighted images.

THE TERMINAL ZONES

Within myelinating white matter there are regions which are late to myelinate. These are particularly obvious in the periventricular zones posterior and superior to the lateral ventricles well seen on T2-weighted (Fig. 6.8) and FLAIR images. These regions are seen in normal infants in the second year; they may persist for many years and are called 'terminal zones'. Their sites are similar to those regions (arrowheads) within the white matter, mentioned above, that correspond to cell poor areas on histology. However, these same regions are often obvious in very preterm infants with minor motor signs but without cerebral palsy, and they are the same areas that are most commonly affected in periventricular leucomalacia (PVL). They are also commonly seen in children imaged for global developmental delay for which no specific cause is found. In these situations the ventricular margin is fairly smooth and of normal shape and there is a band of tissue of low signal intensity on T2-weighted images which separates the regions of long T2 from the ventricular margin. In PVL the ventricles have an irregular margin and the abnormal high signal abuts the ventricular margin. The clearly pathological high signal of PVL is usually more marked than seen with normal terminal zones and often accompanied by marked thinning of the posterior portion of the body of the corpus callosum and some thalamic atrophy.

Another differential diagnosis for regions of high signal and low signal intensity on T2- and T1-weighted images respectively is vascular spaces. These generally have a distinct

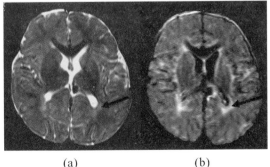

(a)   (b)

Fig. 6.8 Terminal zones. (a) T2-weighted image in a 1-year-old. There is focal increased signal intensity within the terminal zones adjacent to the posterior horns of the lateral ventricles (arrow). (b) The high signal intensity is more obvious on the FLAIR image. This is a relatively common and apparently non-specific finding. It may represent unmyelinated white matter but is particularly frequent in infants born preterm although in isolation it may not be associated with any motor impairment or increased tone in the lower limbs.

Fig. 6.9 Vascular spaces. T2-weighted images in a 2-year-old showing vascular spaces as multiple foci of high signal intensity (arrows).

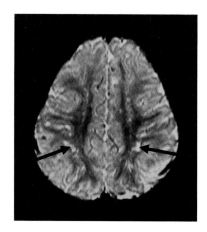

linear appearance on the T1-weighted images (Fig. 6.9) and are best seen on IR (inversion recovery) images. In summary, abnormality in this region is common for a variety of reasons and scan interpretation is very dependent on the clinical situation.

CORPUS CALLOSUM

At term the corpus callosum is thin, even in thickness (about 2 mm), fairly flat and unmyelinated (Fig. 6.2). The genu and splenium do not develop their characteristic shape until later in the first year when they gradually thicken and myelinate (Table 6.1). The body has a more adult appearance around 9 months, often with some focal thinning at the junction between the body and the splenium.

CEREBELLUM

The cerebellar vermis and hemispheres are well developed at term. The cerebellum should rotate anteriorly in the midline and abut the posterior brainstem inferiorly. Myelination is already established in the central regions of the hemispheres and the inferior and superior cerebellar peduncles. By 3 months the appearance is similar to that seen in the adult, but evidence of myelination on T2-weighted images takes longer to develop. More peripheral myelination in the cerebellum, extending to the folia, begins to appear after 4 months on T1-weighted images, and after 8 months on T2-weighted images, and the cerebellum has an adult appearance by 18 months (Fig. 6.10).

THE VENTRICULAR SYSTEM

The lateral ventricles are small and rounded anteriorly and posteriorly and are clearly seen extending into the temporal lobes. The third ventricle is just seen posteriorly between the thalami but the anterior portion may be more obvious as it dips antero-inferiorly towards the pituitary fossa. The aqueduct is narrow but should be visible. The fourth ventricle is slightly wider than it is deep, and about half the diameter of the pons (Figs 6.3c, 6.4b).

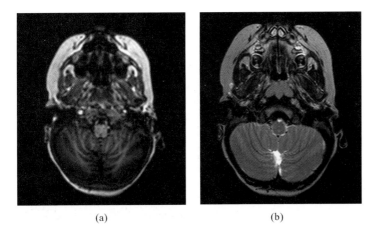

(a)   (b)

Fig. 6.10 The appearance of the cerebellum at 2 years of age showing myelination as high signal on T1-weighted images (a), and as low signal intensity on T2-weighted images (b).

The Extracerebral and Developmental Spaces

The interhemispheric fissure is narrow and regular (Fig. 6.6), but the Sylvian fissures may be prominent, and assessing subtle abnormality in this region can be difficult. The space around the parietal and temporal lobes and the basilar cisterns may appear quite large, up to 5–6 mm, and until 36–37 weeks gestational age wide subarachnoid spaces (12–13 mm) posterior to the parietal lobes can be normal. Enlarged frontal spaces beyond the neonatal period are not uncommon and may be associated with normal development in children scanned in infancy because of macrocephaly (see pages 92–93).

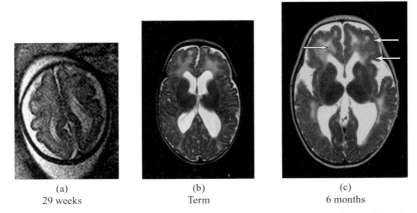

(a)   (b)   (c)
29 weeks   Term   6 months

Fig. 6.11 Evolution of polymicrogyria (a) Fetus of 29 weeks with ventricular dilatation. (b) Term postnatal scan shows ventricular dilatation. There is abnormal high signal intensity within the white matter and a slightly simple appearance to the frontal cortex. (c) At 6 months this is now clearly seen as extensive polymicrogyria (right arrows). The white matter in the frontal lobes still has an abnormally high signal intensity (left arrow)

79

Interpretation of scans

In addition to a thorough knowledge of the normally developing brain, the correct interpretation of images requires an understanding of the range of perinatally acquired lesions and their evolution. Perinatal injury is often symmetrical and may be confused with normal appearances, and vice versa, by those not experienced in imaging the immature brain. It may be appropriate to send images to a centre that regularly performs MR examinations of infants with perinatal injury, for a confirmatory report or second opinion.

Timing of clinical scans

EARLY NEONATAL IMAGING

Antenatal lesions such as haemorrhages, ventricular dilatation and brain malformations are often detected on prenatal imaging, whether this is by ultrasound or MR. In all cases neonatal MR imaging will provide a better definition of the type and extent of the lesion. In some

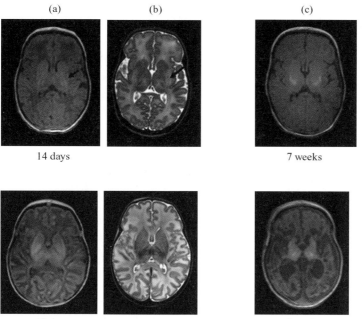

Fig. 6.12 Evolution of perinatally acquired lesions in two separate infants presenting with hypoxic-ischaemic encephalopathy. T1-weighted sequences (a) and (c), and T2-weighted sequences (b). On the top row the lesions are confined to the basal ganglia and thalami, and the abnormal signal intensity within the lentiform is more marked on the T2-weighted images (b). There is residual abnormal increased signal intensity at 7 weeks. On the bottom row the infant has widespread abnormalities within the basal ganglia and thalami and widespread abnormal signal intensity within the white matter consistent with early infarction. At 6 weeks the basal ganglia are markedly atrophied with residual abnormal signal intensity and there are widespread areas of established infarction within the white matter.

cases of abnormal cortical development, such as abnormal migration or pachygyria, however, whilst these abnormalities can be suspected on neonatal imaging, they may be better visualized between 6 and 12 months of age (Fig. 6.11) (Longman et al 2004).

Acquired lesions in the immature brain evolve rapidly from the outset (Figs 6.12, 6.13). Imaging of the preterm infant is probably best done at term equivalent age when the

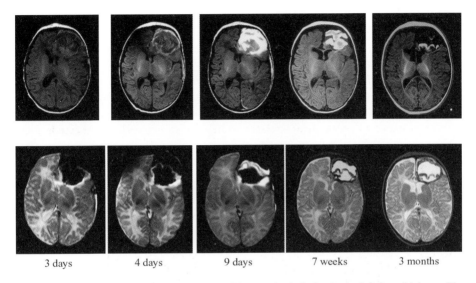

| 3 days | 4 days | 9 days | 7 weeks | 3 months |

Fig. 6.13 Evolution of large perinatally acquired haemorrhagic lesion in the left frontal lobe on T1-weighted images (top row) and T2-weighted images (bottom row).

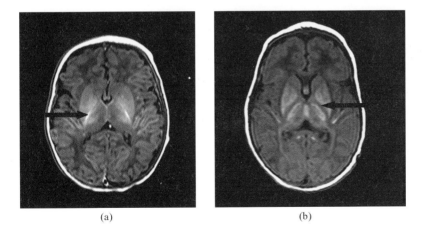

(a)   (b)

Fig. 6.14 T1-weighted images of a normal term infant showing (a) high signal intensity within the normally meylinated posterior limb of the internal capsule (arrow); (b) loss of the normal signal intensity within the posterior limb of the internal capsule in an infant with hypoxic-ischaemic encephalopathy (arrow).

81

appearances of the posterior limb of the internal capsule may be used to help predict outcome (Fig. 6.14) (de Vries et al 1999).

- Infants with abnormal ultrasound examination or with abnormal neurological signs should be referred for MR imaging whenever possible.
- Infants with rapidly developing ventricular dilatation may need to be imaged more acutely, particularly if there is no evidence of haemorrhage on cranial ultrasound.
- Haemorrhagic lesions will be obvious early on and evolve in a fairly predictable manner (Fig. 6.13).
- Lesions consistent with periventricular leucomalacia may only become visible with conventional imaging one to two weeks after their onset, although the timing may not always be accurate (Fig. 6.16). Imaging with diffusion-weighted sequences may identify abnormal tissue before it becomes cystic (Fig. 6.15) (Inder et al 1999).
- A majority of very preterm infants have a diffuse signal abnormality within their white matter when imaged at term equivalent age. This has a high signal intensity (DEHSI) on T2-weighted images and a low signal intensity on T1-weighted images (Fig. 6.17). This appears to be associated with a lower DQ at 2 years of age. The aetiology of this white matter disease of preterm birth is poorly understood at present. It is probably not yet justifiable to image at term just to detect DEHSI.

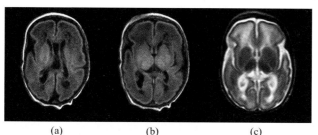

(a)   (b)   (c)

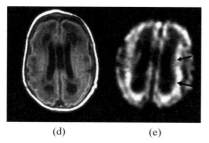

(d)   (e)

Fig. 6.15 Periventricular leucomalacia. Preterm infant at 30 weeks' gestation. There are bilateral cysts in both anterior and posterior periventricular white matter. These are easier to distinguish from the ventricles on the T1-weighted images (a) and (b). On diffusion-weighted images (e) there is abnormal high signal intensity consistent with reduced diffusion (arrows) and early ischaemia in areas that are not yet cystic on conventional T1-weighted images (d).

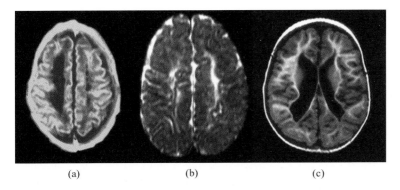

(a)   (b)   (c)

Fig. 6.16 Periventricular leucomalacia. Cystic lesions within the periventricular white matter in an infant aged 35 weeks (arrows) (a), and findings at 15 months of age in (b) and (c). There is irregular ventricular dilatation (c) and increased signal intensity consistent with gliosis in the periventricular white matter seen superior to the ventricles on the T2-weighted image (b).

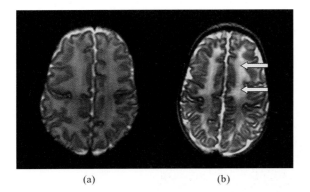

(a)   (b)

Fig. 6.17 T2-weighted images at the level of the centrum semiovale in a term born infant (a) and a preterm infant imaged at term equivalent age (b). There is excessive high signal intensity within the white matter in the preterm infant (arrows). The extracerebral space is also slightly widened and the cortical folding less convoluted.

In the full-term infant, as for the preterm infant, haemorrhagic lesions acquired around the time of delivery will be obvious from symptom onset.

- Perinatally acquired hypoxic-ischaemic brain lesions at term are at their most visually obvious between one and two weeks from delivery. This is true of global injuries seen in infants with hypoxic-ischaemic encephalopathy (HIE) and in infants with perinatal stroke. In some infants with HIE earlier imaging may be required to make a diagnosis or to assist in clinical management. Imaging within the first couple of days may show only subtle abnormalities in the presence of significant brain injury, particularly to the inexperienced radiologist. Early image examinations should always include a diffusion-weighted sequence. Diffusion-weighted imaging (DWI), which is available on most

83

modern scanners, should identify any infarcted white matter (Fig. 6.5, 6.18), but is not so reliable at detecting significant injury to the basal ganglia and thalami (Rutherford et al 2004). The DWI visual appearances of infarcted tissue are obvious very early and last for approximately a week.

- In infants with suspected kernicterus, increased signal intensity on T1-weighted images within the globus pallidus may be relatively subtle in the neonatal period. By 6 months

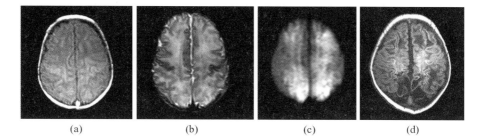

(a)   (b)   (c)   (d)

Fig. 6.18 Diffusion-weighted imaging in white matter infarction. Term born neonate aged 5 days presenting with seizures. Parasagittal injury. (a) T1-weighted spin echo with minimal loss of grey white matter differentiation only. (b) T2-weighted spin echo with loss of grey white matter differentiation most obvious posteriorly. (c) Diffusion-weighted imaging showing very obvious high signal intensity consistent with restricted diffusion and impending infarction. (d) Later T1-weighted imaging at 2 weeks showing widespread cystic breakdown of tissue in the distribution of the previous diffusion abnormalities.

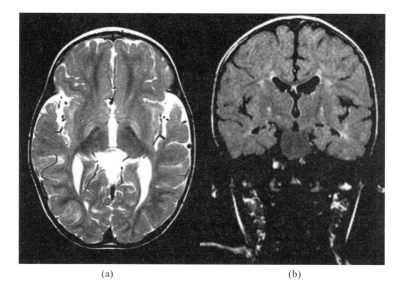

(a)   (b)

Fig. 6.19 Kernicterus in 2-year-old child. (a) T2-weighted sequence shows high signal intensity in the globus pallidus consistent with kernicterus. On the FLAIR image (b) there is additional abnormal signal intensity within the subthalamic nuclei.

of age the abnormalities become more obvious but with a low signal intensity on T1-weighted images and a high signal intensity on T2-weighted images. There may be similar abnormalities within the subthalamic nuclei (Fig. 6.19)

EVOLUTION OF PERINATAL LESIONS: EARLY

There is a predictable evolution of perinatally acquired brain lesions, and so serial conventional imaging may allow the timing of injury to be assessed. Serial diffusion imaging will provide additional information for timing lesions. Haemorrhagic lesions evolve rapidly as blood is broken down (Fig. 6.13), but the exact signal intensity seen on either T1- or T2-weighted images will depend on the site, size and exact nature of the haemorrhagic lesions. Large haemorrhages develop a high signal intensity on T2-weighted images at around 10 days; smaller lesions do not. Repeat imaging may also be useful to document atypical evolution of imaging abnormalities, particularly when an additional or different diagnosis such as a metabolic disorder is suspected. In some metabolic disorders there are additional congenital malformations of the brain, such as agenesis or hypoplasia of the corpus callosum in non-ketotic hyperglycinaemia. A normal scan or an isolated delay in myelination in an infant with persisting seizures should raise the possibility of a metabolic disorder.

EVOLUTION OF PERINATAL LESIONS: LATE

Images performed after the neonatal period can still provide useful information but may be more difficult to interpret. Haemorrhagic lesions may look very dramatic on MR imaging in the neonatal period, but may resolve to leave relatively little in the way of atrophy.

In some cases significant basal ganglia and thalamic lesions may be difficult to detect during the first year after birth (Fig. 6.20). White matter infarction may result in atrophy

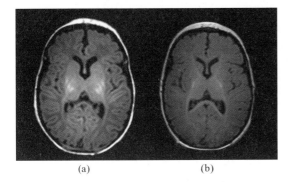

(a)   (b)

Fig. 6.20 Focal basal ganglia abnormalities in an infant presenting with hypoxic-ischaemic encephalopathy. T1-weighted sequence. (a) One month of age. There are small focal abnormal high signal intensities either side of the posterior limb of the internal capsule and some flattening of the lateral lentiform border. (b) Four months of age. There is some probable atrophy of the lentiform nuclei and myelination within the internal capsule is slightly thin. No other abnormalities are obvious but the infant was already showing an abnormal tone pattern.

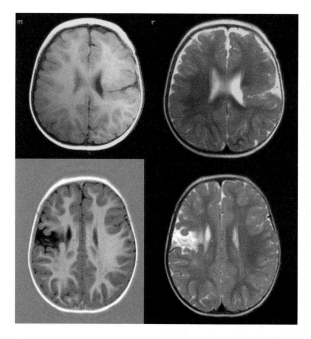

Fig. 6.21 Infants presenting with hemiplegia. White matter clefts. Top row: schizencephaly. Fifteen-month-old infant presenting with a hemiplegia. There is a cleft consistent with a congenital schizencephaly on the left. This is lined with abnormally thick cortex consistent with polymicrogyria. This infant had a sibling who was born extremely preterm and found to have bilateral schizencephaly on ultrasound. Bottom row: in contrast in this infant with a hemiplegia there is a wider opening; whilst this could be consistent with an open schizencephaly the cleft is not lined with abnormally appearing cortex. This infant had a perinatally acquired middle cerebral artery infarction documented on neonatal MR imaging.

which is difficult to detect, particularly if there was little initial involvement of the cortex. In some cases perinatal infarction may evolve and resemble a developmental abnormality such as a schizencephaly (Fig. 6.21).

LESIONS ASSOCIATED WITH PRETERM BIRTH
Periventricular haemorrhages evolve to give a porencephalic dilatation of the ventricle (Fig. 6.22). PVL evolves to give dilated angulated posterior horns, decreased white matter volume, thin corpus callosum and increased T2 in the white matter (Fig. 6.16, 6.22).

Patterns of injury and prediction of outcome
MR imaging provides detailed information about the evolution of brain lesions observed in the neonatal period. Serial MR studies using conventional sequences may provide excellent predictions of outcome. Particular attention has been devoted to the pattern of lesions following perinatal brain injury.

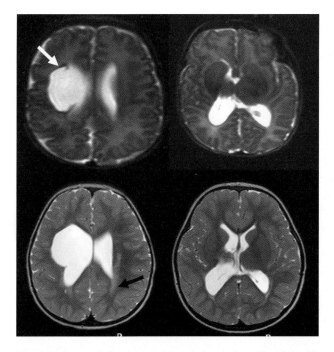

Fig. 6.22 Preterm infant born at 26 weeks' gestation. T2-weighted images (top row) acquired at term equivalent show a right-sided porencephalic cyst from a previous haemorrhagic venous infarction. On these T2-weighted images the cyst has a low signal intensity lining consistent with the presence of haemosiderin (arrow). There is marked thalamic atrophy and involvement of the posterior limb of the internal capsule. At 2 years of age (bottom row) there is some increase in ventricular and cyst size. There is additional increased signal in the periventricular white matter (arrow).

NEONATAL ENCEPHALOPATHY WITH GLOBAL HYPOXIC-ISCHAEMIC
INSULT

Infants with a global hypoxic-ischaemic insult generally have low Apgar scores and low cord pH and clinical signs of neonatal encephalopathy. Their lesions are usually detected on early scans, but are better visualized on the scans performed after the first week. The most frequently observed lesions in infants with criteria fulfilling HIE are basal ganglia and thalamic (BGT) lesions (Figs 6.12, 6.14, 6.20) (Cowan et al 2003a), which are often associated with abnormal signal intensity in the intervening posterior limb of the internal capsule (Fig. 6.14) (Rutherford et al 1998). Lesions in the BGT are often accompanied by injury to the cortex and subcortical white matter, most typically around the central sulcus and in the medial temporal lobe. These changes are most obvious after the first week from injury (Fig. 6.23). In approximately 50 per cent of neonates with BGT lesions there will be more extensive white matter abnormalities (Fig. 6.12).

The severity of the BGT lesions dictates the severity and nature of the cerebral palsy. In children with associated severe white matter changes the motor outcome is still dictated by the BGT lesions but white matter involvement may exacerbate any cognitive deficit.

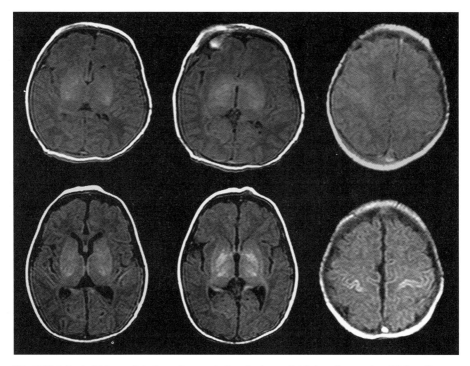

Fig. 6.23 Infant with hypoxic ischaemic encephalopathy imaged at 2 days (top row) and 9 days (bottom row). There are bilateral abnormal high signal intensities within the basal ganglia and thalami and abnormal high signal intensity in the cortex around the central sulcus. The lesions are more obvious at 9 days.

However, infants with severe BGT lesions have severe cognitive impairment regardless of the severity of additional white matter involvement.

In a proportion of infants who present with global hypoxic-ischaemic insult there is no BGT involvement but only white matter lesions (Fig. 6.18). These may be haemorrhagic (Fig. 6.24). These lesions give rise to tissue atrophy and later cognitive impairment. The more severe the white matter lesions, the worse the cognitive outcome (Cowan et al 2003b).

It is important to note that in some children with isolated cognitive impairment this may have arisen as a result of a perinatal injury. However, there would normally be an abnormal perinatal history, usually with seizures, and the child is likely to be micro-cephalic. In addition, in children who have a term perinatally acquired white matter injury, later follow-up images are indistinguishable from what would normally be called periven-tricular leucomalacia. The injury may then be wrongly attributed to antenatal damage at an earlier gestation. In an infant with signs of PVL, on imaging and/or clinically, who was born at term, it is probably only reasonable to implicate perinatal events if there were neonatal symptoms such as encephalopathy or seizures.

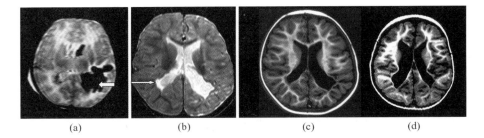

(a)   (b)   (c)   (d)

Fig. 6.24 Haemorrhagic lesions in a term born infant presenting with hypoxic-ischaemic encephalopathy. T2-weighted sequences: (a) There are large haemorrhagic lesions seen as low signal intensity. At 16 months the appearances of the brain are difficult to distinguish from a preterm infant (b) with periventricular leucomalacia with irregular ventricular dilatation, loss of white matter with some high signal intensity consistent with glial tissue (arrow), and decreased myelination. T1-weighted images: (c) The appearances in this infant at 16 months are almost identical to those of a preterm infant (d) with periventricular leucomalacia.

FOCAL LESIONS/CEREBRAL INFARCTION

Infants who present with neonatal seizures but without severely depressed Apgar scores and a necessity for resuscitation usually sustain focal ischaemic or haemorrhagic lesions (Mercuri et al 1995). Focal ischaemia is usually in the form of a middle cerebral artery infarction, most frequently affecting the left hemisphere. The extent of the lesion is generally better appreciated on the scans performed at the end of the first week. In a few infants, abnormalities on early conventional images may be quite subtle (Fig. 6.5a). Diffusion-weighted imaging, in contrast, will be able to highlight infarcted areas already on the scans performed on the same day (Fig. 6.5c). The abnormalities on diffusion-weighted imaging become less obvious by the end of the first week, by which time the abnormalities are more obvious on the conventional T1- and T2-weighted images.

From 2 weeks onwards there may be break-down of infarcted tissue. The extracerebral space may widen. A porencephalic cyst may form, although there may be some tissue visible within it. The affected hemisphere usually looks smaller than the non-affected one, with a generalized decrease in myelination most obvious around the site of the infarct (Fig. 6.21). In some cases, as the brain grows the infarct may appear to decrease in size, and in some infants the original lesion may be difficult to identify (Fig. 6.27). After 6–8 weeks changes in the brainstem due to Wallerian degeneration may also become evident, and are even more evident at 6 months and later.

The extent of the initial lesion has been shown to dictate outcome. Where there is involvement of three sites – namely, the hemispheres, the basal ganglia and the posterior limb of the internal capsule – infants are very likely to develop a hemiplegia (Figs 6.25, 6.26) (Mercuri et al 2001). Factor V Leiden heterozygosity was found more commonly in infants with three-site involvement (Mercuri et al 2001). Three-site involvement is usually obvious on late as well as early images (Figs 6.25, 6.26).

Infants with primarily haemorrhagic lesions probably represent a group with mixed aetiologies (Fig. 6.28), which may dictate outcome. Perinatal white matter damage is

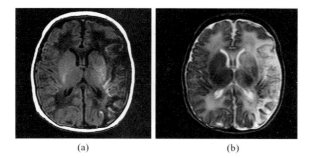

(a)   (b)

Fig. 6.25 Middle cerebral artery infarction. Three-site involvement. Term born infant presenting with seizures. T1-weighted (a) and T2-weighted (b) images at 10 days of age. There is abnormal signal intensity within the hemisphere, lentiform nucleus, thalamus and internal capsule on the left. This triple site involvement is strongly predictive of a later hemiplegia.

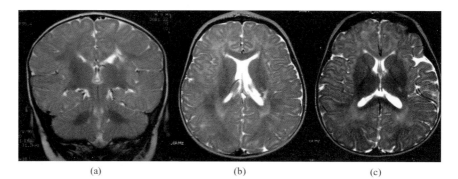

(a)   (b)   (c)

Fig. 6.26 Middle cerebral artery infarction. Three-site involvement. T2-weighted images. Infant aged 1 year with no obvious perinatal symptoms. There is a very small left-sided infarction – involving hemispheric tissue (a), basal ganglia (b) and the posterior limb of the internal capsule (c) resulting in a hemiplegia.

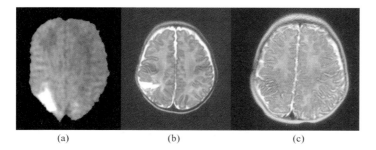

(a)   (b)   (c)

Fig. 6.27 Infant with perinatal right-sided middle cerebral artery infarction. (a) Aged 4 days. Diffusion-weighted imaging showing abnormal high signal intensity within the region of the right middle cerebral artery infarction. (b) Aged 6 weeks. T2-weighted imaging showing a cleft of infarcted tissue on the right. (c) Same infant aged 6 months showing asymmetry of cortical folding but no obvious infarct. There is less myelin and a smaller hemisphere on the right. There is no abnormal increased signal intensity consistent with glial tissue at this level.

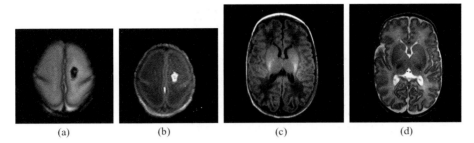

(a)	(b)	(c)	(d)

Fig. 6.28 Small periventricular haemorrhage in a preterm infant at 28 weeks' gestation. (a) and (b) Images at term equivalent age at the level of the basal ganglia. (c) and (d) Images showing symmetrical signal intensity within the posterior limb of the internal capsule.

associated with cognitive deficits; the more severe the damage, the greater the deficit (Cowan et al 2003b). Motor impairment may occur if there is additional involvement of the corticospinal tracts and/or basal ganglia and thalami.

The infant presenting with neurological abnormalities

In some infants a neurological abnormality is only detected later in the first year of life. Imaging at this time is extremely useful.

Infants presenting with a hemiplegia may have a porencephalic cyst consistent with PVH (Fig. 6.22). This may have occurred antenatally in infants born at term with unremarkable perinatal histories. The appearances should be distinguishable from those produced by a neonatal stroke, i.e. a middle cerebral artery infarct. This would be more typical of a term injury, although it is possible that, again, the perinatal history appears blameless or that subtle seizures may have been missed (Fig. 6.26). It is important to exclude a congenital abnormality, resulting in a hemiplegia such as a schizencephaly (Fig. 6.21) or a perisylvian polymicrogyria. These are conditions that may recur in subsequent pregnancies, and careful counselling of the parents will be necessary (Fig. 6.21).

Infants presenting with a diplegia may have imaging findings consistent with periventricular leucomalacia (PVL). Again this may be the result of an antenatal injury in a term born neonate with a normal perinatal history. However, if the term born infant had signs of encephalopathy, late PVL may be the result of a term injury (Fig. 6.24). Imaging may occasionally reveal abnormalities elsewhere in the brain, e.g. cerebellum.

Infants presenting with a quadriplegia may have evidence of extensive PVL or of basal ganglia and thalamic abnormalities. These may look relatively subtle between 6 weeks and 1 year (Fig. 6.20). Severe basal ganglia and thalamic lesions are associated with white matter atrophy, which appears to be a secondary, or delayed, effect. The white matter atrophy is not preceded by overt infarction. On late images the aetiology behind severe white matter atrophy may not be distinguishable. However, if the injury was primarily to the central grey matter, then this will appear atrophied, often with persisting abnormal signal intensity. In infants with white matter atrophy as a consequence of PVL the thalami may appear atrophied but the basal ganglia are usually of normal size and shape.

Occasionally findings consistent with kernicterus may be encountered unexpectedly in infants who present with motor delay or quadriplegia with or without hearing loss. There is usually a history of jaundice requiring intervention, but this may not have been considered severe at the time (Fig. 6.19).

Infants presenting with large heads may have familial large head, a widened extra-cerebral space, large ventricles or a large brain. Initial assessment should include assessment of head growth since birth, and measurement of parental head size. Imaging should always be performed if the child is neurologically abnormal, but may also serve to reassure if a relatively benign cause is found. This would include widened extracerebral spaces or so-called benign hydrocephalus, which usually resolves during the second year of life and needs no intervention (Fig. 6.29). Ultrasound may be useful to assess ventricular size and, if these show progressive dilatation, should also be followed by MR imaging. Dilatation

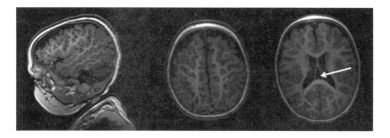

Fig. 6.29 Widened extracerebral space or 'benign external hydrocephalus'. One-year-old ex-preterm infant with head centile increasing over first four months from delivery. T1-weighted images. There is widening of the anterior extracerebral space. There is mild dilatation of the ventricles and a patent cavum vergum (arrow).

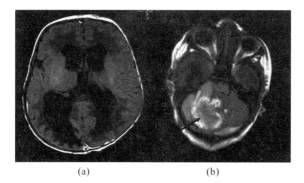

(a)   (b)

Fig. 6.30 Seven-day-old infant with increasing head circumference. T1-weighted images in transverse plane. (a) There is marked ventricular dilatation with abnormal low signal intensity in the periventricular white matter. This may represent oedema but if prolonged can lead to ischaemia within the tissue. (b) There is a large right-sided cerebellar haemorrhage (arrow) causing midline shift and obstruction of the ventricular system.

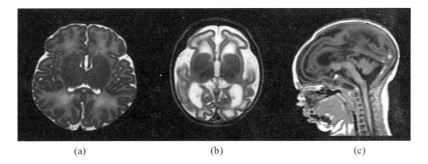

(a)   (b)   (c)

Fig. 6.31 Microcephaly. Cortical migration disorder. (a) A normal pattern of cortical folding at term is shown. (b) Term born infant with microcephaly. T2-weighted image shows a simple gyral pattern and marked dilatation of the ventricles. (c) Sagittal T1-weighted image. There is some additional cerebellar vermis hypoplasia.

may result from obstruction following a perinatal haemorrhage. In infants born at term this may have arisen in the choroid plexus, the thalamus or cerebellum (Fig. 6.30). Many congenital causes of cerebrospinal fluid obstruction may present in infancy, childhood or even adulthood with the late onset of ventricular dilatation, e.g. aqueduct stenosis.

Occasionally an enlarged head is secondary to the presence of a subdural haemorrhage. This may be spontaneous or follow an accidental fall, but further radiology will usually be necessary to rule out other injuries, which may indicate non-accidental aetiology. There are several rare disorders characterized by macrocephaly, such as Alexander's disease and Canavan's disease. These infants are likely to show neurological impairments and may already display overt developmental regression.

Infants presenting with small heads. A small head implies poor brain growth. Once again it is important to assess head growth since delivery and to document parental head circumferences. Early serial head circumference measurements will help distinguish primary from secondary microcephaly. A detailed family history may identify the presence of familial microcephaly although the clinical phenotypes may not always be identical. MR imaging may show overt areas of infarction or atrophy consistent with a previous insult, or identify a genetic or congenital cause of the microcephaly (Fig. 6.31).

Conclusions

Magnetic resonance imaging has become an invaluable technique for investigating the neurologically abnormal infant. Images at any time can usually distinguish between congenital or acquired disorders and will normally provide information on the aetiology and timing of the brain abnormality. These findings may then be used to predict outcome and to counsel the family.

ACKNOWLEDGEMENTS

We would like to thank all the staff of the Robert Steiner MR Unit, Hammersmith Hospital and the neonatal units of Hammersmith and Queen Charlottes Hospital. We are also grateful to the Medical Research Council, the Academy of Medical Sciences, the Health Foundation and Philips Medical Systems for their support.

REFERENCES

Ajayi-Obe M, Saeed N, Cowan FM, Rutherford MA, Edwards AD (2000) Reduced development of cerebral cortex in extremely preterm infants. *Lancet* 356(9236): 1162–1163.

Cowan FM (1998) Sedation for magnetic resonance scanning of infants and young children. In: Whitwam JG, McCloy RF, editors. *Principles and Practice of Sedation*. London: Blackwell Healthcare, 15.3, pp 206–213.

Cowan F, Rutherford M, Groenendaal F, Eken P, Mercuri E, Bydder GM, Meiners LC, Dubowitz LM, de Vries LS (2003a) Origin and timing of brain lesions in term infants with neonatal encephalopathy. *Lancet* 361(9359): 713–714.

Cowan F, Dubowitz L, Mercuri E, Counsell S, Rutherford M (2003b) White matter injury can lead to cognitive without major motor deficits following perinatal asphyxia and early encephalopathy. *Dev Med Child Neurol* 45(Suppl 93): 14.

de Vries LS, Groenendaal F, van Haastert IC, Eken P, Rademaker KJ, Meiners LC (1999) Asymmetrical myelination of the posterior limb of the internal capsule in infants with periventricular haemorrhagic infarction: an early predictor of hemiplegia. *Neuropediatrics* 30(6): 314–319.

Inder T, Huppi PS, Zientara GP, Maier SE, Jolesz FA, Di Salvo D, Robertson R, Barnes PD, Volpe JJ (1999) Early detection of periventricular leukomalacia by diffusion-weighted magnetic resonance imaging techniques. *J Pediatr* 134(5): 631–634.

Longman C, Mercuri E, Cowan F, Allsop J, Brockington M, Jimenez-Mallebrera C, Kumar S, Rutherford M, Toda T, Muntoni F (2004) Antenatal and postnatal brain magnetic resonance imaging in muscle–eye–brain disease. *Arch Neurol* 61(8): 1301–1306.

Mercuri E, Cowan F, Rutherford M, Acolet D, Pennock J, Dubowitz L (1995) Ischaemic and haemorrhagic brain lesions in newborns with seizures and normal Apgar scores. *Arch Dis Child Fetal Neonatal Ed* 73: 67–74.

Mercuri E, Cowan F, Gupte G, Manning R, Laffan M, Rutherford M, Edwards AD, Dubowitz L, Roberts I (2001) Prothrombotic disorders and abnormal neurodevelopmental outcome in infants with neonatal cerebral infarction. *Pediatrics* 107(6): 1400–1404.

Pennock J (2002) Patient preparation; safety and hazards in imaging infants and children. In: Rutherford WB, editor. *MRI of the Neonatal Brain*. London: Saunders.

Rutherford MA, Pennock JM, Counsell SJ, Mercuri E, Cowan FM, Dubowitz LM, Edwards AD (1998) Abnormal magnetic resonance signal in the internal capsule predicts poor neurodevelopmental outcome in infants with hypoxic-ischemic encephalopathy. *Pediatrics* 102: 323–328.

Rutherford MA, Counsell S, Allsop J, Boardman J, Kapellou O, Larkman D, Hajnal J, Edwards AD, Cowan F (2004) Diffusion weighted MR imaging in term perinatal brain injury: a comparison with site of lesion and time from birth. *Pediatrics* 114: 1004–1014.

7
DIAGNOSTIC AND PROGNOSTIC VALUE OF ELECTROPHYSIOLOGY

Enrico Biagioni, Andrea Guzzetta and Giovanni Cioni

Introduction

Electrophysiological techniques provide useful information in all neonatal and infantile diseases of the central nervous system (CNS). These techniques are usually not invasive and can be used directly at the infant's bedside. They are based on the direct recording of cerebral electrical activity, the electroencephalogram (EEG), or on an off-line processing of the raw signal, as for the evoked potentials (EP), corresponding to the changes of cerebral electrical activity evoked by an external stimulus, or the amplitude-integrated EEG, also known as cerebral function monitoring (CFM), a highly compressed and filtered trace suitable for very long recordings. In this chapter these techniques will be illustrated and some information on normal and abnormal findings in the first two years of life will be provided. It is very important to underline that in this early stage of development CNS electrical activities undergo rapid modifications; it is therefore mandatory to correctly evaluate the maturational features of EEG activity, in order to relate the findings to what is expected according to the patient's age.

The EEG

TECHNICAL ASPECTS

To record an EEG in an infant or in a neonate is much more difficult than at other stages of life. These patients are obviously not able to cooperate and, particularly as far as newborns are concerned, the recording is frequently carried out in an intensive care unit, where the presence of other electrical instruments can give rise to artefacts, making the tracing poorly readable. Nowadays new computer-aided electroencephalographs, equipped with battery-operated amplifiers and A/D converters, have significantly improved the EEG quality in these extreme conditions.

In neonates, electrodes are usually applied to the scalp using ring-shaped double-adhesive plasters or directly with a conductive-adhesive paste. Since these techniques allow reliable recordings for many hours, more invasive techniques, such as needle electrodes or the use of toxic substances such as collodion, are generally not necessary at this age. In infants the EEG is recorded with the same technique as in adults (collodion-applied electrodes, latex-cups, etc.), but it is important to make sure that the infant is allowed to rest and sleep safely and comfortably.

The number of electrodes varies according to age. In neonates no more than 8–10 active electrodes are generally applied (Fp1-2, C3-4, O1-2, T3-4 + Cz and Pz or Fz of the International 10–20 System). After the neonatal period, a complete montage is usually possible. Polygraphic channels are also used in both neonates and infants: they generally include electromyography (EMG) of different muscles (deltoid, chin, other muscles of legs and arms, etc.), pneumography (PNG – recorded by means of a nasal thermistor or a strain gauge transducer applied to the chest or to the abdomen), electrocardiogram (ECG) and electro-oculogram (EOG – recorded by means of a piezoelectric accelerometer applied to the eyelid, or electrodes applied at the outer canthi). As some of these additional channels can significantly disturb the young patient, they should be limited to cases where they have effective usefulness for both clinical and research purposes. Recordings must include an entire sleep–wake cycle in newborns and should therefore last at least 45–90 minutes. In infants it is also generally necessary to record some phases of both wakefulness and sleep, either to better appreciate maturational features or to detect possible paroxysmal abnormalities of drowsiness, sleep and arousal.

NORMAL EEG MATURATIONAL FINDINGS IN NEONATES

Cerebral electrical activity undergoes rapid modifications in the early phases of life. In the neonate these changes are particularly fast and do not depend on the interval since birth, but, rather, on the postmenstrual age (PMA) at recording. Hence, EEG features of all healthy neonates at a specific PMA are similar, irrespective of the postnatal age (Anders et al 1971, Dreyfus-Brisac and Monod 1972, Nolte and Haas 1978, Anderson et al 1985, Lombroso 1985, Ferrari et al 1992, Stockard-Pope et al 1992, Biagioni et al 1994, 2000b). This finding strongly indicates that the maturation of cerebral electrical activity in preterm infants, as well as other aspects of CNS functioning, is related to the infant's corrected age (CA), within a developmental *continuum* from conception to childhood. In this section normal features of neonatal EEG activity will be illustrated for each stage of PMA, from early preterm birth to the end of the first month post-term.

In recent years significant improvements in neonatal care have permitted many young preterm infants to survive, despite their low birthweight and their very low gestational age (up to 22–23 weeks' gestation). These tiny neonates give us the opportunity to explore brain electrical activity in a very early phase of development, when cortical foldings are completely undeveloped and glial cells are still migrating from germinal matrix to cortex (Battin et al 1998). At this age (around 23–25 weeks PMA) the EEG activity is constantly discontinuous: bursts of activity are interposed with long (up to 40–50 seconds) periods of flattening (Biagioni et al 2000a, Vecchierini et al 2003, Lamblin et al 2004). This pattern is detectable in healthy newborns up to the end of the neonatal period, although progressively replaced by continuous activity. In very young preterm infants (23–25 weeks PMA) bursts consist of high-amplitude (up to 450 μV), very slow (up to 0.5 Hz) waves, often asynchronous between the two hemispheres. These delta waves are sometimes superimposed on low-amplitude (generally less than 60–70 μV) 8–22 Hz rhythms and, much more clearly, on trains of high-amplitude (up to 200 μV) 3.5–7 Hz activities, characterized by an almost sinusoidal appearance and by a larger representation in the occipital regions. This often asynchronous theta rhythm constitutes the first rhythmic activity detectable in humans and is generally called the 'occipital sawtooth' pattern (Fig. 7.1) (Biagioni et al 2000a, Hughes et al 1990).

In 26–28-week-old preterm infants the temporal organization of brain electrical activity is still constantly discontinuous. Fast 8–22 Hz rhythms are now higher in amplitude and superimposed on slow waves, giving rise to a waveform called 'delta brush' (Stockard-Pope et al 1992, Biagioni et al 1994). Occipital sawtooth is still present but now moves to temporal areas, the so-called 'temporal sawtooth' pattern (Fig. 7.2a) (Anderson et al 1985, Biagioni et al 1994).

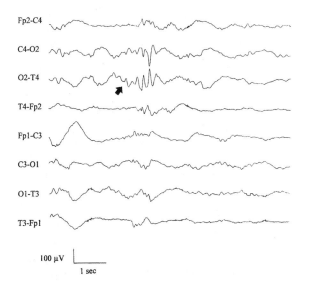

Fig. 7.1 Tracing recorded at 24 weeks PMA in an infant with normal outcome. Occipital sawtooth (arrow) is represented on right posterior region.

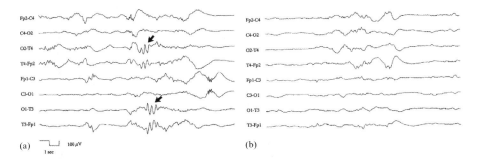

Fig. 7.2 Tracings recorded at 28 weeks PMA. (a) Infant with normal outcome: note the presence of temporal sawtooth (arrows). (b) Infant with severely unfavourable outcome: note the poor representation of temporal sawtooth.

From 29–30 weeks PMA, in periods generally corresponding to behaviourally active phases, bursts of slow waves are much longer and intervals are much shorter, so that a beginning of continuous activity becomes observable. Delta brushes increase their amplitude and their representation, whereas temporal sawtooth activity is less predominant.

This trend continues throughout the following two weeks (31–32 weeks PMA). When the neonate is active, EEG tracing tends to be almost continuous (Nolte and Haas 1978). This last pattern is characterized by medium- to high-amplitude (up to 200 µV) delta waves with superimposed low-amplitude 8–22 Hz activities; a certain 'bursting tendency' (i.e. short periods of relative amplitude decrease) is generally still detectable. When the infant is quiet, EEG tracing is constantly discontinuous: within bursts both slow waves and fast activity are higher than in previous stages of PMA; temporal sawtooth activity is still observable. It is important to take into account that at this age it is possible to detect for the first time a certain organization of behavioural states: hence, a reliable concordance among different physiological parameters (such as body movements, eye movements, regularity of respiration and, of course, EEG activity) is now detectable (Curzi-Dascalova and Mirmiran 1996).

At 33–34 weeks PMA a bursting tendency is no longer observable in continuous patterns during phases of wakefulness and active sleep. During quiet sleep the detectable discontinuous EEG is characterized by shorter intervals (generally less than 20 seconds) and longer bursts than in the earlier stages; delta brushes are now very evident (their amplitude reaches 200 µV), whereas temporal sawtooth activity definitively disappears (Fig. 7.3a) (Biagioni et al 1994).

At around 35–36 weeks a differentiation of a new continuous pattern can be observed, characterized by a relatively lower (less than 50–60 µV) amplitude and by irregular theta and delta band activity with superimposed very low-amplitude 8–22 Hz rhythms. This last pattern generally relates to phases of wakefulness and to those phases of active sleep following quiet sleep. During the phases of active sleep which precede quiet sleep, we observe a continuous pattern with a larger representation of delta band (up to 100 µV-high)

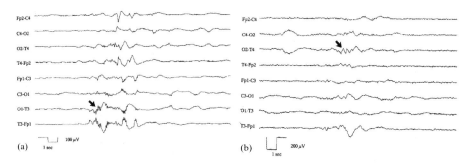

Fig. 7.3 Tracings recorded at 33 weeks PMA. (a) Infant with normal outcome: note the presence of delta brush (arrow), and the absence of temporal sawtooth. (b) Infant with severely unfavourable outcome: note the poor representation of rapid activity and the persistence of temporal sawtooth (arrow).

and 8–22 Hz activities (Nolte and Haas 1978, Stockard-Pope et al 1992). Some polyphasic high-amplitude sharp waves appear in frontal regions, often synchronous between the two hemispheres: these waveforms are known as 'frontal sharp transients' or '*encoches frontales*' (Stockard-Pope et al 1992).

Approaching term age, the neonatal EEG includes five different classical patterns (Dreyfus-Brisac and Monod 1972, Nolte and Haas 1978, Ferrari et al 1992, Stockard-Pope et al 1992). During wakefulness a continuous low-amplitude (less than 50–60 µV) pattern is observable, characterized by irregular theta and delta frequencies (*activité moyenne*); 8–22 Hz rhythms are no longer observable during wakefulness after 37–38 weeks PMA. In the active sleep periods that precede quiet sleep, a medium-amplitude (up to 90–100 µV) mixed theta–delta continuous pattern is detectable (*mixed*); in this pattern it is possible to detect superimposed 8–22 Hz activities until 38–39 weeks. Conversely, phases of active sleep following quiet sleep are characterized by a low-voltage (less than 50–60 µV) predominant theta continuous pattern, with short trains of regular 4–5 Hz activities (*low voltage irregular*); no fast rhythm is detectable in this pattern. Quiet sleep still predominantly relates to a discontinuous pattern (*tracé alternant*): at term age bursts are characterized by up to 200 µV-high delta waves superimposed by low-amplitude 8–22 Hz activities; intervals are short (generally less than 10 seconds) and relatively rich in activity. At around 40 weeks PMA, a new continuous pattern appears in quiet sleep phases, characterized by high-amplitude (up to 200 µV) delta activity (*high voltage slow*).

During the first month of post-term age the progressive disappearance of 8–22 Hz activities (delta brushes) in quiet sleep can also be observed. A high-voltage, slow pattern becomes predominant in this behavioural state, although it is possible to recognize a bursting tendency in quiet sleep until 44 weeks PMA (Nolte and Haas 1978). Moreover, the mixed pattern tends to disappear as the infants more frequently fall asleep in quiet sleep (and therefore phases of active sleep preceding quiet sleep are no longer observable).

NORMAL EEG FINDINGS AT 1–24 MONTHS CORRECTED AGE (CA)
After the fast and dramatic changes of the neonatal period, EEG activity gradually acquires features of more mature ages. In the first two years of life, wakefulness patterns are characterized by predominant low-voltage (up to 50–60 µV) theta activities. EEG reactivity to eye closure generally appears at around 4 months CA (Kellaway 1987): rhythmic activities in posterior regions are much slower than in adults and are included in the lower theta band (4–4.5 Hz) (Fig. 7.4). The frequency of the posterior rhythm is around 6.5–7 Hz at 1 year CA (Biagioni et al 2002), and often reaches the limits of alpha band at the age of 2 years (Kellaway 1987). Rhythmic activity in rolandic regions during quiet wakefulness also appears and develops in this same period, with similar frequencies.

Phases of drowsiness (both before getting to sleep and after arousal) are characterized from the third month CA by high-amplitude (up to 200 µV), regular 3.5–5.5 Hz diffuse activities, the so-called hypnagogic hypersynchrony (Kellaway 1987).

Sleep EEG features at 1–24 months CA are much more similar to those detected in adults than those observable in neonates. Discontinuous patterns are no longer detectable after 1 month CA. The 'low-voltage, irregular' pattern described above, typical of active

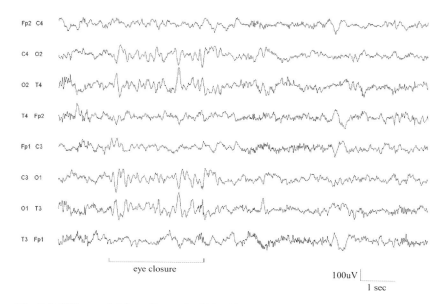

Fp2 C4	
C4 O2	
O2 T4	
T4 Fp2	
Fp1 C3	
C3 O1	
O1 T3	
T3 Fp1	

eye closure

100uV

1 sec

Fig. 7.4 EEG recorded in a 12-month-old healthy infant during wakefulness. The tracing shows normal activity with good response to eye closure (appearance of 7 Hz rhythmic activity) in posterior regions.

sleep, generally disappears within the second month CA. At around 44 weeks PMA, the first 11–16 Hz low-voltage activities, represented more in central regions, are already detectable during sleep: they constitute the 'pre-spindles', precursors of the more mature waveforms observed at older ages (Nolte and Haas 1978). In infancy and up to the second year of life, spindles are sometimes asynchronous in the two hemispheres, and are represented – more often than in childhood – even in deep phases of sleep (Fig. 7.5).

Vertex sharp waves and K-complexes also appear within the first 2–3 months CA. It is important to stress that K-complexes are usually constituted only by a high-amplitude diffuse polyphasic sharp wave at this age (i.e. they are rarely followed by a spindle as in older patients). Moreover, vertex sharp waves, typical of the first sleep phases, usually show a very sharp appearance (so that sometimes it is not easy to distinguish them from epileptiform abnormalities). As far as sleep organization is concerned, the differentiation of classical sleep states according to EEG criteria (i.e. I, II, III, IV and REM) is much less clear than at older ages.

BACKGROUND EEG ABNORMALITIES IN NEONATES

Background EEG abnormalities have been shown to have the highest significance for both diagnosis and prognosis in all CNS diseases of neonates (Monod et al 1972, Pezzani et al 1986, Holmes and Lombroso 1993, Biagioni et al 1996a, Hayakawa et al 1997, Biagioni et al 1999, Lamblin et al 2004). An accurate examination of amplitude, temporal organization and morphology of EEG activities is therefore mandatory for a precise assessment

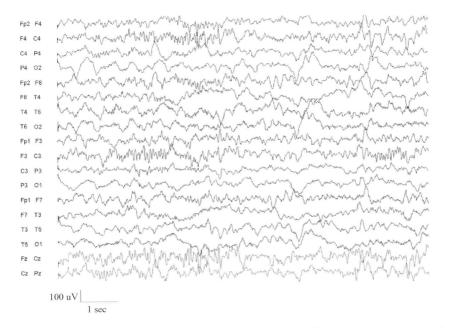

Fig. 7.5 EEG recorded in a 12-month-old healthy infant during sleep. The tracing shows normal activity with symmetrical and partially asynchronous spindles, represented more in fronto-central regions.

of brain function. Some background EEG abnormalities observed in newborns are very similar to those of older patients, while others are very specific for this age.

Constant low voltage constitutes a very severe abnormality. This definition includes tracings constantly characterized by low-voltage activity, without any state-related pattern differentiation. According to some authors (Monod et al 1972, Lombroso 1985), it is possible to distinguish between inactive EEG (amplitude < 2 µV) and low-voltage (< 5–10 µV). It is important to keep in mind that, when EEG amplitude is very reduced, it is often hard to distinguish between residual cerebral activity and artefacts. Moreover, EEG amplitude can also depend on inter-electrode distances and filtering. This very pathological pattern can be detected both in preterm and in full-term infants in association with a severe hypoxic-ischaemic brain insult. Of course, as in the early preterm period inactive intervals can be very prolonged even in normal individuals (see above); in these infants an EEG can be classified as low-voltage only when this feature lasts for a very long time. It is also important to consider that in some cases a constant low voltage is only observable within the first hours of life (e.g. after a severe insult) and is subsequently replaced by other pathological EEG patterns (Biagioni et al 2001), such as constantly discontinuous tracing (see below).

Constantly discontinuous tracings, also known as *burst-suppression patterns*, are characterized by medium- to high-voltage bursts separated by low-activity intervals (Fig. 7.6). As discontinuous patterns are normal not only in preterm but also in full-term neonates, it is important to define this entity precisely, in order to distinguish between normal

101

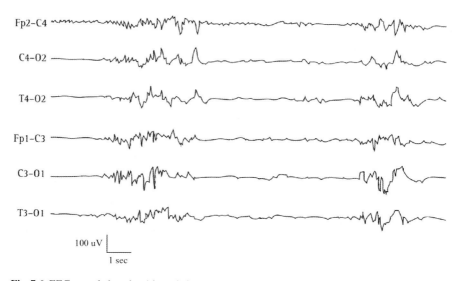

Fp2-C4

C4-O2

T4-O2

Fp1-C3

C3-O1

T3-O1

100 uV

1 sec

Fig. 7.6 EEG recorded on day 1 in an infant born at 40 weeks PMA with birth asphyxia. The tracing is constantly discontinuous with intra-burst paroxysmal abnormalities (sharp waves).

and abnormal findings. Two main rules should be followed. First, no tracing can be classified as constantly discontinuous (or burst-suppression) before 37 weeks PMA. Second, a term-age EEG can be considered as constantly discontinuous only when a discontinuous pattern is present in all phases of sleep and even during wakefulness, unless the infant is so seriously sick that no behavioural state is observable (e.g. comatose patients). In all cases the tracing must be long enough to be sure that the discontinuous pattern is not related to a particular sleep phase (e.g. a normal *tracé alternant*, typical of quiet sleep).

A constantly discontinuous EEG is a frequent finding in hypoxic-ischaemic encephalo-pathy in full-term neonates. This finding carries a severe prognosis (only constant low voltage is probably worse), especially when it persists after the very first days of life (Biagioni et al 1999, Menache et al 2002).

Some quantitative characteristics of constantly discontinuous patterns in neonates are believed to be particularly significant from a prognostic point of view. Very low-amplitude intervals ($< 10 \mu V$ or even $< 5 \mu V$) predict a severe outcome, so that some authors define a constantly discontinuous pattern as 'burst-suppression' only when interval activity is very depressed. According to some recent data (Biagioni et al 1999, Menache et al 2002), interval length is the most reliable parameter to predict subsequent evolution (intervals lasting more than 20–30 seconds always relate to a bad outcome).

Timing of recording is also significant. Full-term infants with perinatal asphyxia should have an EEG as soon as possible after birth: if this first tracing is constantly discontinuous (or low-voltage), it should be repeated during the following days. Rapid EEG normalization (i.e. appearance of continuous activity and state-related EEG patterns) can also lead to a normal outcome. Conversely, when constantly discontinuous patterns persist until the eighth or ninth day of life, the evolution is always unfavourable (Biagioni et al 1999).

Besides perinatal asphyxia, constantly discontinuous patterns can also be observed in other diseases of the central nervous system, such as early infantile epileptic encephalopathies (Ohtahara and Yamatogi 2003). In these severe neonatal syndromes the constantly discontinuous pattern acquires a specific paroxysmal significance (*tracé paroxystique*) and is always accompanied by prolonged EEG discharges. Finally, a discontinuous pattern is also sometimes detectable in other metabolic, genetic and degenerative disorders of the neonate, or may be due to the effect of high doses of anticonvulsant drugs (Ferrari et al 2001).

Interhemispheric asymmetry also constitutes a background abnormality carrying a serious prognosis. Nevertheless, before formulating unfavourable prognostic hypotheses, it is important to exclude technical reasons that could account for such an EEG finding. First, malfunctioning of electrodes on one side can give rise to flattening of traces on some leads. Second, some frequent neonatal conditions can increase the electrical resistance on one side and therefore reduce the amplitude of EEG signal (e.g. scalp oedema or cephalohaematoma). Third, it is well known that a slight asymmetry is normal in neonates, especially at low PMAs (Anderson et al 1985). However, when the asymmetry is significant (i.e. > 50 per cent) and the above-mentioned problems are excluded, this EEG pattern is generally an expression of an underlying pathology (cerebral infarction, haemorrhage, etc.). In the case of underlying pathology we observe a reduced amplitude in the affected hemisphere (Ferrari et al 2001). In other conditions, such as cortical dysplasia and, in particular, hemimegaloencephaly, EEG activity in the affected hemisphere is higher and slower, with interposed frequent paroxysmal EEG discharges (Wertheim et al 1994).

EEG dysmaturity constitutes a specific neonatal background abnormality. This definition includes EEG tracings showing maturational features that are not appropriate for the PMA at recording. The rapid changes in the maturational characteristics of brain electrical activity during the neonatal age were described earlier (see page 96). At a certain PMA, EEG recordings are considered as dysmature when age-specific criteria are not respected (Lombroso 1985, Biagioni et al 1996a). For example, the EEG of a 28-week-old preterm infant with scarce representation of temporal sawtooth activity, and that of a 34-week-old neonate with marked persistence of the same waveform, are both dysmature (Figs 7.2b and 7.3b).

It is important to stress that dysmaturity does not mean having characteristics overlapping those of normal tracings recorded at a previous age but, rather, a general alteration of maturational features. EEG dysmaturity is not frequent in full-term neonates and in these infants it generally constitutes a minor anomaly. In contrast, it is a frequent finding in preterm infants with brain damage (Ferrari et al 1992, Biagioni et al 1996a, Hayakawa et al 1997). The prognostic significance of EEG dysmaturity is generally high: in a study of ours (Biagioni et al 1996a) almost all preterm infants who had normal EEG maturational features also had a normal outcome, whereas some neonates with mildly dysmature EEG and most of those with severely dysmature EEG had an unfavourable evolution.

Some authors (Hayakawa et al 1997, Watanabe et al 1999, Kato et al 2004) distinguish between an acute phase of disorganization of maturational aspects (i.e. increased discontinuity, modifications of amplitude, etc.) and chronic-stage maturational abnormalities (i.e. representation and shape of age-specific waveforms, etc.). In fact, timing of recording is crucial: when the EEG is performed during the very first days of life, it may frequently appear abnormal even in relatively healthy preterm infants, probably because of the neonate's unstable condition (Eaton et al 1994). In contrast, at a postnatal age of above 2 weeks it is possible to find re-organization of brain electrical activity (also from a maturational point of view) in infants with severe brain damage (e.g. periventricular leukomalacia). Therefore, to get the best prediction of neurological outcome, we suggest recording the EEG between the fourth and the thirteenth day of life (Biagioni et al 1996a).

ABNORMAL EEG TRANSIENT FEATURES IN NEONATES
In neonates, as in other stages of life, it is possible to detect some abnormal EEG transient features. These abnormalities (spikes and sharp waves, delta and theta sharp rhythmic activities, alpha discharges) must be distinguished from the above-described physiological waveforms that constitute typical maturational findings at different PMAs (i.e. occipital and temporal sawtooth pattern, delta brushes, *encoches frontales*, etc.). Neonatal abnormal EEG transient features can be observed as interictal abnormalities or can give rise to more or less diffuse EEG discharges in correspondence with epileptic phenomena (neonatal seizures). In this last case, as well as in other stages of life, we can detect a sequence of different epileptiform transient activity (e.g. an alpha discharge, first followed by prolonged theta/delta sharp rhythmic activities and finally by a degrading train of sharp waves). A detailed description of electroclinical findings in neonatal seizures is beyond the scope of this chapter.

Spikes and sharp waves are frequently observable as interictal abnormalities in neonates (Biagioni et al 1996b) and have been considered as quasi-normal features (Monod et al 1972), especially when they are infrequent and represented more in the context of discontinuous patterns. Spikes are obviously shorter in duration (< 80–100 ms) and are less frequent than sharp waves in neonates.

A particular kind of sharp wave is the so-called *positive rolandic sharp wave*, characterized by predominant positive polarity, large amplitude and specific localization in central regions (Dreyfus-Brisac and Monod 1972, Marret et al 1992, Aso et al 1993, Baud et al 1998, Vermeulen et al 2003) (Fig. 7.7). These transient features have been associated with different brain lesions in preterm infants, such as intraventricular haemorrhages, hydrocephalus and white matter lesions. In our experience these abnormalities are more frequently detectable in cases of severe periventricular leukomalacia and occur some weeks after the hypoxic-ischaemic insult (i.e. at around the time cysts are observable on ultrasound scan). *Positive temporal sharp waves* also relate to brain lesions in preterm infants, although their prognostic significance is still debated (Castro et al 2004).

Delta and theta sharp rhythmic activities certainly have an epileptic significance (both ictal and interictal). It is important to distinguish these activities from other physiological maturational transient patterns such as the preterm infant's temporal or occipital theta (temporal and occipital sawtooth). First, the preterm infant's theta activity is characteristic

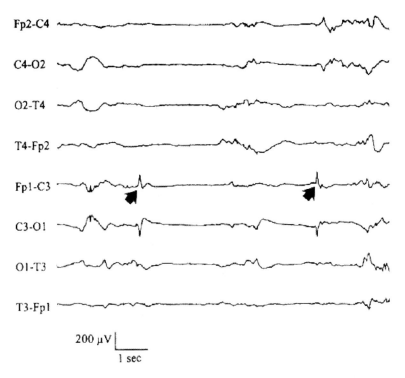

Fp2-C4

C4-O2

O2-T4

T4-Fp2

Fp1-C3

C3-O1

O1-T3

T3-Fp1

200 μV

1 sec

Fig. 7.7 Tracings recorded at 33 weeks PMA: note the sharp waves with largely predominant positive phase in left central region (arrows).

of specific PMAs (whereas theta sharp rhythmic activities are more frequent at around term age). Second, occipital-temporal sawtooth activity shows a very regular (almost sinusinguish) appearance, whereas these epileptiform abnormalities are generally sharp, sometimes with interposed spikes, giving rise to something similar to spike–wave complexes (Biagioni et al 1996b). Finally, *alpha discharges* are generally characterized by low-amplitude activity within the alpha band. Distinguishing between this waveform and the 8–22 Hz activity that constitutes the rapid component of 'delta brush' is often not easy. Lack of underlying slow waves, regular appearance (delta brush is usually sharp) and associated representation of other epileptiform abnormalities (sharp waves, etc.) in the same location can help the diagnosis (Biagioni et al 1996b).

ABNORMAL EEG FINDINGS AT 1–24 MONTHS CA

As stressed above, there is a significant change in the normal organization of cerebral electrical activity after the end of the first month CA. This same change is also observable in infants with pathology. Obviously, in this age-range it is also possible to distinguish between background EEG abnormalities on the one hand, and ictal-interictal (or epilepti-form or, even better, paroxysmal) abnormalities on the other. Nevertheless, in infancy, changes in background activity and paroxysmal waveforms are often so strictly linked to each other (particularly in infantile epileptic encephalopathies) that it is hard to define a precise border between them.

Major background EEG abnormalities, such as *constant low voltage, interhemispheric asymmetry* and a *constantly discontinuous pattern,* can also be identified after the neonatal period, in the case of acute hypoxic-ischaemic insults or in other severe CNS diseases (such as trauma, intoxication, encephalitis, metabolic disorders, tumours, etc.). The characteristics and also the prognostic significance of these EEG abnormalities are similar to those described above for the neonate (Limperopoulos et al 2001). Maturational abnormalities, in contrast, are generally not detectable at this age. In particular, although in some conditions it is possible to register the absence or the abnormal shape of some specific physiological EEG features (e.g. rhythmic activities in posterior regions in correspondence with eye closure, sleep spindles, etc.), in no child is it possible to observe in the same recording activities which are typical of two different age periods (as for the dysmature pattern of the newborn). For example, posterior rhythms are sometimes absent in infants with damage of visual cortex and/or pathways but, when present, these activities have a normal frequency for the age (Biagioni et al 2002).

However, the most frequent background EEG abnormality in infants with previous perinatal hypoxic-ischaemic haemorrhagic encephalopathy is probably the excess of slow waves. This finding is characterized by high-voltage (up to 300 µV) 0.5–3.5 Hz activities, diffuse or localized in some regions of one or both hemispheres, observable during both wakefulness and sleep. Slow waves can be constantly detectable or intermittent (i.e. organized in bursts), and paroxysmal abnormalities (such as sharp waves, spikes, etc.) are always interposed (see above) (Fig. 7.8). When the excess of slow waves is marked, diffuse and constant, with several interposed spikes and poly-spikes, we are faced with a severe disorganization of cerebral electrical activity, giving rise to the so-called hypsarrhythmic pattern (Fig. 7.9) (Randò et al 2004). This last finding is characteristic of the most severe infantile epileptic encephalopathies, such as West syndrome.

A full description of ictal and interictal EEG patterns in infantile spasms or in other epileptic syndromes of infancy is obviously beyond the scope of this chapter. Nevertheless, it is important to stress that serial EEG recordings constitute a mandatory prognostic tool in the follow-up of at-risk newborns, not only for psychomotor development but also for early diagnosis of severe epileptic syndromes. Indeed, in infants with symptomatic infantile spasms there is a long pre-clinical phase preceding the hypsarrhythmic pattern. During this period (generally beginning in the second month post-term) bursts of abnormal slow waves and interposed spikes gradually appear in some cerebral regions (Suzuki et al 2003). Afterwards, these abnormalities increase their amplitude, spread to other locations and become more frequent.

Moreover, besides spikes and poly-spikes, it is possible to detect briefs runs of rapid (10–22 Hz) rhythms, particularly corresponding with awakening and drowsiness (Vigevano et al 2001). When these rhythms become synchronous in the two hemispheres and are accompanied by a short suppression, clinical spasms appear, although generally in a 'subtle' way, such as slight head flexion, slight shoulder movement, eye deviation, staring, arousal, etc. (Biagioni and Cioni 1996). At this stage, the EEG is not yet properly hypsarrhythmic,

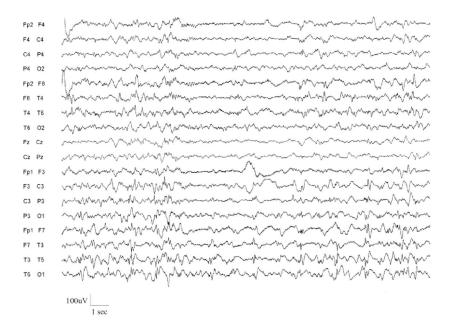

Fig. 7.8 EEG recorded in a 3-month-old infant born at term with severe birth asphyxia. The tracing shows paroxysmal abnormalities (excess of slow activity, spikes, sharp waves), represented more in both temporal and left centro-posterior regions. In the middle of the graph diffuse low-amplitude rapid rhythms are followed by a short flattening.

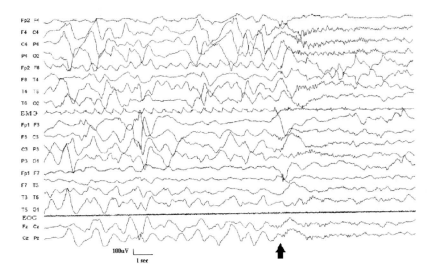

Fig. 7.9 EEG recorded in a 6-month-old infant born at term with severe birth asphyxia. The tracing is characterized by very high-amplitude (up to 600 μV) slow activity. The arrow indicates a diffuse very high slow wave, followed by rapid rhythms (more evident on the right side) and by a flattening. These last abnormalities are accompanied clinically by a spasm.

107

and the psychomotor impairment typical of West syndrome is not yet observed (Randò et al 2004). Hence, serial EEGs in at-risk newborns permit an early diagnosis (and early pharmacological treatment with possibly better results) in symptomatic infantile spasms.

As far as the correlation between neonatal EEG abnormalities and the subsequent occurrence of infantile spasms is concerned, it is probably true that early background EEG abnormalities (e.g. dysmature EEG in preterm infants, and constantly discontinuous pattern in full-term infants) are more predictive than neonatal abnormal EEG transient features (Okumura and Watanabe 2001). Finally, in our experience, there is almost always a 'free' interval between the disappearance of neonatal background EEG abnormalities and the appearance of the excess of slow waves leading to a pre-hypsarrhythmic pattern. Therefore, the prognostic value of EEGs recorded at the end of the first month post-term is generally low.

Techniques of prolonged EEG monitoring: cerebral function monitoring (CFM)

TECHNICAL ASPECTS

Cerebral function monitoring (CFM), also known as amplitude-integrated EEG, is a method of neurophysiological assessment suitable for very long recordings which is very common in neonatal intensive care units. It consists of an amplitude-integrated electroencephalogram, characterized by a single-lead trace (generally P3–P4 of the International 10–20 System). Signal processing consists of amplification, frequency filtration, and amplitude compression and rectification (Thornberg and Thiringer 1990). Frequencies below 2 Hz and above 20 Hz are eliminated and, within this same range, higher frequencies are enhanced. The final result of this process is a very compressed trace; the lower edge of the tracing reflects a possibly stable measurement of non-rhythmic activities, the so-called 'minimum level of cerebral activity', whereas the upper edge reflects both rhythmic and non-rhythmic activities (i.e. the so-called 'maximum level of cerebral activity'). The width of the trace indicates the variability of the signal. Amplitudes are reported on a semi-logarithmic scale and range between 0 and 100 µV.

CFM NORMAL PATTERNS IN FULL-TERM AND PRETERM INFANTS

The normal neonatal CFM tracing usually shows periods characterized by different amplitudes. This finding is also observable in preterm infants but it is more evident at term age (Thornberg and Thiringer 1990), when it is easy to distinguish between phases of broad bandwidth, corresponding to periods of quiet sleep, and phases of narrow bandwidth, corresponding to active sleep or wakefulness. Similar variations are observable from the 31st or the 32nd week of PMA and again probably reflect modifications of the sleep–wake condition (Fig. 7.10a). By comparing CFM traces of full-term and preterm infants, it can be observed that at low PMAs the bandwidth is generally broader and the minimum level of cerebral activity is located at a lower level (1.9 ± 0.5 µV in the low PMA preterm infant). Approaching term age, the CFM trace becomes narrower, especially due to raising of the lower edge, and well-defined, state-related amplitude variations are detectable (Fig. 7.11a) (Thornberg and Thiringer 1990).

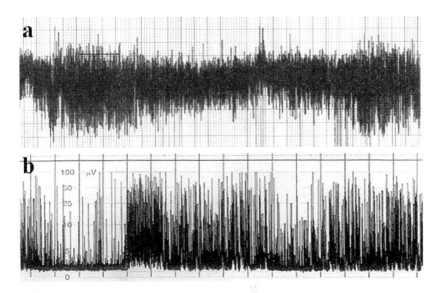

Fig. 7.10 (a) CFM of a 34-week GA preterm infant with prolonged increased echogenicity at ultrasound scan and subsequent normal development. The tracing (adequate for 34 weeks PMA) shows phases of broad bandwidth, corresponding to periods of quiet sleep, alternating with phases of narrow bandwidth, corresponding to periods of active sleep or wakefulness. (b) CFM of a 36-week GA preterm infant with diffuse cerebral oedema at ultrasound scan (this infant subsequently developed cerebral palsy). The tracing shows a discontinuous (not age-adequate) trace with excessive high amplitudes (paroxysmal activity) and low minimum level of cerebral activity (see the lower edge).

Obviously, it is not possible to recognize in the CFM tracing the maturational patterns that characterize the EEG of preterm infants, such as temporal sawtooth or delta brush patterns. This technique of recording rather reflects the development of the general organization of brain electrical activities, such as the differentiation of state-related patterns, the increase in minimum level of cerebral activity (which probably relates to increased amplitudes within inter-burst intervals of discontinuous EEG patterns), and the progressive reduction of maximum voltages.

CFM ABNORMAL PATTERNS AND CLINICAL APPLICATIONS
CFM is now widely used in neonatal intensive care units, as it is easy to use and allows on-line monitoring of cerebral activity (de Vries and Hellstrom-Westas 2005). Its interpretation is also easy, even without specific knowledge of clinical neurophysiology, and therefore it is suitable for paediatricians and neonatologists. Despite the over-simplification of this recording technique, research results indicate a high diagnostic and prognostic value of CFM in neonates, in particular in full-term infants with hypoxic-ischaemic encephalopathy (Eken et al 1995, Hellstrom-Westas et al 1995, al Naqeeb et al 1999, Toet et al 1999).

Specific abnormalities of full-term CFM have been described by various authors; the classification used by Toet et al (1999) is reported below (Fig. 7.11b and c):

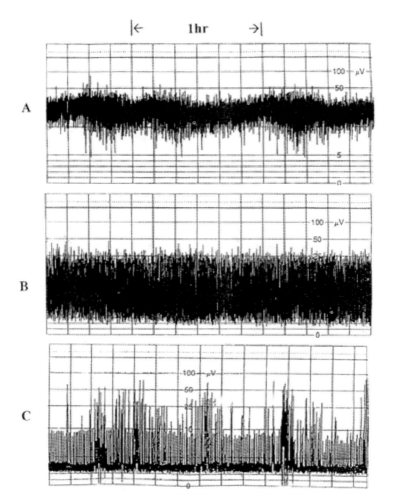

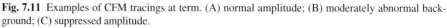

Fig. 7.11 Examples of CFM tracings at term. (A) normal amplitude; (B) moderately abnormal background; (C) suppressed amplitude.

Source: Reprinted from al Naqeeb et al 1999, with permission.

(a) Isoelectric tracing (flat tracing): very low voltage, mainly inactive, with activity below 5 µV.
(b) Continuous extremely low voltage: continuous pattern of very low voltage (around or below 5 µV).
(c) Burst-suppression: discontinuous pattern; periods of very low voltage are intermixed with bursts of higher amplitude.
(d) Discontinuous normal voltage: discontinuous trace where the voltage is predominantly above 5 µV.

Isoelectric tracings and continuous low-voltage patterns consistently relate to a very poor outcome, whereas burst-suppression is also compatible with a normal evolution (Hellstrom-Westas et al 1995), especially when non-persistent in subsequent recordings (Toet et al 1999).

Other authors (al Naqeeb et al 1999) have applied a quantitative classification, based on the voltage of the upper and lower edges of the trace. Moderately abnormal amplitudes (upper margin > 10 μV, and lower margin ≤ 5 μV) relate to a negative outcome in most cases, whereas suppressed amplitudes (upper edge < 10 μV, and lower edge < 5 μV) never result in a normal evolution.

Fewer reports are available on CFM background abnormalities in preterm infants. Indeed, while the most frequent anomalies of the full-term infant's background electrical activity (i.e. what is observable on the EEG as a constant low voltage or a burst-suppression) are recognizable by means of CFM, the specific alterations of maturational features that characterize the EEG of pathological preterm infants do not seem able to modify CFM, nor can specific abnormal transient activity, such as positive sharp waves, be distinguished on such a compressed trace. Nevertheless, there is some evidence that the occurrence of continuous CFM activity and the appearance of differentiated state-related patterns indicate a positive prognosis in low PMA preterm infants, whereas low-voltage traces relate to an unfavourable evolution (Fig. 7.10 b) (Hellstrom-Westas et al 1991, Hellstrom-Westas 1992).

As far as the recognition of neonatal epileptic phenomena is concerned, some descriptions of specific CFM patterns are available in the literature. Al Naqeeb et al (1999) reported that seizures are characterized by a sudden increase in voltage, accompanied by a narrowing of the bandwidth and followed by a period of suppression. Hellstrom-Vestas (1992) described repeated periods of increased voltage activity on the CFM, consisting of the so-called saw-tooth pattern and corresponding to low-voltage discharges on the EEG. Another common CFM correlate of prolonged EEG discharges is long-lasting plateaux of high voltage in both the lower and the upper edges. Nevertheless, it is also widely reported that brief or focal seizure activity can be missed by this technique (Hellstrom-Westas 1992, Toet et al 2002, Rennie et al 2004), necessitating its use in association with standard EEG methods.

Evoked potentials

INTRODUCTION
Essential information on the integrity of the nervous system, and in particular of the central and peripheral sensory pathways, is provided by the study of evoked potentials (EPs), consisting of the electrical responses to repeated visual, auditory or somatosensory stimulation. By averaging a high number of responses it is possible to increase the signal to noise ratio, so detecting low-amplitude electrical potentials generated by the stimulation. EPs have been shown to be of great value in assessing the maturation of the nervous system from birth onwards, and in the prediction of neurodevelopmental outcome after early insult.

All three main types of EPs – i.e. visual EPs (VEPs), brainstem auditory EPs (BAEPs) and somatosensory EPs (SEPs) – can be assessed from birth, even in preterm newborns, although in the latter there are greater technical restrictions and the technique is therefore less often used in clinical practice. A number of adjustments from the adult settings are required in order to apply this technique to newborns and infants, including hardware features, number and frequency of the stimuli, filtering and post-processing. The positive and negative deflections following the stimulus are analysed in terms of general wave morphology, amplitude and latency of the single peaks, and interpeak intervals. All these aspects have different maturational and clinical meanings which have to be carefully assessed in relation to developmental changes and normative data specific to the laboratory and the setting used.

In the following section, the three main types of EPs used in clinical practice during infancy will be considered. In particular, for each technique information will be given concerning the main methodological issues, the maturation profile of the responses and the current clinical value and application.

Visual Evoked Potentials (VEPs)

VEPs are generated by the activation of neuronal populations in the occipital cortex and represent the summation of dendritic synaptic potentials of these neurons (Freeman and Thibos 1975). The exact locations of the generator sources of the VEP are not well defined in humans; however, increasing data seem to support the hypothesis of different circum-scribed neuronal generators in the mesial and lateral occipital cortex, with different latencies of activation and timing of maturation (Arroyo et al 1997).

There are two major classes of VEP stimulation: luminance and pattern. The first is usually delivered as a uniform flash of light, the flash VEP (FVEP); while the second may be presented in either a reversal or an onset–offset fashion, the pattern VEP (PVEP). PVEPs are considered more stable and reliable, and are therefore the criterion standard in collaborative adult patients; however, their use is limited during infancy as they can only be elicited in individuals who are capable of prolonged fixations on the stimulus.

Flash VEPs (FVEPs)

FVEPs are commonly used from birth in infants at risk for neurodevelopmental disabilities. The analysis time is usually set at 1000 ms, as the major components of the response emerge between 200 and 500 ms. The stimulus frequency should be low enough (< 1 Hz) to allow the visual system to return to its resting state. The behavioural state of the infant should be consistent over recordings, as it can affect both amplitude and latency.

The first deflection elicited during development is visible in preterm newborns at around 24 weeks GA, and consists of a large negative wave occurring at approximately 300 ms (N300) (Fig. 7.12). The N300 shortens in latency as the infant matures, at a rate of 4.6–5.5 ms per week (Tsuneishi et al 1995). The second visible component emerges at around 34 weeks GA, consisting of a positive peak occurring at about 200 ms (P200). At term age the response consists of a negative–positive–negative complex which will gradually achieve adult characteristics during the first six months of life, with a progressive decrease of the three main peak latencies.

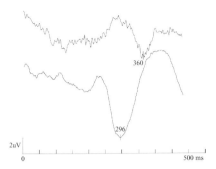

Fig. 7.12 FVEP in a preterm infant born at 32 weeks GA with birth asphyxia who on ultrasound scan showed periventricular flare persisting for 18 days. FVEPs were recorded at 3 days (upper trace), showing a delayed N300 and marked artefacts, and at 3 weeks (lower trace), showing normalization of wave morphology and latency. The outcome at 1 year was normal.

The main clinical application of FVEP in infancy is without doubt related to the early prediction of both visual impairment and neurological outcome in newborns with different types of prenatal and perinatal disorders. This technique has been shown to be a very good predictor of visual impairment of central origin (CVI), both in term infants with perinatal asphyxia (McCulloch and Skarf 1991, McCulloch and Taylor 1992) and in preterm infants with cystic leukomalacia (de Vries et al 1987, Eken et al 1996). Good correlation between FVEP responses and behavioural assessment of visual acuity (e.g. acuity cards) has been shown in these infants, with an overall increase in predictive power with the combined use of the two approaches.

The clinical value of FVEP in the prediction of neurodevelopment has been shown to be different in preterm and full-term infants. Several studies have failed to show a clear-cut correlation between abnormal FVEP and outcome in preterm infants (Beverley et al 1990, Shepherd et al 1999). Nevertheless, two main features of the response have been shown to be often associated with adverse outcome: a delayed N300 before term, and an absent P200 at term. Conversely, a very strong correlation with neurodevelopmental outcome has been consistently shown in studies in the term infant with birth asphyxia (Whyte et al 1986, McCulloch and Skarf 1991, Muttitt et al 1991, Taylor et al 1992). A persistent abnormality of the FVEP during the first week of life has been shown to be the best predictor for an abnormal outcome, while a normal response by the end of the first week is usually associated with normal development. This type of profile is similar to what has been shown in similar populations with EEG background activity, and probably shares with it the same patho-physiological bases. Other types of EPs have been used in this type of patient and an even stronger predictive value has been shown, in particular by the somatosensory EPs (see below).

Pattern VEPs
Different types of PVEP can be used during infancy. The pattern reversal VEP, based on black and white checkerboards, has been the most widely studied both in children and in adults, showing a relatively low intra- and inter-subject variability of waveform and peak latency. However, its use early in infancy has been limited by poor cooperation at this age, particularly in infants with neurological problems.

This technique has been used in preterm infants with inconsistent results, as the morphology of the waveform becomes more stable only as the infant approaches term age. For this reason its application during the neonatal period for prognostic purposes in at-risk newborns has been limited. During the first months of life a rapid decrease in the latency of all peaks occurs. The adult-like latency of the P100 peak is reached by about 1 year of age with large checkerboards, and later with smaller ones. The variability in the maturational profile is, however, extremely high. This gradual decrease in latency might have a potential application as an index of neuronal development, but full evidence is not yet available (Porciatti et al 2002).

Another type of PVEP which has recently been applied in early infancy is the orientation-reversal steady-state VEP. It is based on high-rate stimulations (4 or 8 Hz), generating a sinusoidal waveform which can eventually undergo statistical post-processing analysis of temporal coherence. This technique has been used in particular in the assessment of cortical visual maturation during the first year of life, and has shown a high power in predicting cerebral visual impairment and neurodevelopment in newborns at risk (Mercuri et al 1995, 1998).

BRAINSTEM AUDITORY EVOKED POTENTIALS (BAEPs)

BAEPs are generated by the activation of neuronal populations within the auditory brainstem pathway in response to an acoustic stimulation. They consist of a relatively stable response composed of seven sequential positive waves arising during impulse transmission between the auditory nerve, pons and midbrain. The most important components of the potential during infancy are waves I, III and V (Fig. 7.13) (Stockard-Pope et al 1992). Wave I is produced in the eighth nerve by the transformation into impulses of tone-specific responses in the hair cells. Wave III is formed at the level of the cochlear nucleus of the brainstem; while wave V is produced at the level of the rostral part of the pons and the caudal part of the midbrain. The I–V interpeak latency has been shown to be unaffected by click intensity after a certain threshold and independent of peripheral auditory function; it has therefore been considered as a reliable measure of central auditory conduction time (Eggermont and Don 1980).

BAEPs are commonly used from birth in infants at risk for sensorial and/or neurodevelopmental disabilities. The analysis time is usually set between 15 and 20 ms, as the waves normally arise in the first ten milliseconds after the stimulus. A repetition rate

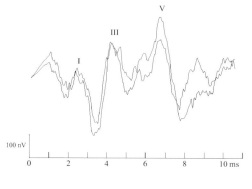

Fig. 7.13 BAEP at 37 weeks PMA in an infant born at 35 weeks GA. Age-adequate latencies and amplitudes are found (click int. 90 dB; freq. 11 Hz; trials 2000).

of 10 per second can be safely used. The stimulus is presented monoaurally and its intensity has to be calibrated above the hearing threshold in order to get a full response. Contralateral masking is advisable to avoid trans-bone conduction to the opposite ear.

The three major waves of the potential can be recognized from 25 weeks GA onwards. All peak latencies decrease gradually with age, with the V wave decreasing faster. This results in an overall reduction of I–V interpeak interval with time. The effect of preterm exposure to auditory stimulation on the maturation of the auditory system has been investigated, with equivocal results, in part due to the different inclusion criteria used and therefore the risk level of the population studied. At term age the morphology of the potential can easily be compared to adult responses, but the latencies are significantly higher. Adult-like responses are reached at about 2 years of age. It has to be noted that a high inter-individual variability has been consistently reported in cross-sectional studies; however, the intra-individual maturation rate is fairly regular.

As a general rule, a prolonged latency of wave I associated with a normal I–V peak interval is suggestive of a peripheral abnormality, while a normal latency of wave I associated with a prolonged I–V interpeak interval indicates a disorder of central conduction time. In both cases an early diagnosis of a hearing defect is mandatory, especially with regard to language development, as it has been shown to be more easily preserved when treatment is started within the first six months of life (Murray et al 1985). For this reason, when abnormal results are detected, repeated assessment once every two months should be performed.

The use of BAEPs as a predictor of neurological outcome in infants with brain insults has also been extensively investigated. The features that are most commonly associated with abnormal development include absence or low amplitude of later peaks and prolonged I–V conduction intervals (Murray et al 1985). The majority of studies investigating the predictive value of this technique, however, stress the presence of a high number of false negatives with respect to neurological outcome. This is mainly due to the frequent sparing of the deep structures explored by BAEPs in many infants with brain lesions and abnormal outcome. This finding, together with the high prognostic value of other neuro-physiological techniques such as EEG, VEPs and SEPs, has limited the application of this type of potential as a predictor of neurological outcome.

SOMATOSENSORY EVOKED POTENTIALS (SEPs)
SEPs are generated by the activation of neuronal populations within the somatosensory pathway in response to a sensory stimulation, i.e. peripheral nerves, the posterior column of the spinal cord and, following decussation, the medial lemniscus, thalamus and parietal cortex. In newborns and infants, the peripheral stimulation most commonly used is electrical stimulation of the median or tibial nerve (Laureau and Marlot 1990, George and Taylor 1991, Boor and Goebel 2000).

The peripheral somatosensory pathways can be assessed reliably over Erb's point (i.e. the site at the lateral root of the brachial plexus 2–3 cm above the clavicle) (Willis et al 1984, Laureau et al 1988) and over the spinal cord (Laureau and Marlot 1990). These subcortical responses are more constantly recordable and stable than the cortical responses during the first six months of life, as the early maturation of peripheral nerve and posterior column fibres is significantly faster than that of the more central structures (Boor and Goebel 2000, Laureau et al 1988).

The cortical responses are assessed by means of contralateral rolandic scalp electrodes. The first cortical response to median nerve stimulation, termed N19 in adults, is called N1 in newborns and young infants. The early N1 deflection is measurable in most normal preterm infants from at least the seventh gestational month, and presents a latency markedly longer than in term infants and adults (Taylor and Wynn-Williams 1986). From birth and up to about 3 years of age, there is a developmental trend of shortening of the peak latencies, increase in the amplitudes, and decrease in the duration of the waveform (Desmedt et al 1976, Willis et al 1984, Laureau et al 1988). This increased conduction velocity is secondary to the myelination and maturation of the pathways; while after the age of 3 years an opposing mechanism is more dominant, i.e. the elongation of the pathway due to physical growth causes the latencies to start to lengthen. A similar general pattern of maturation can also be shown after tibial nerve stimulation.

One of the major clinical applications of SEPs during infancy concerns the prediction of neurodevelopmental outcome of preterm and term infants at neurological risk. The prognostic power of SEPs in preterm newborns with brain lesions has been widely studied, with unclear results. When the median nerve was assessed, either a low sensitivity or a low specificity was reported in the various studies, possibly reflecting differences in methodology and an overall limited prognostic value of the technique. In this population a higher prognostic value has been shown by studies assessing the tibial nerve, probably as a consequence of the frequency of lower limb involvement following preterm lesions.

Another important field of application of infant SEPs is the asphyxiated term infant. General agreement has been reached by different authors on the high value of this technique in predicting an abnormal outcome in newborns with hypoxic-ischaemic encephalopathy. A high sensitivity has been shown in particular during the first 72 hours after delivery, when this technique appears to be more powerful than ultrasound or other types of EPs (Eken et al 1995).

REFERENCES

al Naqeeb N, Edwards AD, Cowan FM, Azzopardi D (1999) Assessment of neonatal encephalopathy by amplitude-integrated electroencephalography. *Pediatrics* 103(6 Pt 1): 1263–1271.

Anders T, Emde R, Parmelee A (1971) A manual of standardized terminology, techniques and criteria for scoring of the states of sleep and wakefulness in newborn infants. Los Angeles: UCLA Brain Information Service/BRI Publications Office, NINDS Neurological Infant Network.

Anderson CM, Torres F, Faoro A (1985) The EEG of the early premature. *Electroencephalogr Clin Neurophysiol* 60(2): 95–105.

Arroyo S, Lesser RP, Poon W-T, Webber WRS, Gordon B (1997) Neuronal generators of visual evoked potentials in humans: visual processing in the human cortex. *Epilepsia* 38(5): 600–610.

Aso K, Abdab-Barmada M, Scher MS (1993) EEG and the neuropathology in premature neonates with intraventricular hemorrhage. *J Clin Neurophysiol* 10(3): 304–313.

Battin MR, Maalouf EF, Counsell SJ, et al (1998) Magnetic resonance imaging of the brain in very preterm infants: visualization of the germinal matrix, early myelination, and cortical folding. *Pediatrics* 101(6): 957–962.

Baud O, d'Allest AM, Lacaze-Masmonteil T, et al (1998) The early diagnosis of periventricular leukomalacia in premature infants with positive rolandic sharp waves on serial electroencephalography. *J Pediatr* 132(5): 813–817.

Beverley DW, Smith IS, Beesley P, Jones J, Rhodes N (1990) Relationship of cranial ultrasonography, visual and auditory evoked responses with neurodevelopmental outcome. *Dev Med Child Neurol* 32(3): 210–222.

Biagioni E, Cioni G (1996) Arousal seizures in subjects with infantile spasms. *J Sleep Res* 5(Suppl 1): 15.

Biagioni E, Bartalena L, Boldrini A, Cioni G, Giancola S, Ipata AE (1994) Background EEG activity in preterm infants: correlation of outcome with selected maturational features. *Electroencephalogr Clin Neurophysiol* 91(3): 154–162.

Biagioni E, Bartalena L, Biver P, Pieri R, Cioni G, et al (1996a) Electroencephalographic dysmaturity in preterm infants: a prognostic tool in the early postnatal period. *Neuropediatrics* 27(6): 311–316.

Biagioni E, Boldrini A, Bottone U, et al (1996b) Prognostic value of abnormal EEG transients in preterm and full-term neonates. *Electroencephalogr Clin Neurophysiol* 99(1): 1–9.

Biagioni E, Bartalena L, Boldrini A, et al (1999) Constantly discontinuous EEG patterns in full-term neonates with hypoxic-ischaemic encephalopathy. *Clin Neurophysiol* 110(9): 1510–1515.

Biagioni E, Bartalena L, Boldrini A, et al (2000a) Electroencephalography in infants with periventricular leukomalacia: prognostic features at preterm and term age. *J Child Neurol* 15(1): 1–6.

Biagioni E, Frisone MF, Laroche S, et al (2000b) Occipital sawtooth: a physiological EEG pattern in very premature infants. *Clin Neurophysiol* 111(12): 2145–2149.

Biagioni E, Mercuri E, Rutherford M, et al (2001) Combined use of electroencephalogram and magnetic resonance imaging in full-term neonates with acute encephalopathy. *Pediatrics* 107(3): 461–468.

Biagioni E, Cioni G, Cowan F, et al (2002) Visual function and EEG reactivity in infants with perinatal brain lesions at 1 year. *Dev Med Child Neurol* 44(3): 171–176.

Boor R, Goebel B (2000) Maturation of near-field and far-field somatosensory evoked potentials after median nerve stimulation in children under 4 years of age. *Clin Neurophysiol* 111(6): 1070–1081.

Castro Conde JR, Martinez ED, Campo CG, et al (2004) Positive temporal sharp waves in preterm infants with and without brain ultrasound lesions. *Clin Neurophysiol* 115(11): 2479–2488.

Curzi-Dascalova L, Mirmiran M (1996) *Manuel des techniques d'enregistrement et d'analyse des stades de sommeil et de veille chez le prématuré et le nouveau-né à terme.* Paris: Inserm.

Desmedt JE, Brunko E, Debecker J (1976) Maturation of the somatosensory evoked potentials in normal infants and children, with special reference to the early N1 component. *Electroencephalogr Clin Neurophysiol* 40(1): 43–58.

de Vries LS, Hellstrom-Westas L (2005) Role of cerebral function monitoring in the newborn. *Arch Dis Child Fetal Neonatal Ed* 90(3): F201–F207.

de Vries LS, Connell JA, Dubowitz LMS, et al (1987) Neurological, electrophysiological and MRI abnormalities in infants with extensive cystic leukomalacia. *Neuropediatrics* 18(2): 61–66.

Dreyfus-Brisac C, Monod N (1972) The electroencephalogram of fulterm newborns and premature infants. In: Remon A, editor. *Handbook of Electroencephalography and Clinical Neurophysiology.* Amsterdam: Elsevier, pp 6–23.

Eaton DG, Wertheim D, Oozeer R, Dubowitz LM, Dubowitz V (1994) Reversible changes in cerebral activity associated with acidosis in preterm neonates. *Acta Paediatr* 83(5): 486–492.

Eggermont JJ, Don M (1980) Analysis of the click-evoked brainstem potentials in humans using high-pass noise masking. II. Effect of click intensity. *J Acoust Soc Am* 68(6): 1671–1675.

Eken P, Toet MC, Groenendaal F, de Vries LS (1995) Predictive value of early neuroimaging, pulsed Doppler and neurophysiology in full term infants with hypoxic-ischaemic encephalopathy. *Arch Dis Child Fetal Neonatal Ed* 73(2): F75–F80.

Eken P, de Vries LS, van Nieuwenhuizen O, et al (1996) Early predictors of cerebral visual impairment in infants with cystic leukomalacia. *Neuropediatrics* 27(1): 16–25.

Ferrari F, Torricelli A, Giustardi A, Benatti A, Bolzani R, Ori L, Frigieri G (1992) Bioelectric brain maturation in fulterm infants and in healthy and pathological preterm infants at term post-menstrual age. *Early Hum Dev* 28(1): 37–63.

Ferrari F, Biagioni E, Cioni G (2001) Neonatal electroencephalography. In: Levene MI, Chervenak FA, Whittle M, editors. *Fetal and Neonatal Neurology and Neurosurgery.* London: Churchill Livingstone.

Freeman RD, Thibos LN (1975) Visual evoked responses in humans with abnormal visual experience. *J Physiol* 247(3): 711–724.

George SR, Taylor MJ (1991) Somatosensory evoked potentials in neonates and infants: developmental and normative data. *Electroencephalogr Clin Neurophysiol* 80(2): 94–102.

117

Hayakawa F, Okumura A, Kato T, et al (1997) Disorganized patterns: chronic-stage EEG abnormality of the late neonatal period following severely depressed EEG activities in early preterm infants. *Neuropediatrics* 28(5): 272–275.

Hellstrom-Westas L (1992) Comparison between tape-recorded and amplitude-integrated EEG monitoring in sick newborn infants. *Acta Paediatr* 81(10): 812–819.

Hellstrom-Westas L, Rosen I, Svenningsen NW (1991) Cerebral function monitoring during the first week of life in extremely small low birthweight (ESLBW) infants. *Neuropediatrics* 22(1): 27–32.

Hellstrom-Westas L, Rosen I, Svenningsen NW (1995) Predictive value of early continuous amplitude integrated EEG recordings on outcome after severe birth asphyxia in full term infants. *Arch Dis Child Fetal Neonatal Ed* 72(1): F34–38.

Hellstrom-Westas L, Klette H, Thorngren-Jerneck K, Rosén I (2001) Early prediction of outcome with aEEG in preterm infants with large intraventricular hemorrhages. *Neuropediatrics* 32(6): 319–324.

Holmes GL, Lombroso CT (1993) Prognostic value of background patterns in the neonatal EEG. *J Clin Neurophysiol* 10(3): 323–352.

Hughes JR, Miller JK, Fino JJ, Hughes CA (1990) The sharp theta rhythm on the occipital areas of prematures (STOP): a newly described waveform. *Clin Electroencephalogr* 21(2): 77–87.

Kato T, Okumura A, Hayakawa F, Kuno K, Watanabe K (2004) Electroencephalographic aspects of periventricular hemorrhagic infarction in preterm infants. *Neuropediatrics* 35(3): 161–166.

Kellaway P (1987) Intensive monitoring in infants and children. *Adv Neurol* 46: 127–137.

Lamblin MD, Andre M, Auzoux M, et al (2004) Indications of electroencephalogram in the newborn. *Arch Pediatr* 11(7): 829–833.

Laureau E, Marlot D (1990) Somatosensory evoked potentials after median and tibial nerve stimulation in healthy newborns. *Electroencephalogr Clin Neurophysiol* 76(5): 453–458.

Laureau E, Majnemer A, Rosenblatt B, Riley P (1988) A longitudinal study of short latency somatosensory evoked responses in healthy newborns and infants. *Electroencephalogr Clin Neurophysiol* 71(2): 100–108.

Limperopoulos C, Majnemer A, Rosenblatt B, et al (2001) Association between electroencephalographic findings and neurologic status in infants with congenital heart defects. *J Child Neurol* 16(7): 471–476.

Lombroso CT (1985) Neonatal polygraphy in full-term and premature infants: a review of normal and abnormal findings. *J Clin Neurophysiol* 2(2): 105–155.

McCulloch DL, Skarf B (1991) Development of the human visual system: monocular and binocular pattern VEP latency. *Invest Ophthalmol Vis Sci* 32(8): 2372–2381.

McCulloch DL, Taylor MJ (1992) Cortical blindness in children: utility of flash VEPs. *Pediatr Neurol* 8(2): 156.

Marret S, Parain D, Jeannot E, Eurin D, Fessard C (1992) Positive rolandic sharp waves in the EEG of the premature newborn: a five year prospective study. *Arch Dis Child* 67(7): 948–951.

Menache CC, Bourgeois BF, Volpe JJ (2002) Prognostic value of neonatal discontinuous EEG. *Pediatr Neurol* 27(2): 93–101.

Mercuri E, Siebenthal K, Tutuncuoglu S, Guzzeta F, Casaer P (1995) The effect of behavioural states on visual evoked responses in preterm and full-term newborns. *Neuropediatrics* 26(4): 211–213.

Mercuri E, Braddick O, Atkinson J, et al (1998) Orientation-reversal and phase-reversal visual evoked potentials in full-term infants with brain lesions: a longitudinal study. *Neuropediatrics* 29(4): 169–174.

Monod N, Pajot N, Guidasci S (1972) The neonatal EEG: statistical studies and prognostic value in full-term and pre-term babies. *Electroencephalogr Clin Neurophysiol* 32(5): 529–544.

Murray AD, Javel E, Watson CS (1985) Prognostic validity of auditory brainstem evoked response screening in newborn infants. *Am J Otolaryngol* 6(2): 120–131.

Muttitt SC, Taylor M, Kobayashi JS, MacMillan L, Whyte HE (1991) Serial visual evoked potentials and outcome in term birth asphyxia. *Pediatr Neurol* 7(2): 86–90.

Nolte R, Haas G (1978) A polygraphic study of bioelectrical brain maturation in preterm infants. *Dev Med Child Neurol* 20(2): 167–182.

Ohtahara S, Yamatogi Y (2003) Epileptic encephalopathies in early infancy with suppression-burst. *J Clin Neurophysiol* 20(6): 398–407.

Okumura A, Watanabe K (2001) Clinico-electrical evolution in pre-hypsarrhythmic stage: towards prediction and prevention of West syndrome. *Brain Dev* 23(7): 482–487.

Pezzani C, Radvanyi-Bouvet MF, Relier JP, et al (1986) Neonatal electroencephalography during the first twenty-four hours of life in full-term newborn infants. *Neuropediatrics* 17(1): 11–18.

Porciatti V, Pizzorusso T, Maffei L (2002) Electrophysiology of the postreceptoral visual pathway in mice. *Doc Ophthalmol* 104(1): 69–82.

118

Randò T, Bancale A, Baranello G, et al (2004) Visual function in infants with West syndrome: correlation with EEG patterns. *Epilepsia* 45(7): 781–786.

Rennie JM, Chorley G, Boylan GB, et al (2004) Non-expert use of the cerebral function monitor for neonatal seizure detection. *Arch Dis Child Fetal Neonatal Ed* 89(1): F37–F40.

Shepherd AJ, Saunders KJ, McCulloch DL, Dutton GN (1999) Prognostic value of flash visual evoked potentials in preterm infants. *Dev Med Child Neurol* 41(1): 9–15.

Stockard-Pope J, Werner SS, Bickford RG (1992) *Atlas of Neonatal Electroenchephalogrphy, 2nd edn*. New York: Raven Press.

Suzuki M, Okumura T, Watanabe T, et al (2003) The predictive value of electroencephalogram during early infancy for later development of West syndrome in infants with cystic periventricular leukomalacia. *Epilepsia* 44(3): 443–446.

Taylor M.J, Murphy WJ, Whyte HE (1992) Prognostic reliability of somatosensory and visual evoked potentials of asphyxiated term infants. *Dev Med Child Neurol* 34(6): 507–515.

Taylor PK, Wynn-Williams GM (1986) A modified mirror projection visual evoked potential stimulator for presenting patterns in different orientations. *Electroencephalogr Clin Neurophysiol* 64(1): 81–83.

Thornberg E, Thiringer K (1990) Normal pattern of the cerebral function monitor trace in term and preterm neonates. *Acta Paediatr Scand* 79(1): 20–25.

Toet MC, Hellstrom-Westas L, Groenendaal F, Eken P, De Vries LS (1999) Amplitude integrated EEG 3 and 6 hours after birth in full term neonates with hypoxic-ischaemic encephalopathy. *Arch Dis Child Fetal Neonatal Ed* 81(1): F19–F23.

Toet MC, van der Meij W, de Vries LS, et al (2002) Comparison between simultaneously recorded amplitude integrated electroencephalogram (cerebral function monitor) and standard electroencephalogram in neonates. *Pediatrics* 109(5): 772–779.

Tsuneishi S, Casaer P, Fock JM, Hirano S (1995) Establishment of normal values for flash visual evoked potentials (VEPs) in preterm infants: a longitudinal study with special reference to two components of the N1 wave. *Electroencephalogr Clin Neurophysiol* 96(4): 291–299.

Vecchierini MF, d'Allest AM, Verpillat P (2003) EEG patterns in 10 extreme premature neonates with normal neurological outcome: qualitative and quantitative data. *Brain Dev* 25(5): 330–337.

Vermeulen RJ, Sie LT, Jonkman EJ, et al (2003) Predictive value of EEG in neonates with periventricular leukomalacia. *Dev Med Child Neurol* 45(9): 586–590.

Vigevano F, Fusco L, Pachatz C (2001) Neurophysiology of spasms. *Brain Dev* 23(7): 467–472.

Watanabe K, Hayakawa F, Okumura A (1999) Neonatal EEG: a powerful tool in the assessment of brain damage in preterm infants. *Brain Dev* 21(6): 361–372.

Wertheim D, Mercuri E, Faundez JC, et al (1994) Prognostic value of continuous electroencephalographic recording in full term infants with hypoxic ischaemic encephalopathy. *Arch Dis Child* 71(2): F97–F102.

Whyte HE, Taylor M, Menzies R, Chin KC, MacMillan LJ (1986) Prognostic utility of visual evoked potentials in term asphyxiated neonates. *Pediatr Neurol* 2(4): 220–223.

Willis J, Seales D, Frazier E (1984) Short latency somatosensory evoked potentials in infants. *Electroencephalogr Clin Neurophysiol* 59(5): 366–373.

8
ASSESSMENT OF THE DEVELOPMENT OF HIGH-RISK INFANTS IN THE FIRST TWO YEARS

Samantha Johnson and Neil Marlow

Babies who are at high risk of developmental problems comprise two main groups: term infants following perinatal hypoxia, and the much greater population of babies born preterm, particularly those born at very low gestational ages. For particular research projects other populations may be assembled but for these studies the research questions will drive the choice of developmental measures. Term infants who recover from severe perinatal hypoxic insults without developing cerebral palsy tend to have normal developmental trajectories over the first two years, but may have more subtle deficits at later ages. By far the most challenging group to understand in developmental terms are preterm infants, in whom multiple developmental problems may be identified and in whom developmental trajectories may be altered by the interruption in their intrauterine development caused by preterm birth and acquired brain injuries. Our discussion will therefore focus mainly on this group.

For the clinician, a developmental assessment is an essential part of any routine clinic visit in order to inform clinical management and parental counselling, to identify individuals eligible for early intervention services, and to monitor progress throughout these efforts. Optimizing the accuracy of early identification is particularly important for more subtle developmental delays that may result in more intrusive conditions at school age. Information regarding developmental outcomes is also required for routine audit and service development. For the researcher, accurate outcome evaluations are critical for epidemiological studies and randomized trials, and for informing the continuing debate regarding the ethics of treatment of babies born at the limits of viability.

More preterm babies are now graduating from neonatal services as a result of improvements in obstetric and neonatal care, the use of antenatal steroids, exogenous surfactant therapy, technological advances, and the developing formalized structure of NICU services (Allen 2002). There is continuing concern regarding the quality of outcome for these survivors. Despite many studies, the prediction of long-term developmental outcome from neonatal course remains difficult as developmental, genetic, social and environmental factors also interact to affect outcome. Given the high risk of disability, particularly in the extremely preterm child (Wood et al 2000, Marlow et al 2005), and the high cost of modern neonatal care, it is important to offer follow-up services in order to screen for disability, organize timely intervention, and monitor the prevalence of poor outcome following perinatal care. Such systems are part of national (BAPM 2001) and European recommendations, and will include a developmental assessment. Understanding and monitoring development, at least over the first two years, are therefore critical functions of a neonatal service, even if other arrangements are made for later assessment.

In this chapter we discuss the assessment of developmental outcome over the first two years after birth. We outline a number of assessment tools which aid the clinician and researcher in the early identification of children with developmental delays, and outline issues surrounding the utility of developmental testing in infancy.

Why should we perform a developmental assessment?

Preterm birth can have adverse effects on a child's development which may persist into adolescence and adulthood (Bhutta et al 2002, Hack et al 2002, Marlow 2004). The prevalence of disability and mean cognitive scores are inversely related to gestational age (Hack and Fanaroff 1999, Bhutta et al 2002), particularly in those born at less than 32 weeks (Wolke et al 2001, Marlow 2005). Different populations have been studied and thus the prevalence of significant developmental disability ranges from 6 to 8 per cent of low-birthweight infants (LBW (< 2500g)), 14 to 17 per cent of very low-birthweight infants (VLBW (< 1500g)), and 20 to 25 per cent for those born extremely preterm (< 26 weeks) or of extremely low birthweight (ELBW (< 1000g)) (Aylward 2002). Boys are also found to be more vulnerable to developmental problems than girls (Hindmarsh et al 2000, Wood et al 2000, Marlow et al 2005).

A number of adverse outcomes are clearly associated with preterm birth: cerebral palsy (CP; typically spastic diplegia), deafness, blindness, and severe cognitive impairment. At borderline viability the prevalence of these conditions, broadly ranging from 15 to 20 per cent, has remained relatively stable over the last decade (Aylward 2003, Marlow et al 2005). As not all high-risk newborns will go on to develop difficulties or impaired quality of life (Werner 1994, Tideman 2000, MacCormick 2002), the monitoring, and reduction in rates, of serious impairment are important goals. Follow-up studies should follow a basic protocol (Mutch et al 1989), and there are recommendations for the definition of health status (i.e. disability) at 2 years (NPEU 1995).

Despite appropriate concern regarding the frequency of these major disabling conditions, the most common area of poor functioning among preterm children is cognition. This is mirrored in the fact that developmental impairment is the most common finding at 2 years (Wood et al 2000, Marlow 2004). At later ages deficits in cognitive, perceptual-motor and visuospatial ability, language and behaviour may be present in as many as 50 to 70 per cent of VLBW infants (Taylor et al 2000). When IQ test results are compared with those of classmates, 41 per cent of 6-year-old extremely preterm children have moderate/severe cognitive impairment (scores less than -2 SD), and a further 31 per cent have mild impairments (-1 to -2 SD) (Marlow et al 2005); at 2½ years only 30 per cent of children had developmental scores -2 SD (Wood et al 2000). A developmental test would thus be most useful if it could identify those at highest risk of later learning difficulties.

Screening or detailed assessment?

Assessment therefore has to *quantify* infant morbidity and *identify* individuals with developmental delays or disability. 'Developmental screening tests' (Box 8.1) are often employed in routine surveillance programmes of whole populations to identify those 'at risk' for unsuspected deviations from normal development; for this purpose screening measures are quick, inexpensive, and easy to administer and so may appear useful for monitoring outcomes. However, the discrimination of abnormality and accuracy of classification using such tests may be relatively poor as they are designed to identify children who require more detailed assessments; their predictive value for later difficulties may also be poor, except in those with the most severe impairment. More detailed comprehensive tests are therefore required for outcome measurement.

Box 8.1 Examples of tester-administered developmental screening tests

- Bayley Infant Neurodevelopmental Screener (BINS) (Aylward 1995).
- Clinical Adaptive Test/Clinical Linguistic Auditory Milestone Scale (CAT/CLAMS) (Rossman et al 1994, Wachtel et al 1994).
- Denver Developmental Screening Test II (DENVER II) (Frankenburg et al 1990, 1992).
- Revised BRIGANCE Diagnostic Inventory of Early Development (BRIGANCE) (Brigance 1991, Glascoe 1995).
- Schedule of Growing Skills, 2nd edition (SGS) (Bellman et al 1996).

Formal standardized measures of development

Standardized tests are psychometric measures designed to inventory an infant's skills against a 'normal' population within a specific assessment paradigm. They usually comprise tester-administered measures in which a trained and competent examiner observes a child's response to a structured set of tasks and activities. These tests require the examiner to follow a strict administration and scoring protocol, deviation from which invalidates scores obtained on the test. This rigorous standardization is designed to reduce measurement error by precluding subjective interpretation of the child's responses. Although test scoring may seem harsh and the tests 'difficult', their uniformity and objectivity are their strength and reflect how the test was used during the standardization process; to deviate from this procedure – for example, because the child is said to 'usually' be able to perform the required tasks – weakens the objectivity and thus the value of the assessment.

Standardized tests are designed to yield numerical results, which are amenable to statistical analysis and thus ideal for use in research studies. One of the key characteristics of standardized tests is the derivation of *norm-referenced* or *standardized* scores. During the standardization process a test is administered to a large population of children of the age range for whom the test is designed. It is important that this population is well chosen and representative. These children form the *normative sample*, and an individual child's score on the test is in effect a comparison to the normative data to determine how he or she is developing in relation to the normal population; classifications of an individual's developmental level are then made on the basis of the deviation of his or her score from that of the mean of the normative sample; conventionally, a score of 2 SD below the normative mean has been used as a cut-off to identify abnormality in preterm populations. Challenging this practice, a consensus statement has suggested that a cut-off of -3 SD may be more appropriate (NPEU 1995) and may be more predictive of later poor performance (Marlow et al 2005).

Standardized tests may also yield 'age equivalent scores' and 'percentile ranks'; although these can be used to make comparisons between an individual's performance and that expected of his or her peers, classifications of developmental level are not made using these scores as they are based on raw rather than standardized scores (Salvia and Ysseldyke 1991).

The standardization of a test does not ensure its psychometric integrity. Properties such as validity and reliability vary widely between tests, and standardization alone does not guarantee the selection of a normative sample that is representative of the population for whom the test is designed. Furthermore, any test used should ideally have a recent standardization: the well described upward drift in standardized scores over time, often referred to as the Flynn effect (Flynn 1999), may result in overestimations of a child's developmental level if older normative data are applied (Campbell et al 1986, Wolke et al 1994, Goldstein et al 1995, Gagnon and Nagle 2000, Marlow et al 2005). The selection of any individual measure should therefore take account of information regarding its standardization and psychometric integrity (Box 8.2).

In practice, individual clinicians will use tests with which they have experience and which have face value in their discipline. Some might therefore prefer a test with less impressive psychometric properties if it guides clinical management. However, standardized tests are also widely used experimentally and by professionals involved in outcome evaluations, and thus lend themselves well to comparison across disciplines and between research protocols. The need for uniformity in test methods across studies is particularly important, as the selection and use of outcome measures can be a major source of bias in research trials (Aylward 2002).

Although developmental tests are available for use with infants from birth through the first two years of life, the utility of these instruments for reporting outcomes for preterm infants might be optimized by use at 2 years. A number of common conditions and syndromes are not evident or resolved until 2 years, and milder dysfunctions may become more evident at this age (NPEU 1995, Bracewell and Marlow 2002). A problem with the use of repeated sequential testing is that the scores of a particular child may vary greatly over the early years (Largo et al 1990). This may represent random variation in performance and application in particular testing situations rather than underlying trends, even in a child who has evolving disability. Reporting assessments made closer to school age may also optimize their predictive value for academic performance by reducing the interval between measures.

Box 8.2 Assessing the psychometric properties of standardized tests

Reliability: this refers to the consistency of a scale – the extent to which a test will yield the same results when administered repeatedly. Differences in scores obtained using the same test under the same conditions should reflect genuine differences in development rather than measurement error.

- **Internal consistency:** the correlation between items within a scale or subscale.
- **Test–retest reliability:** the correlation between scores obtained by the same examiner administering the test on several occasions to the same persons.
- **Inter-rater reliability:** the correlation between scores obtained by two different examiners administering the test to the same persons.

Validity: the extent to which a test measures what it purports to measure. Differences in test scores between individuals should reflect genuine differences in the specific abilities or skills the test is designed to assess.

- **Content validity:** a systematic examination of test items to determine whether the test contains a representative sample of the abilities or domain that the test is designed to measure.
- **Construct validity:** an assessment of whether the test measures the underlying theoretical constructs or traits it is designed to measure – often assessed by comparing the test performance of different groups of individuals, children of different ages, or confirmatory factor analyses.
- **Concurrent validity:** the correlation between the scores obtained on the test and scores obtained on another well-validated measure of the same construct – the 'criterion measure' – administered at the same time.
- **Predictive validity:** the correlation between the scores obtained on the test and scores obtained on another well-validated (criterion) measure administered at a later date. (Concurrent and predictive validity are also referred to as criterion-referenced validity.)

The use of corrected age in assessing preterm children can be contentious given the potential result of the under-identification of children with developmental delays and impairments (Lems et al 1993, Aylward 2002). Corrected age should be used when assessing very preterm children (< 32 weeks), particularly during infancy when the effects of preterm birth are more significant. Although some confusion remains as to the age at which to cease correction for preterm birth, it is generally recommended that correction be applied until at least 2 years (NPEU 1995).

Developmental assessment tools

MULTI-DOMAIN DEVELOPMENTAL ASSESSMENTS

The interpretation of specific facets of development is difficult in infancy given the interdependence of developmental skills during this period. Meisels and Atkins-Burnett (2000) provide the example of a picture naming task. The correct response is the production of the corresponding name, requiring the integration of sensory, cognitive and oral motor abilities in addition to the scored expressive vocabulary output. Similarly, the 'cognitive' task of building a tower of blocks requires the integration of cognitive ability, perceptual awareness, and gross and fine motor skills.

Losch and Dammann (2004) recently attempted to quantify the effect of motor skills on VLBW preschoolers' performance on standardized tests of cognitive development. Using principal component factor analysis, two factors emerged which jointly explained 53 to 70 per cent of the variance in test scores: cognitive/language skills and motor skills. Whilst tests of 'cognition' have validity in measuring language and cognitive abilities, a significant proportion of the variance in test scores can be explained by the child's motor abilities, even for those children in whom motor impairment is not obvious. Within very preterm populations this observation may have great importance, as motor and cognitive impairments may have very different aetiologies, which is reflected in the different patterns of associations and antecedents found in the cognitive and motor scores of preterm children (Wood et al 2005).

For research and longitudinal studies, it may therefore be expedient to combine the assessment of multiple domains in infancy, particularly for optimizing the prediction of later outcome. Multi-domain developmental assessments are ideally suited to this purpose, providing an efficient measure of global development. Despite the difficulty in isolating specific skills, some assessments have been designed to provide standardized measures of functioning in (often artificially) separate domains of development to identify specific patterns of deficits influencing overall functioning; these 'subscales' are typically reviewed after a developmental deficit is identified from a global assessment.

There are many standardized tests for use in early childhood, a number of which assess development in children aged 24 months and above (Box 8.3). Many of these are standardized from 2 years of age, but this is usually the lowest detectable performance for the test and their use at 2 years is not recommended due to the difficulty in establishing a basal performance, particularly in a sample of preterm infants for whom significant impairment might be expected.

Early developmental assessment tools were essentially clinically based, to aid in the accurate identification of patterns of impairment. The 1980s witnessed an increasing interest in the development of standardized assessments, and a number of tests now exist for use with infants (Table 8.1). These are typically designed to record attainment of developmental milestones, and thus sample a wide array of skills from multiple domains. In the following sections we outline these tests and review a number of the more widely used assessments in greater detail. (We have provided a comprehensive reference list for readers interested in detailed information regarding standardization and psychometric properties of the tests addressed in this chapter.)

125

Criterion-referenced and norm-referenced tests may appear similar in nature but are different in their construction. The results of norm-referenced tests are used to compare an individual's performance with that of the normal population, to determine his or her standing in relation to peers. In contrast, criterion-referenced tests are used to compare an individual's performance with that of an agreed standard, or criterion, typically to measure the mastery of developmental skills. Criterion-referenced tests are therefore useful for producing a profile of development and for planning or monitoring interventions. However, they do not yield standardized scores and are therefore less well suited for use as stand-alone outcome measures, particularly for research purposes, as they preclude comparisons

TABLE 8.1
Standardized or criterion-referenced ([c]) multi-domain developmental assessments for use in the first two years after birth

Assessment	Age range	Source
Battelle Developmental Inventory II	Birth–8 years	Newborg 2005
Bayley Scales of Infant Development II	1 month–42 months	Bayley 1993
Bayley Scales of Infant and Toddler Development III	1 month–42 months	Bayley 2006
Developmental Assessment of Young Children	Birth–71 months	Voress and Maddox 1998
Developmental Profile II [c]	Birth–7 years	Alpern et al 1986
Early Learning Accomplishment Profile [c]	Birth–3 years	Glover et al 1995
Griffiths Mental Development Scales – Revised	Birth–8 years	Griffiths 1996, Luiz et al 2004
Merrill-Palmer-Revised Scales of Development	Birth–6½ years	Roid and Sampers 2004
Mullen Scales of Early Learning	Birth–68 months	Mullen 1995
Provence Profile [c]	Birth–3 years	Provence et al 1995

between individuals. Whilst all the tests listed in Table 8.1 provide normative data, three of these are criterion-referenced rather than norm-referenced standardized tests:

- The **Provence Birth-to-Three Developmental Profile** (PP) (part of the multi-disciplinary Infant-Toddler Developmental Assessment package (IDA; Meisels and Atkins-Burnett 2000); derived performance age scores are compared with normative data and with the child's chronological age to determine the presence or absence of developmental delay.
- The **Early Learning Accomplishment Profile** (E-LAP; Glover et al 1995) yields age equivalent scores and comprises items sampled from other infant tests to provide an assessment of development over the first three years.
- The **Developmental Profile** (2nd edition (DP-II); Alpern et al 1986) is designed to inventory the development of children from birth to 7 years; age equivalent scores are compared with the normative sample or the child's chronological age. Norm tables are used to determine the magnitude and clinical significance of any discrepancies.

The remaining assessments in Table 8.1 provide standardized outcomes and are established research tools. The BSID-II remains the most widely used test in research studies, although the Griffiths Mental Development Scales (in their previous editions) are widely used in the UK and many other European countries. Details of the standardized tests are summarized in Table 8.5 (see page 149).

The **Bayley Scales of Infant Development** (BSID; Bayley 1969) were revised and re-standardized in 1993 to form the BSID-II (see Box 8.4). The test samples a wide array of abilities and assesses attainment of key developmental milestones in children from 1 to 42 months in two domains: Mental (MDI) and Psychomotor (PDI) Development. A third scale – the Behaviour Rating Scale (BRS) – is used to evaluate aspects of the child's test performance to provide complementary information for test interpretation. The BSID-II is a highly structured test with a stringent administration protocol; parental reports may be recorded but are not permitted as substitutes for tester-observed scores. The BSID-II can be lengthy to administer (25 to 60 minutes to complete), and examiner qualifications are high, requiring graduate or professional training in assessment.

Age-related item sets are administered, within which basal and ceiling limits are established; unlike other tests, the BSID-II requires a cumulative, rather than consecutive, number of passes and failures. Raw scores are converted to age-adjusted *index scores* (*mean* 100, *SD* 15) and developmental ages for both MDI and PDI. Developmental ages may also be derived for four facets – Cognitive, Language, Personal/Social, and Motor – although standardized scores are not available for these subscales. Raw scores on the BRS are only used to derive percentiles; this scale is not implicated in the derivation of overall test scores for the MDI or PDI.

Standardization of the BSID-II is impressive. The normative sample was large (n = 1700 for the test, including an unusually large group of 1300 children aged 0 to 24 months). It was also stringently sampled: stratified by age for gender, race/ethnicity, geographical region, and parental educational level, and representative of the US population according to census data published in 1988. Norms are provided in one-month intervals for children aged 1 to 36 months, and the BSID-II performance for clinical populations (including children born preterm) is described, although normative data are not provided for these groups.

Psychometric properties of the scales are also described. Average internal consistency across all age groups is >.80 for both the MDI and PDI, and coefficients for test–retest reliability for 175 children with a median test interval of four days were .87 and .78 for the MDI and PDI respectively across all ages tested; reliability was highest for children tested at 24 and 36 months. Inter-scorer reliability for 51 assessments produced coefficients of .96 for the MDI and .75 for the PDI. Both test–retest and inter-scorer reliabilities were lower for the BRS (typical of behaviour scales).

The validity of the MDI and PDI is less well detailed and is based largely on the analysis of the BSID. Content validity and construct validity are described. Criterion-related validity is demonstrated by correlations of .62 and .63 between the MDI and PDI of the BSID and BSID-II for 200 children. Correlations between the MDI and PDI and McCarthy Scales of Children's Abilities for 50 children are .79 and .59 respectively. The MDI also correlates .73 with WPPSI scale scores and .49 with the DAS full scale score. Data concerning predictive validity are not provided.

Whilst the BSID-II is widely accepted as a valid and reliable measure of development, there are some disadvantages associated with its use:

1   **Lack of standardized subscale scores.** Unlike other assessments, the BSID-II 'facets' comprise relatively few items and do not yield standardized scores. Whilst age equivalent scores can be used to compare strengths and weaknesses they should be interpreted with caution. Bayley (1993), however, asserts that this was not an intended function of the scale given the interrelated nature of development during infancy.
2   **Language bias.** The MDI incorporates numerous expressive language items and some authors have expressed concern regarding the lack of a standardized score for non-verbal performance, particularly for children with specific language and hearing impairments or disabilities.
3   **Derivation of normative scores.** The derivation of index scores for children at the extreme ends of the one-month age bands must also be treated with caution as the same raw score can result in different index scores in adjacent norms tables.
4   **Use of the Behaviour Rating Scale (BRS).** The psychometric properties of the BRS are weaker and it has less value as a quantifiable outcome measure.
5   **Children with disabilities.** The use of the BSID-II with children with impairments has also been criticized. Normative data were not collected for children with disabilities and there are no guidelines for adaptation of the testing procedure for such groups; indeed, any test adaptations compromise use of the standardized scores.
6   **'Floor effects'.** As the lowest index score is 50, the BSID-II is not recommended for assessing the functioning of individuals with significant disabilities, as a developmental level cannot be quantified for these children; in such cases it would also be inappropriate to use the BSID-II to monitor progress over time, as increments in performance

cannot be quantified in this range. For research purposes and statistical analyses, scores lower than 50 may be assigned a nominal value (e.g. 39) to reflect a score obtained less than –3 SD; other researchers have used extrapolated norms for index scores from 30 to 50 (Robinson and Mervis 1996), or have calculated a Bayley Developmental Quotient (BDQ) facilitating correlational analyses.

7   **The use of 'item sets'.** The unconventional use of 'item sets' has been the focus of much discussion. These were designed to reduce the number of items to be administered during a session. When assessing populations in whom development may be delayed or disordered, their use can be problematic, particularly given the comprehensive nature of the two scales. For example, a child with advanced language may achieve a ceiling on non-verbal items and thus obtain an MDI that does not reflect his or her language skills; similarly, a child with spastic diplegia may satisfy a basal limit on fine motor items and thus receive a PDI that does not reflect his or her gross motor skills (see Black and Matula 2000).

8   **Test entry point.** Because the test requires entry at the child's chronological age, establishing the basal and ceiling limits for a child with developmental delays can result in the administration of a large number of items ultimately drawn from beyond the starting item set, and thus the number of necessary items and failures is increased. However, if testing begins at an estimated developmental age for children with impairments, this may ultimately result in an underestimation of ability and the derivation of index scores that may be widely different from those that would be derived had test entry been at the item set corresponding to the child's chronological age (Washington et al 1998); this has also been shown to occur with normally developing children (Gauthier et al 1999).

9   **Use in preterm infants.** Concerns have been addressed regarding the use of corrected age and the corresponding selection of items sets and norm tables for children born preterm (Matula et al 1997, Ross and Lawson 1997). Although this continues to be a contentious issue, when assessing preterm infants a child's corrected age should be used to determine both the entry point and corresponding norm table as suggested in the manual.

The limitations of the BSID-II may appear numerous, particularly in comparison to other tests. However, this does not necessarily compromise the test. The excess of information regarding this scale stems from its popularity as a research and clinical tool; given its widespread use there is a wealth of information regarding its utility. Despite the limitations outlined, the BSID-II has many properties that make it a valuable assessment tool and thus it remains a popular choice as an outcome measure. It is a rigorously standardized test with adequate psychometric properties, and its widespread use has enabled meta-analyses and cross-disciplinary discourse, an essential element of outcome assessment. As yet there are no standardization data for other countries, although in a sample of over 800 3-year-olds in the UK a normal mean and SD were observed (Wood et al 2000).

In 2006 a much anticipated revision of this test was released by Harcourt Assessment (www.harcourtassessment.com) – the Bayley Scales of Infant and Toddler Development,

Box 8.4 Features of the Bayley Scales of Infant Development II (BSID-II)

Strengths
- The most widely used standardized assessment of infant development.
- Standardized scores for two domains: Mental (MDI) and Psychomotor (PDI).
- A large normative sample of 1300 children aged 0 to 24 months.
- Rigorous standardization stratified by age and representative of the US population.
- Adequate psychometric properties for provision of a valid and reliable assessment.

Limitations
- The use of item sets can be problematic for children with specific impairments or developmental delays, and when correcting for preterm birth.
- Less utility for assessing children with significant impairment or disability.
- Adaptation for children with disabilities is not permitted and invalidates test use.
- Lacks standardized scores for subscales/facets.
- No provision of a separate score for non-verbal abilities.

3rd edition (Bayley-III; Bayley 2006; Box 8.5). This is now the most recently revised and re-standardized developmental test and is heralded as the new criterion standard for infant developmental assessment. While the Bayley-III continues to provide a comprehensive multi-domain assessment of children aged 1 to 42 months for use by experienced professionals, a number of significant improvements have been made in order to produce a more user-friendly test and to address the limitations of the BSID-II.

The Bayley-III comprises three distinct tester-administered scales which yield standardized composite scores (*mean* 100, *SD* 15) for Cognitive, Language and Motor skills. The latter two scales also yield separate scaled scores (*mean* 10, *SD* 3) for Expressive and Receptive Communication and for Gross and Fine Motor skills respectively. Percentile ranks, developmental age equivalents and new growth scores may also be derived. It is interesting that many BSID-II MDI items are spread across these three scales and thus the Cognitive scale now provides a more focused measure of non-verbal cognitive abilities; this has utility for the assessment of cognition in children with early speech, language and hearing impairments.

The Bayley-III also has extended floors and ceilings, with standardized scores ranging from 40 to 160. The extended floor, combined with the derivation of separate standardized scores for each scale, should aid in the assessment of children with lower functioning and disordered or impaired development, and should address many of the problems associated with the lack of subscale scores and language bias of the BSID-II MDI. In addition, test administration is more user-friendly: item scoring procedures have been simplified and the problematic item-set structure of the BSID-II has been abandoned in favour of the establishment of basal and ceiling limits using the more conventional system in which item passes and fails are accumulated consecutively.

The Bayley-III also includes two parent report scales to assess Social-Emotional Development and Adaptive Behaviour. The stimulus materials and manipulatives have been updated and the test items revised, although many BSID-II items are retained. The testing kit itself is less cumbersome and includes a useful training video for examiners. Scoring software can be purchased and the reporting of results is facilitated with growth charts and detailed caregiver feedback forms.

The psychometric integrity of the Bayley Scales is maintained in this 3rd edition. The standardization of the scale remains as good as that of the BSID-II, with updated normative data obtained in 2004 from a standardization sample of 1700 children stratified according to age and representative of the 2000 US population census. The manual includes detailed information about the reliability and convergent and discriminant validity of the Bayley-III, and the results of studies of special groups with high-incidence clinical diagnoses (e.g. SGA, Down syndrome, cerebral palsy, pervasive developmental disorder) to improve the clinical utility of the scales. Interestingly, the Bayley-III is currently being standardized in the UK for the first time.

The revisions included in the Bayley-III undoubtedly serve to address the limitations of the BSID-II, particularly for use with high-risk populations. However, the test is yet in its infancy and researchers and clinicians are only now beginning to adopt the Bayley-III as the instrument of choice. As with all new tests, it will take some time before studies of the Bayley-III are published and detailed information regarding its utility and, potentially, its limitations for use in clinical groups will become available.

In our personal experience and in communications with peers to date, some concerns have arisen. Some examiners have found that the test can be lengthy to administer, particularly for normally developing children. Given the Flynn effect (Flynn 1999), the re-standardized edition of a test typically yields lower mean scores than its predecessor. However, examiners have noted that the Bayley-III yields Cognitive scale scores higher than would be expected on the BSID-II MDI, and which may be developmentally inappropriate, potentially resulting in the under-identification of impairment. Indeed, the test authors note that Bayley-III scores are around seven points higher than corresponding BSID-II index scores (Bayley 2006, Harcourt Assessment Inc. 2007). In addition, the utility of the Bayley-III in identifying impairment in very preterm infants has not yet been adequately assessed. In the coming years studies will undoubtedly ensue which investigate the use of this test in children with both typical and atypical development.

The **Griffiths Mental Development Scales** (Griffiths Scales) comprise the 'baby scales' (Griffiths 1954) for children from birth to 23 months, and the 'extended scales' for children from 24 months to 8 years (Griffiths 1970, Luiz et al 2004). In this chapter we will review the baby scales (Griffiths Scales: 0–2) as the scales most applicable for use with children in their first two years (see Box 8.6).

The Griffiths Scales: 0–2 were originally developed in 1954, and have undergone a necessary and timely revision (Griffiths 1996). The scales comprise 276 items designed to provide a global assessment of functioning in five domains: Locomotor, Personal-Social, Hearing and Language, Eye and Hand Coordination, and Performance. The Griffiths Scales have strict examiner qualifications and may only be used by clinicians and psychologists with experience in developmental assessment. Examiner certification is by a five-day training course. Administration takes approximately 45 minutes. The 1996 manual provides comprehensive guidelines for item administration, although for information regarding the conceptual nature of the scales examiners should refer to the original 1954 publication.

Test entry is at the child's chronological age level and basal and ceiling limits are established conventionally (six consecutive passes and failures respectively). Domain raw scores are converted to standardized scores (*mean* 100, *SD* 16), termed 'Sub-Quotients', percentiles, and developmental age for each domain; the sum of these produces the General Quotient (GQ) – a standardized score for overall developmental level (*mean* 100, *SD* 12) – and corresponding age equivalent scores and percentiles. Norms are given in one-month intervals for the first 24 months.

The Griffiths Scales are the only tests to be developed and standardized in the UK. The normative sample of 665 children aged 0 to 24 months is noteworthy. The process for standardizing the scale, however, is less so: although the sample was examined for subgroups for sex, urban/rural residence, social class, ethnicity, and geographical location, it was not stratified by age. Selection of the sample generally lacks detailed comparison to UK national population statistics; for example, male births and social advantage appear to be over-represented. The years during which the normative data were collected are not provided. Psychometric information is also meagre in comparison to other tests. Internal consistency is good, with an average correlation of .95 for the GQ across 0–2 years. Test–retest reliability is poor, particularly for the first year: for 28 children tested on two occasions correlation between GQ scores is .48. Information regarding inter-scorer reliability and the validity of the revised scale is not provided. (The Griffiths Extended Scales provide more information regarding the standardization and psychometric properties of the scale, see Luiz et al 2004.)

Limitations of the Griffiths Scales: 0–2 can be summarized as follows:

1 **Poor standardization details** (see above).
2 **Children with disabilities.** As with the majority of standardized tests the scales have less utility for children with disabilities as modifications to the administration procedure invalidate test norms and are not permitted.
3 **Structure of the scales.** Use of the scales can be problematic for children whose ages fall around the 23-month cut-off. Whilst the baby scales are designed for use with children aged 0–2 years, and the extended scales for children aged 2 to 8 years, they are not directly comparable. The extended scales include a sixth subscale (Practical Reasoning) and either scale must be used separately as both produce separate GQs based on different normative data sets. One is left with the question of potential problems establishing a basal performance on the extended scales, particularly for preterm children, and encountering ceiling effects on the baby scales.
4 **Caregiver reports.** Although the test is examiner-administered, this test differs from the BSID-II in that caregiver reports may be elicited and scored on specified items, thus potentially compromising objectivity.

Despite these weaknesses the Griffiths Scales are well accepted as a useful developmental tool. Although less well recognized in the US, they are widely used in the UK, the rest of Europe (after local standardization), South Africa, Australia, New Zealand and Hong Kong. Given that the tests were recently re-standardized, a body of evidence regarding their psychometric properties and function as outcome measures will naturally evolve and may serve to strengthen the integrity of the scales.

The **Mullen Scales of Early Learning** (MSEL; Mullen 1995) combine the Infant (Mullen 1989) and the Preschool (Mullen 1992) Mullen Scales and thus span a wide age range from birth to 68 months (see Box 8.7). Although designed to measure cognitive functioning, the MSEL can be used to provide a more global assessment for infants in five domains: Gross Motor (for children from birth to 33 months only), and four 'cognitive' domains of Fine Motor, Visual Reception, Receptive Language, and Expressive Language. The test should be used by professionals with training in developmental assessment and the full scale may be administered in 30 to 40 minutes.

Administration requires adherence to a strict protocol, although caregivers' help may be enlisted in eliciting the child's performance on some items. Basal and ceiling limits are established using the conventional protocol (three consecutive passes and failures respectively) and raw scores are converted to age-adjusted normalized *T* scores (*mean* 50, *SD* 10), percentiles, and age equivalents for each subscale. The four cognitive subscales are combined to derive the Early Learning Composite (ELC) standardized score (*mean* 100, *SD* 15), percentile, and age equivalent. The large normative sample (n = 1849) was stratified by age and grouped into two-month intervals for children aged 1 to 14 months, and six-month intervals for children aged 15 to 68 months; the sample comprised between 84 and 156 children per group.

Internal consistency of the ELC is high (r = .91); correlations for test–retest reliability for children 1–24 months (n = 50) are >.80; and inter-scorer reliability is >.90. Construct validity is described and criterion-related validity is demonstrated by moderate correlations between the ELC and the MDI of the BSID (r = .70), the Gross Motor subscale and the PDI of the BSID (r = .76), and the Fine Motor scale and the Peabody (PDMS) Fine Motor subscale (r = ≥.65).

Limitations of the MSEL can be summarized as follows:

1   **Composite score.** The ELC does not reflect gross motor functioning. The score for motor development does not encompass fine motor skills and is based on a small number of test items (subscale total = 35).
2   **Item gradients.** The steep item gradient of the cognitive scales, particularly in infancy, may result in a lack of discrimination between individual levels of functioning (Bradley-Johnson 2001).
3   **Standardization.** The normative data, although large, are not wholly representative of the US population. The normative data are now rather outdated, having been collected between 15 and 23 years ago. Use of the MSEL has been overtaken by more

contemporary tests and thus a revision and re-standardization of the scales would be advantageous.

The **Battelle Developmental Inventory** (BDI; Newborg et al 1984, 1987) is an older developmental test for children from birth to 8 years. Although the BDI has recently been revised and re-standardized (BDI-II) and had become available for purchase at the time of preparation of this chapter, our discussion will initially focus on the first edition of the test as this has been widely used and cited to date. This will also provide a basis for a description of the features of the revised scale.

The original BDI was designed to assess development across five domains: Personal-Social, Adaptive, Motor, Communication and Cognition. It is examiner-administered, although it can also be scored through caregiver interview or observation, and requires an administration time of approximately one hour for children up to the age of 3 years. Originally intended for use by teachers, the BDI is also one of the few standardized tests that can be administered by individuals without training in developmental assessment, and has thus become popular as an instrument for assessing school readiness and special needs.

Each of the five scales is divided into sub-domains (n = 22) from which raw scores are converted to standardized z scores (*mean* 0, *SD* 1), T scores (*mean* 50, *SD* 10), percentiles, age equivalents, deviation quotients, and normal curve equivalents for the five scales, four additional sub-domains (Fine Motor, Gross Motor, and Expressive and Receptive Language) and a composite score for the full scale. The BDI was standardized in 1982–1983 with a sample of 800 children, approximately 100 per year, and thus 200 children aged 0 to 24 months. Demographic characteristics were similar to the 1981 US census data and the sample was stratified by age for geographical region, ethnicity and gender; information regarding rural/urban residence and socio-economic status of the sample is not provided. The original norms published in 1984 were recalibrated in 1987 using median rather than mean age group performance due to skewed normative data.

Coefficients for test–retest reliability of the full scale, assessed over a four-month interval for children in six-month age bands for those aged 0 to 23 months, were high ($r = \geq.98$). Correlation coefficients for inter-scorer reliability were also high, ranging from .81 to 1.0. Content and construct validity are described and the BDI correlates at least moderately ($r = .40$ to .94) with other developmental tests (e.g. Developmental Activities Screening Inventory, DASI (Dubose and Langley 1977); Vineland Social Maturity Scale (Doll 1965); Stanford-Binet Intelligence Scale-Revised, S-B (Terman and Merrill 1960)). Unsurprisingly the BDI also correlates highly with the BDI Screening Test ($r = .99$). Information is not provided regarding predictive validity or internal consistency of the scales.

The BDI has advantages in its provision of a profile of standardized scores across the five domains and additional sub-domains, making it ideal for instructional planning and monitoring intervention efficacy. Unusually for standardized tests it provides guidelines for adaptations of the test for individuals with disabilities without compromising the normative value of the test. The test has some limitations, however:

1 **Sub-domains.** There is reported concern regarding the small number of items in some sub-domains.
2 **Derivation of standardized scores.** Caution must be observed when interpreting standardized scores for children whose age falls at the extremes of an age interval, as these can differ widely.
3 **Limited psychometric information.** Some authors suggest that more information regarding validity of the scale would be beneficial (e.g. Malcolm 1998, Salvia and Ysseldyke 1991).
4 **'Floor effects'.** The lowest standardized score provided in norm tables is 65 and thus, in comparison to the BSID-II, the scale may not discriminate in the lowest performance range. A Developmental Quotient can be calculated for lower scores as advised by the authors.
5 **Purchase of test stimuli.** The full test stimuli must be purchased by the examiner, thus introducing potential bias and effects on standardization procedures.
6 **Standardization.** Although the BDI employed established standardization procedures, the normative sample is small in comparison to other tests. The test permits scoring to be based on caregiver interview, potentially affecting objectivity. More crucially, the norms are now outdated having been collected over 20 years ago, and thus a revision of the BDI would be timely.

At the time of preparation of this chapter a second edition of the BDI was released. The BDI-II (Newborg 2005) retains the structure of the original scale, providing standardized scores in the five domains of Personal-Social, Adaptive, Motor, Communication, and Cognitive skills, and 13 additional sub-domains, thus preserving its properties as a useful tool for instructional planning and the provision of a detailed profile of development (see

Box 8.8). Raw scores are converted to percentiles, age equivalents, and standardized scores for sub-domains (*mean* 10, *SD* 3), for domains, and for overall functioning (*mean* 100, *SD* 15).

The revision also addresses reported limitations of the BDI. The number of items in each sub-domain has been expanded at all ages, and the range of standardized domain and composite scores has been extended to 40–160. The psychometric properties of the test have been improved, and the publisher states that test reliabilities of the domains and sub-domains meet or exceed traditional standards for psychometric scales. The test has been very recently re-standardized on a markedly larger normative sample (n = 2500) closely matching the 2000 US census, thus providing contemporary normative data.

The BDI-II is one of the most recently standardized infant developmental assessments and thus observed limitations of the test are few. Its popularity as a contemporary outcome measure, however, is questionable: clinicians and researchers may continue to use a tool they are familiar with and which has previously become established as a conventional measure. It is unlikely to supersede the Griffiths Scales or the BSID-II as an outcome measure, particularly as revisions and re-standardizations of these tests are also available.

The remaining two tests listed in Table 8.1 represent the most recent multi-domain assessments. First published in 1998, the **Developmental Assessment of Young Children** (DAYC) is designed to measure 'different but interrelated developmental abilities' (Voress and Maddox 1998, p. 3) in children from birth to 6 years across five domains: Cognition, Communication, Social-Emotional, Physical, and Adaptive Behaviour (see Box 8.9). It requires administration in both a test and a naturalistic setting, and obtains information through observation, direct assessment, and parental or teacher interview. Testing follows a conventional procedure, with entry point at the child's chronological age and the

---

Box 8.8 Features of the Battelle Developmental Inventory, 2nd edition (BDI-II)

Strengths
- Spans a wide age range from birth to 8 years.
- Can be administered by individuals without training in developmental assessment.
- Standardized scores are derived for five domains, 13 additional sub-domains, and for overall functioning.
- Provides a profile of development across domains, useful for instructional planning.
- Guidelines are provided for adapting the test for children with physical, hearing, or visual impairments which do not compromise the normative value of the test.
- Standardized on a stratified and representative normative sample.

Limitations
- Items may be scored from caregiver reports, potentially compromising objectivity.

conventional establishment of a basal and ceiling limit for each subscale. Raw scores are converted to standardized scores (*mean* 100, *SD* 15), percentiles, and age equivalents for each subscale and overall to yield a General Development Quotient (GDQ).

Development and standardization of the test appear sound. The large normative sample (n = 1269) includes a moderate number of 441 children from birth to 2 years. Sample selection was sound, with stratification by age and accurate representation of the US population based upon national data published in 1996. Norms are derived at two-month intervals for children aged 0 to 15 months, and three-month intervals for children aged 16 months and above. Unlike other tests the DAYC normative sample includes children with disabilities and those at risk for compromised development.

The test is also psychometrically sound. Reliability is demonstrated with a coefficient of .99 for internal consistency of the GDQ. Test–retest reliabilities for the subscales are >.90, and .99 for the GDQ. Inter-scorer reliability was also demonstrated, with co-efficients of .99 between two independent observers. Test validity is similarly well detailed. Criterion-related validity is weaker, with moderate correlations of .48 and .57 between the DAYC and the Battelle Screening Test and the Revised Gesell and Amatruda Developmental and Neurologic Examination (Knobloch et al 1987) respectively. Further information for concurrent and predictive validity would be advantageous, particularly with respect to other standardized measures, rather than screening tests.

As this is a relatively new test it is as yet rarely referred to in academic literature, and thus observed criticisms of the test are few. The DAYC can be lengthy to administer as the full scale requires between 50 minutes and 1 hour 40 minutes to complete. The authors state that a child's chronological age, rather than corrected age, should be used to derive scores for preterm children; this may be contentious given the accepted use of corrected age for outcome assessment up to at least 2 years. Although the authors also justify the use of caregiver reports for item scoring, there is still concern among researchers regarding measurement error that may occur as a result of deviation from a formal tester-administered measure.

Overall, the DAYC is a well constructed contemporary test providing a detailed profile of development. Its performance in relation to other conventional standardized tests and utility as an outcome measure for preterm infants are yet to be established.

The most recently developed test is the **Merrill-Palmer-Revised Scales of Development** (M-P-R; Roid and Sampers 2004). Similar to the Leiter-R, the M-P-R represents a conceptual departure from other tests of development, being designed to assess the cognitive processes that underlie abilities traditionally measured by tests of intelligence and development, and thus assesses quality of performance in addition to the achievement of developmental milestones (see Box 8.10). The examiner qualifications are high and the test should ideally be conducted by psychologists with graduate or professional training in psychological measurement.

The test is designed for use with children aged from 1 to 78 months. Construction of the test is dictated by the theoretical framework adopted and comprises two major test batteries – Cognitive and Gross Motor – designed to assess skills in the following domains: Cognitive, Fine Motor, Receptive/Infant Language, Memory, Speed of Processing,

Box 8.9 Features of the Developmental Assessment of Young Children (DAYC)

Strengths
- Recently developed and standardized (first published 1998).
- Representative normative sample stratified by age, and including children with impairments.
- Sound psychometric properties, providing a valid and reliable measure.
- Comprehensive assessment of development across five domains.
- Standardized scores for all subscales and for global developmental level.
- Provides a profile of development across domains, useful for instructional planning.

Limitations
- Items can be scored by caregiver/teacher report, potentially compromising objectivity.
- The DAYC can be lengthy to administer in full.
- Yet to be established as a conventional outcome measure.

Visual-Motor skills, Expressive Language, and Gross Motor skills. The Gross Motor scale also includes an assessment of unusual movements and quality of movements, designed to identify atypical performance in cases in which the child has achieved motor milestones. A series of parent reports is also used to assess Social-Emotional Development and Self-Help/Adaptive Behaviour. Parent report is also used in conjunction with an examiner-administered measure of Expressive Language, and is the only measure of this skill for children younger than 13 months.

In contrast to other tests, entry point is based on the examiner's estimate of the child's developmental age level; chronological age is used only when an estimate cannot be made. Raw scores are converted to normalized standardized index scores. Index scores (*mean* 100, *SD* 15), age equivalent scores, and percentiles are derived for the following 12 domains: Cognitive, Fine Motor, Receptive Language, Visual-Motor, Memory, Speed of Processing, Gross Motor, Expressive Language, Overall Language, Social-Emotional Development (parent report), Temperament (parent report), Self-Help/Adaptive Behaviour (parent report); and for a Developmental Index (DI) of cognitive or intellectual functioning derived from the Cognitive, Fine Motor, and Receptive Language subscales (although the number of standardized scores available is reduced for younger infants). Raw scores for each of the index scales are also converted to criterion-referenced 'Growth Scores' which can be used to provide a measure of intra-personal growth over repeated testing (the development and use of these scores are described in detail in Roid and Miller 2003 and Roid and Sampers 2004).

The M-P-R was standardized on a nationally representative sample of 1068 children in the US, but with a relatively small sample of 356 children aged 0 to 24 months. The normative data are stratified by age for gender, ethnicity, parental educational level, and geographical region; a number of the subscales were standardized on smaller samples of 650 to 850 children. Coefficients for internal consistency are >.90 across all age groups for almost all subscales, except Memory and Speed of Processing. Test–retest coefficients for 41 children assessed on two occasions around three weeks apart are >.80 for all subscales.; these correlations are weaker for the Infant Language and Memory tests and for the examiner ratings of test behaviour and parent ratings of temperament.

The major subscales of the M-P-R cognitive battery correlate moderately to strongly with the BSID-II MDI (ranging from .76 for Cognitive Skills to .98 for Expressive Language), and the Gross Motor and Fine Motor indexes correlate .81 and .49 with the PDI. Significant correlations were also shown between the M-P-R cognitive battery subscales and the Leiter-R standardized scores (>.80). Data were also collected on clinical groups from which the mean performance is detailed, including a small sample of 39 children born preterm.

The M-P-R is thus the most recently developed assessment and represents a divergence from the theoretical framework of existing tests. The derivation of standardized scores for 12 domains of development, in addition to the summary scores, is impressive, and the production of 'growth scores' for assessing small increments of improvement is useful for longitudinal monitoring, particularly in impaired populations: improvement in children with significant disabilities may not be picked up with other tests as they will be functioning

---

Box 8.10 Features of the Merrill-Palmer-Revised Scales of Development (M-P-R)

Strengths
- Designed to assess *components* of cognitive abilities.
- Includes measures of gross motor skill, social-emotional, and adaptive behaviour.
- Standardized scores for 12 domains and summary scores for global functioning.
- Designed to measure small increments in improvement over time.
- Guidelines for adaptation of administration for children with impairments.
- A minimal or wholly non-verbal format, useful for children with impairments and whose first language is not English.
- The normative sample (US) is representative and stratified by age.
- Good psychometric properties on most dimensions.

Limitations
- Can be complex to administer and requires high examiner qualifications.
- Can be lengthy to administer, score and interpret.
- Scores must be interpreted with caution when administering the test non-verbally.
- Yet to be established as a conventional outcome measure.

2–3 SD below the mean where the limits of the test are imprecise and the lowest raw scores produce the same standardized scores or categorical descriptions at each test.

The test is also well suited for use with impaired populations on other dimensions. Responses on the cognitive battery require only receptive language ability. Adaptation of the testing procedure is permitted and the authors provide guidelines for adapting the test for children with physical disabilities, hearing impairments and deafness, limited expressive communication (e.g. autism), and those whose first language is not English.

Furthermore, the authors provide specific guidelines as to how the test may be administered in a minimal or wholly non-verbal format. The receptive language items may be omitted to provide a largely non-verbal measure of cognition, although a DI cannot then be derived. Specific guidelines are also provided for some items to be administered wholly non-verbally through the use of mime or gesture, as in the Leiter-R, but domain scores must be interpreted with caution and a DI must be interpreted in this context. Importantly, the M-P-R may provide a means of assessing the more subtle cognitive deficits associated with the residual disability seen in outcomes of preterm infants.

ASSESSMENTS OF MOTOR DEVELOPMENT

Motor development may be assessed in isolation for both clinical and/or research purposes. Whilst 'motor' subscales of multi-domain assessments may be used, these are often based on a small number of items and should be interpreted in the context of the test within which the subscale was standardized. A number of additional tests have been devised to provide more detailed measures of motor development over the first two years (Table 8.2).

TABLE 8.2
Assessments of motor development for use in the first two years

Assessment	Age range	Source
Movement Assessment of Infants (MAI)	Birth to 12 months	Chandler et al 1980
Alberta Infant Motor Scale (AIMS)	Birth to 18 months	Piper and Darrah 1994
Peabody Developmental Motor Scales 2 (PDMS-2)	Birth to 5 years	Folio and Fewell 1983, 2000

Two of these instruments are *criterion-referenced* rather than norm-referenced tests:

- The **Movement Assessment of Infants** (MAI; Chandler et al 1980) is used to assess neuromotor functioning across four scales: Primitive Reflexes, Muscle Tone, Autonomic Reactions, and Volitional Movement. Raw scores are used to derive risk scores for each scale and overall, with higher scores indicating greater degree of risk, or deviation from the norm.
- The **Alberta Infant Motor Scale** (AIMS; Piper and Darrah 1994) is an observational assessment of the components of motor abilities, normed on a sample of 2202 children living in the Canadian Province of Alberta. Information on inter-scorer and test–retest

141

reliabilities and concurrent validity is provided by the authors, and subsequent studies have demonstrated the predictive validity of the scale and its utility for preterm infants (Darrah et al 1998, Jeng et al 2000). Given its ability to detect subtle changes in motor skills the AIMS may be ideally suited to longitudinal use and evaluative monitoring.

In contrast, the **Peabody Developmental Motor Scales 2** (PDMS-2; Folio and Fewell 2000) is a standardized test of motor development from birth to 5 years (see Box 8.11). It assesses interrelated gross and fine motor abilities across five age-determined subscales: Reflexes (birth to 11 months), Object Manipulation (over 12 months), Stationary Skills, Locomotion, Grasping, and Visual-Motor Integration. The full scale requires 45 to 60 minutes to administer and should be used by professionals with a thorough understanding of motor development.

Raw scores are converted to age equivalents, percentiles and scaled scores (*mean* 10, *SD* 3) for each subscale. These are then combined to provide three additional composite scores (*mean* 100, *SD* 15): Gross Motor Quotient (GMQ), Fine Motor Quotient (FMQ) and Total Motor Quotient (TMQ). The authors state that test interpretation should be based primarily at the level of the composite scores and that the TMQ provides the best estimate of overall motor abilities. The authors also state that correction for preterm birth should not be applied beyond 24 months of age.

As the PDMS-2 is designed to provide an instructional programme for remediation of motor deficits, the scales are amenable to testing children with disabilities. Although guidelines are not provided for the adaptation of specific items, the authors provide general instructions on adapting the scales and permit standardized scoring to be completed when an adapted administration is employed.

The PDMS-2 was standardized on a large sample of 2003 children in 1997 and 1998, encompassing a large group of 898 children aged 0–2 years. This normative sample is representative of the national population, is stratified by age for geographical location, gender, race, urban/rural residence, and ethnicity, and includes children with disabilities and impairments. Evidence is also provided for the psychometric properties of the scale. Correlation coefficients for internal consistency are >.90 for composite scores across all ages combined and for children from different ethnic groups and those with speech-language disorders and physical disabilities. Test–retest reliability of composite scores ranges from .73 to .96 for children aged 2 to 11 months, with slightly higher correlations (.93 to .96) for children aged 12 to 17 months. Inter-scorer reliability is high for both subscale and composite scores ($r = \geq .96$). Content and construct validity are well documented, and criterion-referenced validity is confirmed by correlations between the GMQ and FMQ of .84 and .91 respectively between the PDMS-2 and the original PDMS. The PDMS-2 also produced high correlations with the MSEL gross motor and fine motor subscales (.86 and .80 respectively).

The PDMS-2 is the only scale that provides a comprehensive standardized assessment of a child's developing motor abilities. It provides a detailed profile of development in five domains and is thus ideal for instructional planning. Standardization of the test permits reliable and valid comparisons to be drawn, although reliability of the scales is poorer

Box 8.11 Features of the Peabody Developmental Motor Scales 2 (PDMS-2)

Strengths
- Recently revised and re-standardized.
- A comprehensive measure of gross and fine motor abilities across five subscales.
- Standardized scores are derived for each subscale and a further three composite scores.
- Provides a profile of motor abilities, strengths and weaknesses.
- May be adapted for children with disabilities without compromising test norms.
- Includes an instructional programme for intervention and remediation of motor skills.
- Good standardization with normative sample stratified by age.
- Large representative normative sample (898 children aged 0–24 months).
- Good psychometric properties.

Limitations
- Reliability of the scale is poorer for children aged 2–11 months.
- Objectivity may be compromised by the lack of specific guidelines for adapting the test protocol for children with disabilities.
- Examiner must buy a large number of stimuli, potentially affecting standard-ization.

for younger children (2 to 11 months). The authors state that the test is appropriate for use with children with disabilities, for whom it should initially be administered as per protocol, with adaptations made subsequently where necessary. Despite this, the authors do not provide specific guidelines for such adaptations and thus these may vary greatly between examiners and examinees, potentially resulting in a loss of objectivity. The examiner must also individually obtain a large number of test stimuli, again potentially resulting in subtle differences in standardization.

However, these disadvantages are few and the PDMS-2 provides a well standardized and comprehensive measure. It is a recently revised test and the authors acknowledge that a body of empirical work confirming the utility of the test with various samples and methodologies will naturally ensue, and they encourage examiners to share their findings.

ASSESSMENTS OF COGNITIVE DEVELOPMENT
In addition to the comprehensive cognitive structure of the M-P-R, other standardized tests have been designed to provide specific measures of cognitive development in the first two years (Table 8.3); these are discussed briefly in this section.

The oldest measure is the **Cattell Infant Intelligence Scale** (Cattell 1940). Originally standardized on a sample of 274 children, the Cattell norms were published in 1940 and, although this test has much historical significance, it is outdated and rarely used today. The

TABLE 8.3
Assessments of cognitive development for use in the first two years

Assessment	Age range	Source
Cattell Infant Intelligence Scale	2 to 30 months	Cattell 1940
Infant Psychological Development Scale	2 weeks to 2 years	Uzgiris and Hunt 1975
Cognitive Abilities Scale 2 (CAS-2)	Birth to 3 years	Bradley-Johnson 1987, Bradley-Johnson and Johnson 2001

Infant Psychological Development Scale (Uzgiris and Hunt 1975), a criterion-referenced test designed to assess development in eight cognitive domains, is also rarely used today, having been superseded by newer tests.

A recently revised test is the **Cognitive Abilities Scale 2** (CAS-2; Bradley-Johnson and Johnson 2001) (see Box 8.12). The CAS-2 comprises an Infant form (3 to 23 months) and a Preschool form (24 to 47 months) and takes 20 to 30 minutes to administer. The Infant form comprises three subscales: Exploration of Objects, Communication, and Initiation and Imitation. In contrast to other tests, the child is given three trials of each item to obtain an adequate sample of the child's skills, thus accounting for the inconsistent nature of infants' test performance. The test yields a composite General Cognitive Quotient (GCQ; *mean* 100, *SD* 15) and corresponding percentile and age equivalent. The test also yields a Non-vocal Cognitive Quotient (NCQ) which quantifies the child's performance on the non-vocal items, useful for assessing children with limited expressive communication and those who are rendered shy by the test situation.

The CAS-2 has a moderately large normative sample of 1106 children, with 248 to 305 children per year, representative of the US population and including children with impairments. Norms are provided in one-month intervals up to 12 months, and two-month intervals up to 23 months. Internal consistency coefficients are >.80 for all ages, and inter-scorer coefficients are strong, ranging from .95 to .99. Test–retest reliability estimates for children aged 12–47 months range from .95 to .99; these are weaker for children aged from 3 to 11 months (.81 to .79), although still exceeding acceptable limits. The GCQ and NCQ correlate moderately with the BSID-II MDI for the Infant form (r = .66 and .62), and .77 and .87 with the WPPSI Performance subtest. Evidence for predictive validity is provided only for the Preschool form.

The CAS-2 is a well standardized measure of cognitive development. The production of the NCQ is a particular strength of the scale and, like the M-P-R, is useful for assessing children with expressive language difficulties. (For a more detailed review, see Haile Mariam 2004.)

Limitations of standardized tests

The relative merits of standardized assessments are the subject of much debate. In particular, the use of such tests in isolation is criticized by professionals advocating the importance of multi-disciplinary longitudinal approaches and the collection of information from a variety of contexts: assessment is not an end in itself but a method of gathering information to enhance a child's development within the wider influence of the family and community (e.g. Aylward 1994, Meisels and Atkins-Burnett 2000). This is particularly important for children born preterm as preterm birth itself does not produce a single deficit, neither is it the sole aetiological factor: multiple associated factors can serve to compound or protect against developmental deficits (e.g. socio-economic status, maternal education, and maternal mental health). It would be advantageous to integrate in an assessment all these dimensions within the child's rearing environment (Sameroff and Chandler 1975). Although we accept that an assessment must be interpreted in context, in this chapter we have focused on the quantitative nature of outcome assessment – classifying individuals and quantifying developmental outcome. For such 'first line' identification, standardized assessments continue to be important tools.

A further limitation of the use of standardized tests in infancy lies in their often poor predictive validity, particularly given the emphasis in outcome assessment on identifying later disability and on elucidating early predictors of such deficits. Consistent findings indicate that longer-term prediction is improved for children with developmental deficits and for clinical populations, with prediction being most problematic in those children who exhibit borderline or normal performance (Largo et al 1990, Gross et al 1997, Barnett et al 2004). The validity of assessments for predicting school-age outcome improves as the child ages: the correlation between preschool tests and later IQ tests is typically stronger than that between tests in infancy and adulthood.

Explanations for the relatively poor predictive validity have centred around qualitative differences between skills assessed by infant and school-age tests, changes in CNS function, and, not least, the progressive influence of social and environmental factors (Aylward and Kenny 1979). Although predictive validity is improved in clinical populations and in older children, the prediction of an individual's outcome remains difficult. As we have stated above, given the interdependence of development in infancy and the contribution of the assessment of multiple domains in accounting for the variance in later abilities, comprehensive assessment of an infant's *overall* developmental progress may improve the prediction of later outcome.

Parental measures of development

Although standardized tests are the 'criterion standard' for outcome measurement, they can be costly and time consuming: they typically require specialist professionals to administer them, and the tests themselves and associated equipment (e.g. standard record forms) can be costly to purchase. Administration time can also be lengthy and can be prolonged when testing a child with impairments or one who is unwilling to cooperate. This is a particular problem for large-scale usage – for example, in epidemiological studies and multi-centre randomized trials, in experimental studies, and for routine clinical follow-up. In these circumstances an alternative cost- and time-efficient approach may be advantageous. Such an approach may take the form of parent report measures.

The accuracy of parent report questionnaires is generally contentious. Some authors have stressed the benefits of such measures, as parents can be an economical and potentially rich source of information regarding their child's development (e.g. Bates 1993, Dinnebeil and Rule 1994). Whilst tester-administered measures are based upon a snapshot of a child's behaviour observed in a situation that may be new and unsettling for the child, parents' observations are based upon an extensive sample of behaviour in a wide range of everyday contexts. Parents thus have the capacity to report on their child's current abilities rather than what their child is willing to do for a stranger in a short period of time.

However, other authors have suggested that the accuracy of parent reports may be limited, and note that there is a general trend for parental estimates of development to be more favourable than professional estimates made using standardized measures (Glaun et al 1999) – although it may similarly be argued that standardized tests serve to under-estimate abilities. Dale (1991) has suggested that the arguments levelled at parental measures may apply more to the way a parent's assessment is elicited rather than to its intrinsic value as a measure *per se*. As such, an effectively constructed questionnaire has the capacity to elicit accurate information about a child's development, and thus the validity of a questionnaire is ultimately dependent upon the quality of its construction (Dale et al 1989, Dinnebeil and Rule 1994).

Parent reports have the advantage of being short questionnaires which are inexpensive, quick and easy to administer and score, and can be used by a variety of health professionals without the need for intensive training in assessment. In addition, they are acceptable to parents, quick and easy to complete, and can be administered by post or completed in a waiting room. Such measures may also be useful in promoting parent–professional communication and in facilitating parents' involvement in the monitoring of their child.

A number of parent report questionnaires have been constructed to assess development over infancy and early childhood, the more widely used of which are listed in Table 8.4. The content of these questionnaires often appears similar to the tester-administered measures as a result of their having been developed as parent report versions of such tests, or being based on standardized test items.

TABLE 8.4
Parent report questionnaires to assess development in the first two years after birth

Parent report	Age range	Domains assessed	Source
Minnesota Child Development Inventory (MCDI)	1 to 6 years	Gross Motor Fine Motor Expressive Language Comprehension – Conceptual Situation Comprehension Self-Help Personal-Social General Development	Ireton and Thwing 1974
Child Development Inventory (CDI, revision of the MCDI)	15 months to 6 years	Gross Motor Fine Motor Social Self-Help Expressive Language Language Comprehension Letters Numbers General Development	Ireton 1992
Ages and Stages Questionnaires, 2nd edition (ASQ)	19 age intervals: 4–60 months	Communication Gross Motor Fine Motor Problem Solving Personal/Social	Squires et al 1999 (2nd edn)
Developmental Profile II (DP-II)	Birth to 7 years	Physical Self-Help Social Academic Communication	Alpern et al 1986
Parents' Evaluation of Developmental Status (PEDS)	Birth to 8 years	Global developmental status	Glascoe 1998
DENVER II Prescreening Developmental Questionnaire II (PDQ II)	Birth to 6 years	Fine Motor Gross Motor Personal-Social Language	Frankenburg and Bresnick 1998
Kent Inventory of Developmental Skills (KIDS)	Birth to 15 months	Cognitive Language Motor Self-Help Social	Reuter et al 2000
Vineland Adaptive Behavior Scales (VABS)	Birth to 18 years 11 months	Communication Daily Living Skills Socialization Motor Skills	Sparrow et al 1984

147

Parent report	Age range	Domains assessed	Source
Parent Report of Children's Abilities – Revised for Preterm Infants (PARCA-R)	Assess at 24 months corrected age	Non-verbal Cognition Linguistic Skills Parent Report Composite	Saudino et al 1998 Johnson et al 2004

These questionnaires typically yield cut-off or pass-or-fail scores (e.g. ASQ), and others yield additional normative scores such as age equivalents and developmental quotients (e.g. CDI). Such scores are used to classify the presence or absence of developmental delay and identify the need for further monitoring. The validity of these instruments is thus typically determined by degree of congruence between parent and professional estimates of development, and by examining the screening test characteristics (e.g. sensitivity and specificity) of these instruments.

To our knowledge, the Kent Inventory of Developmental Skills (KIDS; Reuter et al 2000) is the only parent report questionnaire to produce standardized scores (*mean* 100, *SD* 15) for five developmental domains (Cognitive, Language, Motor, Self-Help and Social) and for overall functioning, having been standardized in the UK and the rest of Europe. This tool may therefore be more applicable for use as a stand-alone measure in cases in which formal assessment is not practical.

Of note is the Parent Report of Children's Abilities (PARCA; Saudino et al 1998, Oliver et al 2002) which was designed to provide a parental assessment of cognitive and language development in 2-year-old children. We have recently modified and validated this questionnaire (PARCA-R; Johnson et al 2004) for use as an outcome measure for very preterm infants (<30 weeks). This has good concurrent validity (r = .68) with BSID-II MDI scores, and good diagnostic utility (sensitivity 81 per cent and specificity 81 per cent) for prediction of an MDI score <70. Given the reliabilities of the BSID-II, the PARCA-R is probably as accurate as repeating a formal developmental assessment with another examiner.

The PARCA-R has proven a useful tool for assessing cognitive development at 2 years for very preterm children; it is currently used in several large national and international randomized trials, and is included in the planning for a range of new studies.

Parent report questionnaires may therefore provide a relatively accurate alternative to formal tests as outcome measures in cases in which resources are limited. The utility of parent reports lies in classifying the presence or absence of developmental delay; age equivalent scores produced are appropriate for clinical use whilst questionnaire raw scores and standardized scores (KIDS) may be more amenable to statistical experimental use. However, caution should be noted. Whilst parent reports are useful screening measures, they do not provide a substitute for a formal examiner-administered test. A formal standardized test would ideally be performed in all cases in which it is feasible to do so. Parental measures may reduce the frequency of professional tests required and might therefore be best viewed as a method of optimizing developmental assessments rather than as a substitute for them.

TABLE 8.5
Standardized tests for assessing development from birth to 2 years

Assessment	Age range	Administration protocol	Administration time	Domains assessed	Standardization Years	Sample	Norm-referenced scores	Examiner qualification
Bayley Scales of Infant Development, 2nd edition (BSID-II)	1 to 42 months	Direct assessment	25–60 mins	Mental development (MDI) Motor development (PDI) Behaviour rating scale (BRS)	1991–1992	1700 USA	Age-adjusted normalized standardized scores and developmental age equivalents for MDI and PDI (*Mean* 100, *SD* 15); percentiles for BRS Descriptive categories are provided for MDI and PDI scores and for percentiles on BRS	Graduate or professional qualification in individual assessment; experience in testing young children similar to those for whom the test will be used
Bayley Scales of Infant and Toddler Development, 3rd edition (Bayley-III)	1 to 42 months	Direct assessment and parent report	30–90 mins	Cognitive Language Motor Social-Emotional (parent report) Adaptive Behaviour (parent report)	2004	1700 USA	Age-adjusted normalized scaled scores (*Mean 10, SD 3*) for all subtests and the Cognitive and Social-Emotional scales, composite scores (*Mean* 100, *SD* 15) for the Cognitive, Language, Motor and Adaptive Behaviour scales, and percentile ranks for all scales Developmental age equivalents and growth scores are also derived for subtests	Graduate or professional qualification in educational or psychological assessment; training and experience in developmental assessment

TABLE 8.5 continued
Standardized tests for assessing development from birth to 2 years

Assessment	Age range	Administration protocol	Administration time	Domains assessed	Standardization Years	Sample	Norm-referenced scores	Examiner qualification
Griffiths Mental Development Scales – Baby Scales (Griffiths Scales: 0–2)	Birth to 23 months	Direct assessment	35–60 mins	Locomotor Personal-Social Hearing and Language Eye and Hand Co-ordination Performance	(Not stated)	665 UK	Age-adjusted normalized standardized scores (Sub-Quotients, SQ. *Mean* 100, *SD* 16), age equivalents, and percentile ranks for each subscale Subscale raw scores are combined to provide an age-adjusted, normalized standardized score (General Quotient, GQ. *Mean* 100, *SD* 12), age equivalent, and percentile rank for overall functioning	High examiner qualifications: psychologist or clinician with training in developmental assessment Examiners must undergo a five-day training course for certification
Mullen Scales of Early Learning (MSEL)	Birth to 5 years 8 months	Direct assessment; some direct caregiver assessment is permitted	1-year-olds: 15 mins 3-year-olds: 30 mins	Gross Motor (<33 months) Fine Motor Visual Reception Receptive Language Expressive Language	1981–1986 and 1987–1989	1849 USA	Age-adjusted normalized standardized *T* scores (*Mean* 50, *SD* 10), percentile ranks, and age equivalents for each subscale The four cognitive sub-scales are combined to provide an age-adjusted normalized standardized Early Learning Composite (ELC) score (*Mean* 100, *SD* 15), percentile, and age equivalent Descriptive categories provided for all scores	Professionals with training or experience in the clinical assessment of infants and young children

Instrument	Age range	Method	Time	Domains	Year	Sample / Country	Scores	Qualifications
Battelle Developmental Inventory II (BDI-II)	Birth to 8 years	Direct assessment and caregiver interview	1–2 hours	Personal-Social Adaptive Motor Communication Cognitive	2002–2003	2500 USA	Age-adjusted normalized standardized scores for each sub-domain (*Mean* 10, *SD* 3), domain (*Mean* 100, *SD* 15), and an overall Developmental Quotient (*Mean* 100, *SD* 15), and z-scores, percentile ranks, and age equivalents	Psychologists and 'paraprofessionals' (e.g. infant, preschool, primary, special needs teachers)
Developmental Assessment of Young Children (DAYC)	Birth to 5 years 11 months	Direct assessment, observation and/or caregiver interview	50 mins to 1 hr 40 mins (full scale)	Cognitive Communication Socio-emotional Physical Adaptive Behaviour	(Not stated)	1269 USA and Canada	Percentile, age equivalent, and age-adjusted normalized standardized scores for each subtest (*Mean* 100, *SD* 15), and for the full scale – General Development Quotient (GDQ, *Mean* 100, *SD* 15)	Examiners should possess formal training in assessment techniques
Merrill-Palmer-Revised (M-P-R)	1 month to 6 years 6 months	Direct assessment, examiner observation, and parent report	30–40 mins cognitive scales, additional time for Gross Motor and Expressive Language scale and Examiner Report	Cognitive Fine Motor Receptive Language Memory Visual-Motor Speed of Processing Expressive Language Gross Motor Social-Emotional Self-Help/Adaptive Temperament	2000	1068 USA	Age-adjusted normalized standardized scores (*Mean* 100, *SD* 15), age equivalents, and percentiles for 11 domains, overall language ability, and a Developmental Index (DI) derived from the Cognitive Battery Descriptive categories provided for index scores.	High qualifications required: psychologists, child-assessment experts, and clinicians with graduate or professional training in psychological assessment Interpretation should be at psychologist level
Movement Assessment of Infants	Birth to 12 months	Direct assessment	Up to 30 mins	Gross motor skills	–	–	Criterion-referenced test: 'risk scores' only. No standardized scores	Health professionals and psychologists with knowledge of child development. Formal training in MAI administration recommended

TABLE 8.5 continued
Standardized tests for assessing development from birth to 2 years

Assessment	Age range	Administration protocol	Administration time	Domains assessed	Standardization Years	Sample	Norm-referenced scores	Examiner qualification
Alberta Infant Motor Scale (AIMS)	Birth to 18 months	Observation	20–30 mins	Gross motor skills (assessed in four postural positions)	1990–1992	2202 Alberta, Canada	Percentiles for overall gross motor development. No standardized scores	Health professionals with knowledge of components of motor development and experience in infant motor assessment
Peabody Developmental Motor Scales, 2nd edition (PDMS-2)	Birth to 5 years 11 months	Direct assessment	45–60 mins	Gross and fine motor	1997–1998	2003 USA and Canada	Age-adjusted normalized standardized scores (*Mean* 10, *SD* 3), percentiles, and age equivalents for each subscale. Subscales are combined to provide age-adjusted normalized quotients for gross motor skills (GMQ), fine motor skills (FMQ) and total motor skills (TMQ, *Mean* 100, *SD* 15), percentiles, and age equivalents. Descriptive categories provided for all scores	Thorough knowledge of the assessment of motor skills, test statistics, and developmental delays in motor abilities. Practice in administering motor assessments
Cognitive Abilities Scale 2 (CAS-2)	3 months to 3 years 11 months	Direct assessment	20–30 mins	Cognitive	1997–1999	1106	General Cognitive Quotient (GCQ, *Mean* 100, *SD* 15), percentile, and age equivalent. The test also yields a Non-vocal Cognitive Quotient (NCQ, *Mean* 100, *SD* 15)	Psychologists; may be used by educational psychologists

Summary

Standardized norm-referenced tests are widely used by clinicians and researchers for assessing developmental outcome in high-risk infants. They provide highly objective, valid and reliable measures which can be used to determine the extent of developmental delay or impairment. Whilst it is useful to assess development in separate domains for instructional planning, it is difficult to isolate domain-specific functioning in infancy, and the prediction of later outcome may thus be optimized by assessing development across multiple domains. Ultimately, test selection is dependent upon the specific purpose for which the results are intended, but a measure with sound psychometric properties is beneficial in all instances.

A number of multi-domain standardized assessments have become established as conventional outcome measures, of which the BSID-II and the Griffiths Scales continue to be the most widely used. More recently developed tests (DAYC and M-P-R) appear to be sound tests of development, although they need establishing as conventional measures and must compete against contemporary revisions of the more popular measures, such as the recently revised and re-standardized Bayley-III. Tests of specific skills or abilities may be obtained from subscale scores of the above scales, or using a standardized test designed to assess development within one domain – for example, using the PDMS-2 for assessing motor abilities or the CAS-2 or M-P-R for assessing cognition. Although parent report measures may provide cost-efficient alternatives to developmental assessments, standardized tests remain the criterion standard for outcome assessment in high-risk infants.

ACKNOWLEDGEMENTS

Ms Nikki McNarry, Physiotherapist, Queen's Medical Centre, Nottingham, NH7 2UH. Dr Sarah Horrocks, Consultant Community Paediatrician, Rhuddlan Children's Centre, Denbighshire, North Wales.

REFERENCES

Allen MC (2002) Preterm outcomes research: a critical component of neonatal intensive care. *Ment Retard Dev Disabil Res Rev* 8: 221–233.

Alpern GD, Boll TJ, Shearer M (1986) *The Developmental Profile II (DP-II)*. Los Angeles, CA: Western Psychological Services.

Aylward GP (1994) *Practitioner's Guide to Developmental and Psychological Testing*. New York: Plenum Publishing Corporation.

Aylward GP (1995) *The Bayley Infant Neurodevelopmental Screener*. San Antonio, TX: The Psychological Corporation.

Aylward GP (2002) Cognitive and neuropsychological outcomes: more than IQ scores. *Ment Retard Dev Disabil Res Rev* 8: 234–240.

Aylward GP (2003) Cognitive function in preterm infants. No simple answers. *JAMA* 289: 752–753.

Aylward GP, Kenny TJ (1979) Developmental follow-up: inherent problems and a conceptual model. *J Pediatr Psychol* 4: 331–343.

BAPM (2001) *Standards for Hospitals Providing Intensive and High Dependency Care*. London: British Association of Perinatal Medicine.

Barnett AL, Guzzetta A, Mercuri E, Henderson SE, Haataja L, Cowan F, Dubowitz L (2004) Can the Griffiths scales predict neuromotor and perceptual-motor impairment in term infants with neonatal encephalopathy? *Arch Dis Child* 89: 637–643.

Bates E (1993) Comprehension and production in early language development. *Monogr Soc Res Child Dev* 58: 222–242.

Bayley N (1969) *Bayley Scales of Infant Development, 1st edn.* New York: The Psychological Corporation.

Bayley N (1993) *Bayley Scales of Infant Development, 2nd edn.* San Antonio, TX: The Psychological Corporation.

Bayley N (2006) *Bayley Scales of Infant and Toddler Development, 3rd edn.* San Antonio, TX: Harcourt Assessment Inc.

Bellman M, Lingam S, Aukett A (1996) *Schedule of Growing Skills, 2nd edn.* London: NFER-Nelson.

Bhutta AT, Cleves MA, Casey PH, Cradock MM, Anand KJS (2002) Cognitive and behavioral outcomes of school-aged children who were born preterm: a meta-analysis. *JAMA* 288: 728–737.

Black MM, Matula K (2000) *Essentials of Bayley Scales of Infant Development-II Assessment.* New York: John Wiley & Sons.

Bracewell M, Marlow N (2002) Patterns of motor disability in very preterm children. *Ment Retard Dev Disabil Res Rev* 8: 241–248.

Bradley-Johnson S (1987) *Cognitive Abilities Scale.* Austin, TX: Pro-Ed.

Bradley-Johnson S (2001) Cognitive assessment for the youngest children: a critical review of tests. *J Psychoed Assess* 19: 19–44.

Bradley-Johnson S, Johnson CM (2001) *Cognitive Abilities Scale, 2nd edn.* Austin, TX: Pro-Ed.

Brigance AH (1991) *Revised BRIGANCE Diagnostic Inventory of Early Development (Birth to Seven Years).* North Billerica, MA: Curriculum Associates, Inc.

Campbell SK, Siegel E, Parr CA, Ramey CT (1986) Evidence for the need to re-norm the Bayley Scales of Infant Development based on the performance of a population-based sample of 12-month-old infants. *Top Early Child Spec Educ* 6: 83–96.

Cattell P (1940) *Cattell Infant Intelligence Scale.* San Antonio, TX: The Psychological Corporation.

Chandler LS, Andrews MS, Swanson MW (1980) *Movement Assessment of Infants: A Manual.* Rolling Bay, WA (published by the authors).

Dale P (1991) The validity of a parent report measure of vocabulary and syntax at 24 months. *J Speech Hear Res* 34: 565–571.

Dale P, Bates E, Reznick J, Morrisset C (1989) The validity of a parent report instrument of child language at twenty months. *J Child Lang* 16: 239–249.

Darrah J, Piper M, Watt MJ (1998) Assessment of gross motor skills of at-risk infants: predictive validity of the Alberta Infant Motor Scale. *Dev Med Child Neurol* 40: 485–491.

Dinnebeil L, Rule S (1994) Congruence between parents' and professionals' judgements about the development of young children with disabilities: a review of the literature. *Top Early Child Spec Educ* 14: 1–25.

Doll E (1965) *Vineland Social Maturity Scale, rev edn.* Circle Pines, MN: American Guidance Service.

Dubose RF, Langley MB (1977) *Developmental Activities Screening Inventory.* Hingham, MA: Teaching Resources.

Elliott CD (1990) *Differential Ability Scales.* San Antonio, TX: The Psychological Corporation.

Elliott CD, Smith P, McCulloch K (1996) *British Ability Scales II, Administration and Scoring Manual.* Windsor: NFER-Nelson.

Flynn JR (1999) Searching for justice. The discovery of IQ gains over time. *Am Psychol* 54: 5–20.

Folio MR, Fewell RR (1983) *Peabody Developmental Motor Scale and Activity Cards.* Chicago: Riverside Publishing Co.

Folio MR, Fewell RR (2000) *Peabody Developmental Motor Scales, 2nd edn.* Austin, TX: Pro-Ed.

Frankenburg WK, Bresnick B (1998) *DENVER II Prescreening Developmental Questionnaire II (PDQ II).* Denver: Denver Developmental Metrics, Inc.

Frankenburg WK, Dodds JB, Archer P, Bresnick B (1990) *Denver II Screening Manual.* Denver: Denver Developmental Materials.

Frankenburg WK, Dodds JB, Archer P, Bresnick B (1992) The Denver II: a major revision and restandardisation of the Denver Developmental Screening Test. *Pediatrics* 89: 91–97.

Gagnon SG, Nagle RJ (2000) Comparison of the revised and original versions of the Bayley Scales of Infant Development. *School Psychol Int* 21: 293–305.

Gauthier SM, Bauer CR, Messinger DS, Closius JM (1999) The Bayley Scales of Infant Development II: where to start? *J Dev Behav Pediatr* 20: 75–79.

Glascoe FP (1995) *A Validation Study and the Psychometric Properties of the Brigance Screens.* North Billerica, MA: Curriculum Associates.

Glascoe FP (1998) *Collaborating with Parents: Using Parents' Evaluation of Developmental Status to Detect and Address Developmental and Behavioral Problems.* Nashville, TN: Ellsworth & Vandermeer Press LLC.

Glaun D, Cole K, Reddihough D (1999) Mother–professional agreement about developmental delay in preschool children: a preliminary report. *J Appl Res Intellect Disab* 12: 69–76.

Glover EM, Preminger JL, Sanford AR (1995) *Early Learning Accomplishment Profile Revised Edition (E-LAP).* Lewisville, NC: Kaplan Press.

Goldstein DJ, Fogle EE, Wieber JL, O'Shea TM (1995) Comparison of the Bayley Scales of Infant Development – Second Edition and the Bayley Scales of Infant Development with premature infants. *J Psychoed Assess* 13: 391–396.

Griffiths R (1954) *The Abilities of Babies.* London: University of London Press.

Griffiths R (1970) *The Abilities of Young Children.* London: Child Development Research Centre.

Griffiths R (1996) *The Griffiths Mental Development Scales from Birth to 2 Years, Manual. The 1996 Revision.* Henley: Association for Research in Infant and Child Development, Test Agency. (Revised by M Huntley.)

Gross RT, Spiker D, Haynes CW (1997) Helping low birth weight premature babies. *The Infant Health and Development Program.* Stanford, CA: Stanford University Press.

Hack M, Fanaroff AA (1999) Outcomes of children of extremely low birthweight and gestational age in the 1990s. *Early Hum Dev* 53: 193–218.

Hack M, Flannery DJ, Schluchter M, Cartar L, Borawski E, Klein N (2002) Outcomes in young adulthood for very-low-birth-weight infants. *N Engl J Med* 346: 149–157.

Haile Mariam A (2004) Review of the cognitive abilities scale–second edition. *J School Psychol* 42: 171–176.

Harcourt Assessment Inc. (2007) Bayley-III Technical Report 2. Factors contributing to differences between Bayley-III and BSID-II scores.

Hindmarsh GJ, O'Callaghan MJ, Mohay HA, Rogers YM (2000) Gender differences in cognitive abilities at 2 years in ELBW infants. *Early Hum Dev* 60: 115–122.

Ireton HR (1992) *Child Development Inventory.* Minneapolis: Behavior Science Systems.

Ireton HR, Thwing EJ (1974) *The Minnesota Child Development Inventory.* Minneapolis: Behavior Science Systems.

Jeng S, Yau KT, Chen L, Hsiao S (2000) Alberta Infant Motor Scale: reliability and validity when used on preterm infants in Taiwan. *Phys Ther* 80: 168–178.

Johnson S, Marlow N, Wolke D, Davidson L, Marston L, O'Hare A, Peacock J, Schulte J (2004) Validation of a parent report measure of cognitive development in very preterm infants. *Dev Med Child Neurol* 46: 389–397.

Kaufman AS, Kaufman NL (2004) *Kaufman Assessment Battery for Children, 2nd edition.* Circle Pines, MN: American Guidance Service.

Knobloch H, Stevens F, Malone AF (1987) *Manual of Developmental Diagnosis: The Administration and Interpretation of the Revised Gesell and Amatruda Developmental and Neurologic Examination.* Houston: Developmental Evaluation Materials.

Largo RH, Graf S, Kundu S, Hunziker U, Molinari L (1990) Predicting developmental outcome at school age from infant tests of normal, at-risk and retarded infants. *Dev Med Child Neurol* 32: 30–45.

Lems W, Hopkins B, Samsom JF (1993) Mental and motor development in preterm infants: the issue of corrected age. *Early Hum Dev* 34: 113–123.

Losch H, Dammann O (2004) Impact of motor skills on cognitive test results in very-low-birthweight children. *J Child Neurol* 19: 318–322.

Luiz D, Barnard A, Knoesen N, Kotras N (2004) *Griffiths Mental Development Scales – Extended Revised (GMDS-ER).* Amersham: Association for Research in Infant and Child Development.

McCarthy D (1972) *Manual for the McCarthy Scales of Children's Abilities.* New York: The Psychological Corporation.

MacCormick MC (2002) Premature infants grow up. *N Engl J Med* 346: 197–198.

Malcolm KK (1998) Developmental assessment: evaluation of infants and preschoolers. In: Vance H, editor. *Psychological Assessment of Children: Best Practices for School and Clinical Settings, 2nd edn.* New York: John Wiley & Sons.

Marlow N (2004) Neurocognitive outcome after very preterm birth. *Arch Dis Child Fetal Neonatal Ed* 89: F224–F228.

Marlow N (2005) Outcome following preterm birth. In: Rennie JM, editor. *Roberton's Textbook of Neonatology, 4th edn.* London: Elsevier.

Marlow N, Wolke D, Bracewell M, Samara M (2005) Neurologic and developmental disability at 6 years of age after extremely preterm birth. *N Engl J Med* 352: 9–19.

Matula K, Gyurke JS, Aylward GP (1997) Response to commentary: Bayley Scales-II. *J Dev Behav Pediatr* 18: 112–113.

Meisels SJ, Atkins-Burnett S (2000) The elements of early childhood assessment. In: Shonkoff JP, Meisels SJ, editors. *Handbook of Early Childhood Development, 2nd edn*. Cambridge: Cambridge University Press.

Miller LJ (1982) *Miller Assessment for Pre*schoolers. Oxford: The Psychological Corporation.

Mullen EM (1989) *Infant Mullen Scales of Early Learning*. Cranston, RI: TOTAL Child.

Mullen EM (1992) *Preschool Mullen Scales of Early Learning*. Cranston, RI: TOTAL Child.

Mullen EM (1995) *Mullen Scales of Early Learning*. Los Angeles: Western Psychological Services.

Mutch LM, Johnson MA, Morley R (1989) Follow up studies: design, organisation, and analysis. *Arch Dis Child* 64: 1394–1402

NPEU (National Perinatal Epidemiology Unit) and Oxford Health Authority (1995) Report of two working groups. Disability and Perinatal Care: Measurement of health status at two years. Oxford.

Newborg J (2005) *Battelle Developmental Inventory II*. Chicago: Riverside Publishing Co.

Newborg J, Stock JR, Wnek L, Guidubaldi J, Svinicki J (1984) *Battelle Developmental Inventory*. Allen, TX: DLM Teaching Resources.

Newborg J, Stock JR, Wnek L, Guidubaldi JE, Svinicki J (1987) *Battelle Developmental Inventory with Recalibrated Technical Data and Norms: Examiner's Manual*. Chicago: Riverside Publishing Co.

Oliver B, Dale PS, Saudino KJ, Petrill SA, Pike A, Plomin R (2002) The validity of a parent-based assessment of cognitive abilities in three-year olds. *Early Child Care Dev* 172: 337–348.

Piper MC, Darrah J (1994) *Motor Assessment of the Developing Infant*. Pennsylvania: W.B. Saunders Company.

Provence S, Erikson J, Vater S, Palmeri S (1995) *Infant-Toddler Developmental Assessment: IDA*. Chicago: Riverside Publishing Co.

Reuter J, Katoff L, Wozniak JR (2000) *Kent Inventory of Developmental Skills, 3rd edn*. Los Angeles: Western Psychological Services.

Robinson BF, Mervis CB (1996) Extrapolated raw scores for the second edition of the Bayley Scales of Infant Development. *Am J Ment Retard* 100: 666–670.

Roid G, Miller L (2003) *Leiter International Performance Scale–Revised*. Wood Dale, IL: Stoelting Co.

Roid GH, Sampers JL (2004) *Merrill-Palmer-R Scales of Development Manual*. Wood Dale, IL: Stoelting Co.

Ross G, Lawson K (1997) Using the Bayley-II: unresolved issues in assessing the development of prematurely born children. *J Dev Behav Pediatr* 18: 109–111.

Rossman MJ, Hyman SL, Rorabaugh ML, Berlin LE, Allen MC, Modlin JF (1994) The CAT/CLAMS assessment for early intervention services. Clinical Adaptive Test/Clinical Linguistic and Auditory Milestone Scale. *Clinical Pediatr* 33: 404–409.

Salvia J, Ysseldyke JE (1991) *Assessment, 5th edn*. Boston, MA: Houghton Mifflin Co.

Sameroff A, Chandler, M (1975) Reproductive risk and the continuum of caretaking casualty. In: Horowitz F, Hetherington J, Scarr-Salapatek S, Siegel G, editors. *Review of Child Development Research*. Chicago: University of Chicago Press.

Saudino K, Dale P, Oliver B, Petrill S, Richardson V, Rutter M, Simonoff E, Stevenson J, Plomin R (1998) The validity of a parent-based assessment of the cognitive abilities of 2-year-olds. *Br J Dev Psychol* 16: 349–363.

Sparrow SS, Balla DA, Cicchetti DV (1984) *Vineland Adaptive Behavior Scales*. Circle Pines, MN: American Guidance Service.

Squires J, Bricker D, Potter L (1999) *Ages and Stages User's Guide, 2nd edn*. Baltimore: Brookes Publishing.

Taylor HG, Klein N, Hack M (2000) School-age consequences of birth weight less than 750g: a review and update. *Dev Neuropsychol* 17: 289–231.

Terman LM, Merrill MA (1960) *Stanford-Binet Intelligence Scale, 3rd Revision (Form L-M)*. Boston: Houghton Mifflin.

Thorndike RL, Hagen EP, Sattler JM (1986) *Technical Manual: Stanford-Binet Intelligence Scale, 4th edn*. Chicago: Riverside Publishing Co.

Tideman E (2000) Longitudinal follow-up of children born preterm: cognitive development at age 19. *Early Hum Dev* 58: 81–90.

Uzgiris IC, Hunt JM (1975) *Assessment in Infancy: Ordinal Scales of Psychological Development*. Urbana: University of Illinois Press.

Voress JK, Maddox T (1998) *DAYC. Developmental Assessment of Young Children*. Austin, TX: Pro-Ed.

Wachtel RC, Shapior BK, Palmer FB, Allen MC, Capute AJ (1994) CAT/CLAMS: a tool for the pediatric evaluation of infants and young children with developmental delay. *Clin Pediatr* 33: 410–415.

Washington K, Scott DT, Johnson KA, Wendel S, Hay AE (1998) The Bayley Scales of Infant Development-II and children with developmental delays: a clinical perspective. *J Dev Behav Pediatr* 19: 346–349.

Werner EE (1994) Overcoming the odds. *J Dev Behav Pediatr* 15: 131–136.

Wechsler D (1989) *Wechsler Preschool and Primary Scale of Intelligence*. San Antonio, TX: The Psychological Corporation.

Wolke D, Ratschinski G, Ohrt B, Riegel K (1994) The cognitive outcome of very preterm infants may be poorer than often reported: an empirical investigation of how methodological issues make a big difference. *Eur J Pediair* 153: 906–915.

Wolke D, Schulz J, Meyer R (2001) Entwicklungslanzeitfolgen bei ehemaligen, sehr unreifen Fruhgeborenen. *Monatsschrift fur Kinderheilkunde* 149: 53–61.

Wood NS, Marlow N, Costeloe K, Chir B, Gibson AT, Wilkinson AR, for the EPICure Study Group (2000) Neurologic and developmental disability after extremely preterm birth. *N Engl J Med* 343: 378–384.

Wood NS, Costeloe K, Gibson AT, Hennessy EM, Marlow N, Wilkinson AR, for the EPICure Study Group (2005) The EPICure Study: associations and antecedents of neurological and developmental disability at 30 months of age following extremely preterm birth. *Arch Dis Child Fetal Neonatal Ed* 90: F134–F140.

9
COGNITIVE DEVELOPMENT IN THE FIRST TWO YEARS OF LIFE

Francesco Guzzetta, Chiara Veredice and Andrea Guzzetta

Introduction

Although developmental tests have been used as an essential part of the routine examination for over 50 years (see Chapter 8 for a systematic review), there are still a number of unresolved questions concerning their accuracy in discriminating specific aspects of development. One of the most problematic questions is if and how the available scales discriminate between cognitive function and other closely related aspects of development, and how early cognitive development can be evaluated.

It is well known that the extent of neurodevelopmental abnormalities is generally not obvious soon after birth in infants who have suffered early insults, either genetically transmitted or acquired in intrauterine, perinatal or neonatal life. This 'latency' period, observed for example for motor skills, appears to be particularly long for cognitive abilities due to the fact that these are normally achieved at a late stage. The study of the so-called cognitive prerequisites, i.e. the primary skills from which cognitive development originates, represents a relevant target for the prediction of possible developmental difficulties, even in early cognitive development.

In this chapter we will review the value of tests designed to assess specific aspects of cognitive function, and the value of other techniques that can be used in the first two years of life.

Development of cognitive competence

Sensory-motor behaviours expressing a cognitive component can already be identified at birth. Neonatal assessment techniques such as the Brazelton Neonatal Behavioural Assessment Scale (NBAS) (Brazelton 1984), or more sophisticated scales such as the NICU Network Neurobehavioral Scale (NNNS) (Lester et al 2004), include several items exploring 'pre-cognitive' behaviours. Among them are all the items regarding habituation, visual and auditory animate and inanimate orientation, cuddliness, consolability and self-quieting activity. Although habituation and orientation may be considered at birth as 'subcortical' behaviours, they may already be sustained by emergent selective attention and memory abilities. These skills can already be detected in the newborn by autonomic changes (Montagner et al 2002).

The same evolution from a 'reflex' to a 'cognitive' behaviour can be observed in the early modification of sucking as a non-specific sucking into differentiated nutritive and non-nutritive sucking. However, the best method of following the cognitive maturation of infant behaviour is based on observation of responses to sensory stimulation, and in particular visual behaviour.

In the first three to four months of life there is a gradual shift from visuo-perceptual function due to activity in subcortical networks already operational at birth, to proper cortical executive control (Atkinson 1984). This mature cortical function is based on a number of cortical streams which begin to operate at different postnatal ages during the first three to four months of life. Two are the main streams grossly related to two anatomically distinct networks, the parvocellular and magnocellular: the parvocellular system (ventral stream) subserves detailed form vision and colour vision; while the magnocellular system (dorsal stream) subserves spatial and movement perception.

This 'perceptual' visual maturation is followed by the development of integrations that allow actions to be performed: first, manual action (control of reach/grasp) at 4–5 months, then locomotor action at 12 months, up to the production of speech and automation of visuo-motor programs (Atkinson 2000).

This neurobiological (anatomo-physiological) approach corresponds to behavioural features assessed by the analysis of ocular responses and by developmental scales. The first kind of assessment concerning early ocular behaviour (the first three months of life) can properly examine the visual maturation of perception, comprising categorizing and storing visual information in visual memory. As soon as dependence on pure sensory experience fades, the birth of representation is observed: the maturation of scanning ability, becoming free from an initial reflex fixation, assessed by the fixation shift test (Atkinson et al 1992), is a relevant stage for the future acquisition of representation.

Sensory-motor intelligence occurs from the fifth month up to the second year of life, with the acquisition or completion of several abilities such as (a) object constancy, i.e. the ability to evoke objects that are not present in the sensory fields of the infant, the basis of representative intelligence; (b) symbolic function, on which language is founded; and (c) logical operations through motor actions, such as operation causality, means of obtaining desired environmental events, and construction of object relations in space.

The old scales of cognitive development were purely descriptive. The first systematic approach to early cognitive development was proposed by Jean Piaget: his model of the so-called 'psychologie génétique', i.e. a psychological (cognitive) ability of the nervous system to generate its own development, and its post-Piagetian evolutions, represents a more solid framework in which to consider the psychological features of early cognitive development.

As Piaget stressed, cognitive abilities during the sensory-motor period of life are defined by lack of thought and language: mental 'operations' that mark intelligent behaviour are simply motor 'actions'. This has two important consequences: first, it is difficult to distinguish between motor and cognitive competence and thus between a perceptual-motor and a cognitive disorder. Thus, cognitive assessment techniques may be strongly impaired by the presence of a perceptual or motor disorder, not a rare occurrence in early brain-injured infants. The other relevant effect of the sensory-motor character of cognitive competence at this age is the discontinuity with the cognitive behaviour of the successive developmental stages. This makes it difficult to make connections between cognitive assessments performed at these two distinct periods. It may partly explain the low correlation between developmental tests administered in the first months of life and those administered at 2–4 years: 0.21, which falls to near zero at 5–7 years, both in normal infants and in infants at risk or with abnormal outcome (McCall et al 1972, Kopp and McCall 1982). So, the poor predictive value of the results of cognitive assessment performed with the usual assessment techniques is obvious.

Assessment techniques

Cognitive Prerequisites
The building blocks of cognition may be detected from birth through the study of neurovegetative behaviours using habituation paradigms. With these procedures, moderate but significant correlations have been found between early performance and later cognitive development (Lewis and Brooks-Gunn 1981, Fagan and Singer 1983). Sensory perception appears to be an important determinant of neurodevelopment, and the observation of *visual behaviour* is one of the most commonly used methods for assessing early cognitive ability at a time when representative and language abilities, as well as finalized motor schemas (praxias), are not yet observable. Visual 'grasping' (fixation and pursuit), scanning, attention and selection are already present in the first months of life and are largely used by young infants to explore the world around them. The study of the maturation of visual function, and disorders, in the first months of life therefore represents an essential tool to understand the possible roots of cognitive deficits and to predict eventual delays in the development of cognitive function (Atkinson 2000).

A few studies have reported an increased risk of impaired cognitive development both in infants with severe congenital disorders of the peripheral visual system (Sonksen and Dale 2002) and in those with abnormalities of the post-chiasmatic part of the visual pathway, affected by cerebral visual impairment (CVI). Infants with CVI, however, frequently show extensive brain lesions which may also be responsible for more global neurodevelopmental difficulties, making it difficult to establish the possible role played by visual dysfunction in determining cognitive delay. Recent studies, however, have reported a stronger association between developmental quotients (DQ) and abnormalities of visual function, such as acuity, visual field, fixation shift and VEPs, than between DQ and brain lesions or motor impairment (Mercuri et al 1999, Cioni et al 2000).

In this respect, specific aspects of visual function that mature and become prominent after the first four to five months after birth, such as the ability to shift fixation, and the evoked responses to high-frequency orientation reversal stimuli, may play a more relevant role as markers of cortical maturation and DQ prediction (Mercuri et al 1999). These findings are consistent with the results of other studies which highlight the role of visual function in the early stages of infant neurodevelopment (Tröster et al 1994, Shumway-Cook and Woollacott 1995).

Not only visual functions have been considered as early predictors of development. The assessment of *auditory attention* in infancy has been used for understanding and predicting cognitive disorders (Gomes et al 2000). Different components of auditory attention can be analysed in order to monitor its development. *Arousal* can be analysed from birth, although it becomes more stable and predictable only after the first few weeks of life, when sleep/wake cycles are clearly differentiable. The *orienting response* is largely driven by the physical characteristics of the stimulus in the first weeks, but eventually becomes more related to its novelty and not to its intrinsic features. A proper *attentional response* in young infants can be exhibited initially for limited periods in selected circumstances. Further development involves improved automatic auditory discrimination, possibly due to more precise representations of stimuli in memory, and increased duration of the response.

Several studies have reported that both peripheral and central abnormalities of the auditory pathway are associated, to some extent, with some abnormalities of cognitive development. Schlumberger et al (2004) studied 54 children with severe or profound bilateral congenital deafness, without neurological or cognitive impairment, concluding that an early cochlear implantation is associated with good verbal development but might also improve non-verbal capacities, such as spatial integration, motor control, and attention. Benasich and Tallal (2002) examined a group of infants with family history positive for specific language impairment, showing a significant correlation between rapid auditory processing at 7.5 months (assessed by means of a forced-choice paradigm), and emerging language at 24 months.

DEVELOPMENTAL ASSESSMENT IN THE FIRST TWO YEARS OF LIFE: FROM
ECLECTIC TO INFORMATION PROCESSING MODELS

Even though the neurodevelopment of infants has been studied since the eighteenth century, the first systematic study was carried out by Gesell (Gesell and Thompson 1934), who proposed developmental scales which were subsequently widely accepted and used, and which have been successively revised and published (Knobloch and Pasamanick 1960). Five developmental fields are included in the revised Gesell Developmental Schedules: gross motor, fine motor, language, personal/social, and adaptive scales that represent the early problem-solving ability of the infant. The items of the Gesell scales were defined on the basis of accurate and systematic observation of infant behaviour and are founded on an eclectic model of development. The same principle has been followed by other diffusely used scales in recent decades, such as the Bayley Scales of Infant Development, the Griffiths Mental Development Scales, or, perhaps less well known, the Cattell or Brunet and Lézine scales.

A new original approach was the 'psychologie génétique' of Piaget, which led to the construction of a model-oriented scale. The founding principle of Piaget's doctrine is that development continues through successive adaptive (intelligent) behaviours by organizing new cognitive abilities at a higher and higher level. The scales that were inspired by the Piagetian model, and others based on similar principles such as Uzgiris and Hunt's Infant Psychological Development Scale, include different series of items aimed at monitoring single cognitive functions such as object permanence, gesture or vocal imitation, operation causality, means of obtaining desired environmental events, and construction of object

161

relations in space. (For more detailed descriptions and criticism of all these scales, see Chapter 8.)

A completely different approach is represented by the information processing model, on which several new techniques are now based. This approach is founded on the principle that an incoming stimulus goes through different sensorial modalities and is processed by the brain network. This allows its recognition and prepares the individual for a more or less elaborated response. In infants assessed during the sensory-motor stage, the response is a motor response.

This model has several benefits. First of all, it makes the study of specific processes of cognition easier, making it possible to follow the maturation of specific biological hardware by monitoring the analysis of single perceptual processes such as visual function. This information, combined with other techniques such as neuroimaging, can improve the anatomo-functional investigation of the impaired ability. Finally, longitudinal evaluation of a specific function, capturing the continuity of cognitive development, enhances the predictive value of the assessment.

The main fields in which the information processing model may be applied in infancy are the examination of visual recognition memory, visual attention and stimulus processing speed.

Visual recognition memory (VRM) is based on the preference that infants have for a new stimulus compared to another 'older' stimulus, already seen. VRM is generally assessed by using the paired-comparison paradigm (Fantz 1964, Fagan 1970). The main index of VRM is the novelty score, i.e. the percentage of time the infant spends looking at the novel stimulus compared to the time spent looking at both (familiar and novel) stimuli. The only test of VRM published so far, the Fagan Test of Infant Intelligence (FTII; Fagan and Sheperd 1989), has not been fully standardized, but data confirming its reliability and validity are available (Rose et al 2003).

In normal infants VRM increases significantly during the first year of life (Ross-Sheehy et al 2003). The test has also been used in different risk groups, including preterm infants, infants with neonatal respiratory distress syndrome and infants exposed *in utero* to different teratogenic factors such as alcohol, cocaine, nutritional deficiency, etc.

VRM appears to be highly predictive for both general cognitive function and specific aspects of information processing abilities such as memory or speed of processing. From a meta-analysis of the literature, the correlation of infant VRM with later cognitive function was shown to be higher than that of any other psychological test used in early infancy (McCall and Carriger 1993). Significant predictive correlations between VRM at 7 months and IQ at later assessments, even up to 11 years, were also found in two different groups of very low birthweight preterm infants and term infants (Rose and Feldman 1995). It has also been reported that a cut-off of 54 per cent novelty preference at 7 months can reliably identify children who later develop intellectual disability, and that the results have both good sensitivity and specificity (Rose et al 1988, Fagan and Haiken-Vasen 1997). There is also some evidence that these measures have a predictive power for IQ scores even at later ages, up to the end of adolescence (Sigman et al 1997).

The relationship between infant VRM and later global intellectual development appears to be strongly correlated with specific measures of ability of information processing, as demonstrated by Rose et al who reported a good correlation between VRM and specific cognitive tests assessing memory and speed of processing at 11 years (Rose et al 2003).

A few studies have reported that the maturation of visual *attention* throughout infancy may also provide some information regarding the maturation of VRM, and cognitive development more generally. Gaze duration and shift rate, which become respectively shorter and more frequent with age, are associated with VRM maturation (Colombo 1993).

Processing speed is another aspect of cognitive function that can be assessed in the first two years of life. It is now possible to measure processing speed in infancy with tests that are based on the assessment of the reaction times to initiate saccades in a visual expectation paradigm (Haith et al 1988), or those relying on measure of the time needed to encode information within a 'continuous familiarization' task (time of familiarization) (Rose et al 2002).

The processing speed measure also seems to have predictive value for later cognitive development (Vernon 1987, Dougherty and Haith 1997).

NEUROPHYSIOLOGICAL AND NEUROIMAGING TECHNIQUES

More sophisticated techniques have been introduced in recent decades in an attempt to obtain an objective evaluation of specific aspects of cognitive function, such as working memory or behavioural inhibition, even in infancy.

Several **neurophysiological studies** have used event-related potentials (ERP), which involve recording and averaging brain electrical activity in response to a specific stimulus. The principle used for ERP is the same as for the evoked potentials routinely used to assess the integrity of specific sensorial pathways (visual, auditory, somatosensory), but the attention in ERP is focused on the ability of the brain to perform specific cognitive processes. Differences in the timing and scalp topography of ERP components allow inferences about the temporal and spatial characteristics of brain activity involved in processing of cognitive elements involved in the stimuli.

Exposing an infant to a recognized visual stimulus (e.g. parent's face) will produce a large positive peak occurring with a latency of 300 milliseconds after stimulus presentation (P300 wave). This peak is thought to reflect the process of updating the working memory after the presentation of the stimulus, and can be broadly localized in the brain by analysing the electrode recording the strongest response (Thomas 2003). In order to obtain a more precise brain localization of the generated activity, more sophisticated mathematical analysis, such as dipole source localization, is required. However, these types of study are very hard to perform during infancy as they require a large number of trials and very low noise levels.

ERP techniques have also proven useful in infancy for the exploration of other domains. Carver et al (2000) assessed long-term explicit memory by means of behavioural and electrophysiological measures in 9-month-old infants, showing how the capacity for long-term recall, emerging near the end of the first year of life, is mirrored by the ability for long-term recognition, as measured by ERPs. Richards (2000) analysed covert attention in infants as young as 14 weeks, showing evidence of covert attention as expressed by larger ERP responses when visual stimuli were preceded by valid cue targets.

163

Another possible application was shown by Molfese et al (2003) in early prediction of preschool linguistic performance. They assessed sound discrimination during neonatal age by means of the analysis of ERP responses to different sounds (/bi/ vs /gi/), showing a significant correlation between ERP results and verbal IQ scores at 5 years. Sound discrimination was also studied by Black et al (2004) in intrauterine growth-restricted (IUGR) newborns with head-sparing, tested with both a speech/non-speech paradigm to assess auditory sensory processing, and a novel (stranger's voice) and familiar (mother's voice) paradigm to assess recognition memory. IUGR newborns showed a much stronger response to mother's voice, as opposed to controls, suggesting that IUGR newborns with head-sparing may have an accelerated but atypical process of cognitive development.

A new means of early exploration of cognitive processes is represented by functional neuroimaging. In the last few years, this technique has played an increasing role in studies of normal and abnormal development during infancy. In comparison with the ERPs, it provides much more accurate information on brain localization, but its use in infancy is still very limited due to the complexity of technical adaptations required for its application in this age range.

A few studies have reported the use of fMRI in the assessment of the functional organization of the visual (Born et al 2000, Morita et al 2000) and auditory system (Altman and Bernal 2001, Anderson et al 2001). More recently, functions requiring a higher cognitive competence, such as language, have also been explored with fMRI (Dehaene-Lambertz et al 2002). To determine which brain regions support language processing at this young age, these authors measured the brain activity evoked by normal and reversed speech in awake and sleeping 3-month-old infants, showing that left-lateralized brain regions, similar to those of adults, were already active in infants well before the onset of speech production.

Overall, these studies seem to open up important new perspectives in the investigation of early cognitive development both in the normal infant and in those with congenital or early acquired brain damage.

Clinical role of developmental assessment in the first two years of life

One of the most challenging tasks during the follow-up of newborns at neurological risk is the early assessment of cognitive development. The estimation of cognitive prerequisites, i.e. the primary skills from which cognitive development originates, represents a fundamental means of early prediction of later development.

Developmental cognitive assessment may have two main clinical targets: (1) early detection of developmental abnormalities in order to enable early intervention; and (2) the provision of useful information for prediction of developmental outcome.

Prediction of later cognitive performance seems better for children classified as delayed or neurologically impaired than for 'normal' children; this could be because cerebral impairment may increase the longitudinal 'stability' of cognitive functions with the limitation of the variability in development over time (Largo et al 1990). Predictive value of developmental performance from 9 to 24 months (according to some authors, even before 9 months in severely intellectually disabled infants) is reliable enough both for normal and intellectually disabled children, but not for borderline patients. Subscores and specific clusters seem to predict IQ even better than total scores. Using the Griffiths scales, for example, a cluster of the subscales D (performance), E (eye–hand coordination) and C (hearing and speech) relates very strongly to later cognitive development. Gross motor development seems a weak predictor of cognitive development (infants with motor deficit may show good cognitive development, while advanced motor skills may be associated with poor cognitive development).

Cognitive impairment is often detected only by analysis of cognitive development curves, which show a dissociated development, e.g. in relation to language variability (temporary delay during the second and third year of life); there is thus a need for detailed analysis of single developmental features (language, performance, motor).

Development deviation may be caused by organic brain impairment or major life events (severe illness, admission to hospital, separation from the family, etc.). Among the different fields of clinical interest in the evaluation of cognitive development in infancy, such as non-progressive brain injuries, degenerative or metabolic diseases or unfavourable social context, we will briefly deal with a paradigmatic condition, the early onset epilepsies.

A MODEL OF DISRUPTION OF EARLY DEVELOPMENT: THE EARLY ONSET EPILEPSIES
A good and 'spontaneous' model of early disruption of cognitive development is represented by the early onset epilepsies, and in particular West syndrome, which has among its clinical markers arrest or deterioration of global development. From the seminal observations of Illingworth (1955), cognitive involvement in early onset epilepsies has become the object of accurate studies aimed at understanding its possible mechanisms and, consequently, eventual treatment strategies.

Early onset epileptic encephalopathies but also early onset epilepsies are frequently associated with cognitive stagnation or deterioration. Different pathogenic mechanisms of cognitive delay are now considered, whether linked to the epileptic disorder *per se* or to other causes (Deonna, 1999). The difficulty in performing a cognitive assessment at an early age, in particular when an epileptic disorder is concomitantly present, explains the poor reports in the literature.

The typical perceptual involvement in some epileptic syndromes, and particularly in West syndrome, could be the key to the possible mechanism by which the cognitive consequence of the epileptic disorder manifests itself (Guzzetta et al 1993, Jambaqué et al 1993, Guzzetta et al 2002). It has been consistently reported that various aspects of visual function are impaired during the active stage of West syndrome. Visual abnormalities can already be detected by means of behavioural and electrophysiological tests during the first weeks of the disease and even before (Iinuma et al 1994, Okumura and Watanabe 2001, Guzzetta 2002), including poor visual responsiveness (Guzzetta et al 1993, Jambaqué et al 1993, Castano 2000, Brooks 2002), abnormal visual evoked potentials (Taddeucci et al 1984, Wenzel 1987), and deficits in other aspects of visual function such as fixation shift (Guzzetta et al 2002). These perceptual abnormalities appear to be related not only to the brain lesion, but also to the epileptic disorder *per se*, as in most cases the improvement of seizures is followed by a recovery of visual functions (Randò et al 2004). Moreover, the organization of the sleep pattern on EEG may show a good association with visual findings, further suggesting a specific role of the disrupted brain activity on visual behaviour (Randò et al 2004).

Similar findings supporting a close relationship between perceptual impairment and epileptic disorder in West syndrome have emerged when investigating the auditory function. Several authors have described abnormalities of brainstem evoked potentials during the acute phase of the syndrome (Kaga et al 1982, Curatolo et al 1989, Miyazaki et al 1993).

More recently, we have investigated auditory function longitudinally in a group of infants with West syndrome, from its onset and for the following two months (Baranello et al 2006). In our series, auditory function was significantly impaired in the early stages of the syndrome, as a consequence of both low-level arousal dysfunction and high-level cortical processing. Although we failed to show a significant correlation between auditory function and different aspects of the EEG, the presence of abnormalities in infants with cryptogenic epilepsy and the improvement after offset of seizures seem to support at least partially an influence of the epileptic disorder *per se* on the genesis of the sensorial impairment.

The integrity of the perceptual system is considered highly significant in early cognitive development and its derangement is therefore strongly associated with developmental delay. This has been confirmed in infants with West syndrome, particularly when visual behaviour is involved (Randò et al 2005). It is important to identify abnormalities in order to be able to plan an adequate treatment (rehabilitation) strategy. Moreover, investigation of early cognitive development in epileptic diseases of the first two years of life can help identify surgical candidates among drug-resistant infants with epilepsy. The detection of cognitive deterioration in such infants represents a key factor in the decision to attempt surgical intervention in order to prevent other major consequences of epilepsy.

REFERENCES

Altman NR, Bernal B (2001) Brain activation in sedated children: auditory and visual functional MR imaging. *Radiology* 221: 56–63.
Anderson AW, Marois R, Colson ER, Peterson BS, Duncan CC, Edhrenkranz RA, et al (2001) Neonatal auditory activation detected by functional magnetic resonance imaging. *Magn Reson Imaging* 19: 1–5.
Atkinson J (1984) Human visual development over the first 6 months of life. A review and a hypothesis. *Hum Neurobiol* 3(2): 61–74.
Atkinson J (2000) *The Developing Visual Brain*. Oxford: Oxford University Press.
Atkinson J, Hood B, Wattam-Bell J, Braddick O (1992) Changes in infants' ability to switch visual attention in the first three months of life. *Perception* 21(5): 643–653.
Baranello G, Randò T, Bancale A, D'Acunto MG, Epifanio R, Frisone MF, et al (2006) Auditory attention at the onset of West syndrome: correlation with EEG patterns and visual function. *Brain Dev* 28(5): 293–299.
Bayley N (1936) *California Infant Scale of Mental Development*. Berkeley: University of California Press.
Benasich AA, Tallal P (2002) Infant discrimination of rapid auditory cues predicts later language impairment. *Behav Brain Res* 136: 31–49.
Black LS, de Regnier RA, Long J, Georgieff MK, Nelson CA (2004) Electrographic imaging of recognition memory in 34–38 week gestation intrauterine growth restricted newborns. *Exp Neurol* 190(Suppl 1): S72–S83.
Born AP, Miranda MJ, Rostrup E, Toft PB, Peitersen B, Larsson HB, et al (2000) Functional magnetic resonance imaging of the normal and abnormal visual system in early life. *Neuropediatrics* 31: 24–32.

Brazelton TB (1984) *Neonatal Behavioral Assessment Scale*. Clinics in Developmental Medicine 88. Philadelphia: JB Lippincott.

Brooks BP, Simpson JL, Leber SM, Robertson PL, Archer SM (2002) Infantile spasms as a cause of acquired perinatal visual loss. *J AAPOS* 6(6): 385–388.

Carver LJ, Bauer PJ, Nelson CA (2000) Associations between infant brain activity and recall memory. *Dev Sci* 3: 234–246.

Castano G (2000) Cortical visual impairment in children with infantile spasms. *J AAPOS* 4(3): 175–178.

Cattell P (1940) *The Measurement of Intelligence of Infants*. New York: Psychological Corporation.

Cioni G, Bertucelli B, Boldrini A, Canapicchi R, Fazzi B, Guzzetta A, et al (2000) Correlation between visual function, neurodevelopmental outcome, and magnetic resonance imaging findings in infants with periventricular leucomalacia. *Arch Dis Child Fetal Neonatal Ed* 82: F134–F140.

Colombo J (1993) *Infant Cognition: Predicting Later Intellectual Functioning*. Newbury Park, CA: Sage.

Curatolo P, Cardona F, Cusmai R (1989) BAEPs in infantile spasms. *Brain Dev* 11(5): 347–348.

Dehaene-Lambertz G, Dehaene S, Hertz-Pannier L (2002) Functional neuroimaging of speech perception in infants. *Science* 298(5600): 2013–2015.

Deonna T (1999) [Dysphasias of development.] *Arch Pediatr* 6(Suppl 2): S383–S386.

Dougherty TM, Haith MM (1997) Infant expectations and reaction time as predictors of childhood speed of processing and IQ. *Dev Psychol* 33: 146–155.

Fagan JF (1970) Memory of the infant. *J Exp Child Psychol* 9: 217–226.

Fagan JF, Haiken-Vasen JH (1997) Selective attention to novelty as measure of information processing. In: Burack JA, Enns JT, editors. *Attention, Development, and Psychopathology*. New York: Guilford Press.

Fagan JF, Sheperd P (1989) *The Fagan Test of Infant Intelligence*. Cleveland, OH: Infantest Corporation.

Fagan JF, Singer LT (1983) Infant recognition memory as a measure of intelligence. In: Lipsitt LP, Rovee-Collier CK, editors. *Advances in Infancy Research*, Norwood, NJ: Ablex, vol 2, pp 31–78.

Fantz RL (1964) Visual experience in infants: decreased attention to familiar patterns relative to novel ones. *Science* 146: 668–670.

Gesell A, Thompson H (1934) *Infant Behaviour: Its Genesis and Growth*. New York: McGraw-Hill.

Gomes H, Molholm S, Christodoulou C, Ritter W, Cowan N (2000) The development of auditory attention in children. *Front Biosci* 5: 108–120.

Griffiths R (1954) *The Abilities of Babies*. High Wycombe, UK: The Test Agency.

Griffiths R (1970) *The Abilities of Young Children*. High Wycombe, UK: The Test Agency.

Guzzetta F, Crisafulli A, Isaya Crino M (1993) Cognitive assessment of infants with West syndrome: how useful is it for diagnosis and prognosis? *Dev Med Child Neurol* 35(5): 379–387.

Guzzetta F, Frisone MF, Ricci D, Rando T, Guzzetta A (2002) Development of visual attention in West syndrome. *Epilepsia* 43(7): 757–763.

Haith MM, Hazan C, Goodman GS (1988) Expectation and anticipation of dynamic visual events by 3.5-month-old babies. *Child Dev* 59: 467–479.

Iinuma K, Haginoya K, Nagai M, Kon K, Yagi T, Saito T (1994) Visual abnormalities and occipital EEG discharges: risk factors for West syndrome. *Epilepsia* 35(4): 806–809.

Illingworth RS (1955) Sudden mental deterioration with convulsions in infancy. *Arch Dis Child* 30: 529–537.

Jambaqué I, Chiron C, Dulac O, Raynaud C, Syrota P (1993) Visual inattention in West syndrome: a neuropsychological and neurofunctional imaging study. *Epilepsia* 34(4): 692–700.

Kaga M, Azuma C, Imamura T, Murakami T, Kaga K (1982) Auditory brainstem response (ABR) in infantile Gaucher's disease. *Neuropediatrics* 13(4): 207–210.

Knobloch H, Pasamanick B (1960) An evaluation of the consistency and predictive value of the 40 week Gesell Developmental Schedule. In: Shagass C, Pasamanick B, editors. *Child Development and Child Psychiatry*. Psychiatric Research Reports of the American Psychiatric Association 13, pp 10–31.

Kopp CB, McCall RB (1982) Predicting later mental performance for normal, at-risk, and handicapped infants. In: Bates PB, Brin OG, editors. *Life Span Development and Behavior*. New York: Academic Press, pp 33–61.

Largo RH, Graf S, Kundu S, Hunziker U, Molinari L (1990) Predicting developmental outcome at school age from infant tests of normal, at-risk and retarded infants *Dev Med Child Neurol* 32: 30–45.

Lester BM, Tronick EZ, Brazelton TB (2004) The Neonatal Intensive Care Unit Network Neurobehavioral Scale procedures. *Pediatrics* 113(3 Pt 2): 641–667.

Lewis M, Brooks-Gunn J (1981) Visual attention at three months as a prediction of cognitive functioning at two years of age. *Intelligence* 5: 181–190.

167

McCall RB, Carriger MS (1993) A meta-analysis of infant habituation and recognition memory performance as predictors of later IQ. *Child Dev* 64: 57–79.

McCall RB, Hogarty PS, Hurlburt N (1972) Transitions in infant sensori-motor development and the prediction of childhood IQ. *Am Psychol* 27: 728–748.

Mercuri E, Braddick O, Atkinson J, Cowan F, Anker S, Andrew R, et al (1998) Orientation-reversal and phase-reversal visual evoked potentials in full-term infants with brain lesions: a longitudinal study. *Neuropediatrics* 29(4): 169–174.

Mercuri E, Haataja L, Guzzetta A, Anker S, Cowan F, Rutherford M, et al (1999) Visual function in term infants with hypoxic insults: correlation with neurodevelopment at 2 years of age. *Arch Dis Child Fetal Neonatal Ed* 80: F99–F104.

Miyazaki M, Hashimoto T, Tayama M, Kuroda Y (1993) Brainstem involvement in infantile spasms: a study employing brainstem evoked potentials and magnetic resonance imaging. *Neuropediatrics* 24(3): 126–130.

Molfese DL, Molfese VJ, Key AF, Kelly SD (2003) Influence of environment on speech sound discrimination: findings from a longitudinal study. *Dev Neuropsychol* 24(2–3): 541–548.

Montagner H, Deliac P, Bordes JP, Cazenave M, Bensch C (2002) Heart rate variations in five-month-old children during interactions in a controlled environment. *Acta Paediatr* 91(6): 641–648.

Morita T, Kochiyama T, Yamada H, Konishi Y, Yonekura Y, Matsumura M, et al (2000) Difference in the metabolic response to photic stimulation of the lateral geniculate nucleus and the primary visual cortex of infants: a fMRI study. *Neurosci Res* 38: 63–70.

Okumura A, Watanabe K (2001) Clinico-electrical evolution in prehypsarrhythmic stage: towards prediction and prevention of West syndrome. *Brain Dev* 23(7): 482–487.

Randò T, Bancale A, Baranello G, Bini M, De Belvis AG, Epifanio R, et al (2004) Visual function in infants with West syndrome: correlation with EEG patterns. *Epilepsia* 45: 781–786.

Randò T, Baranello G, Ricci D, Guzzetta A, Tinelli F, Biagioni E, et al (2005) Cognitive competence at the onset of West syndrome: correlation with EEG patterns and visual function. *Dev Med Child Neurol* 47(11): 760–765.

Richards JE (2000) Localizing the development of covert attention in infants using scalp event-related potentials. *Dev Psych* 36: 91–108.

Rose SA, Feldman JF (1995) Prediction of IQ and specific cognitive abilities at 11 years from infancy measures. *Dev Psychol* 31: 685–696. *J Pediatr* 116: 19–26.

Rose SA, Feldman JF, Wallace JF (1988) Individual differences in infants' information processing: reliability, stability, and prediction. *Child Dev* 59: 1177–1197.

Rose SA, Jankowski JJ, Feldman JF (2002) Speed of processing and face recognition at 7 and 12 months. *Infancy* 3: 435–455.

Rose SA, Feldman JF, Jankowski JJ (2003) The building blocks of cognition. *J Pediatr* 143: S54–S61.

Ross-Sheehy S, Oakes LM, Luck SJ (2003) The development of visual short-term memory capacity in infants. *Child Dev* 74(6): 1807–1822.

Schlumberger E, Narbona J, Manrique M (2004) Non-verbal development of children with deafness with and without cochlear implants. *Dev Med Child Neurol* 46: 596–606.

Shumway-Cook S, Woollacott M (1995) *Motor Control: Theory and Practical Applications.* New York: Williams and Wilkins.

Sigman MD, Cohen SE, Bechwith L (1997) Why does infant attention predict adolescent intelligence? *Inf Behav Dev* 20: 133–140.

Sonksen PM, Dale N (2002) Visual impairment in infancy: impact on neurodevelopmental and neurobiological processes. *Dev Med Child Neurol* 44: 782–791.

Taddeucci G, Fiorentini A, Pirchio M, Spinelli D (1984) Pattern reversal evoked potentials in infantile spasms. *Hum Neurobiol* 3(3): 153–155.

Thomas KM (2003) Assessing brain development using neurophysiologic and behavioural measures. *J Pediatr* 143: S46–S53.

Tröster H, Hecker W, Brambing M (1994) Longitudinal study of gross-motor development in blind infants and preschoolers. *Early Child Dev Care* 104: 61–78.

Vernon PA (1987) *Speed of Processing and Intelligence.* Norwood, NJ: Ablex.

Wenzel D (1987) Evoked potentials in infantile spasms. *Brain Dev* 9(4): 365–368.

10
HEARING, LANGUAGE AND COMMUNICATION

Anna Chilosi, Paola Cipriani, Sandra Maestro and Elisabetta Genovese

This chapter will illustrate the main tools and results of hearing screening programmes in high-risk newborns. It will also review the development of language and communication in the first two years of life and the main instruments for assessment, validated for different languages. The chapter will end with a brief description of early signs of autism, which represents the most severe disorder of communication, detectable during the same period.

Hearing screening methods in high-risk newborns

In high-risk newborns the incidence of hearing impairment is high (1–3 per cent of surviving newborns) and is always associated with perception and language disorders.

The overall prevalence of bilateral hearing loss in children is estimated to be between 0.5 per 1000 live births (Pabla et al 1991) and 1.2/1000 (Davis et al 1995) up to 2.1/1000 (Vartainien et al 1997) in different studies, depending on factors such as methods of hearing loss detection, degree of hearing loss targeted, geographical area and period of the study. Investigation of hearing impaired children aims to identify the cause of the hearing loss, and to provide information relevant to hearing loss management, co-existing medical problems and prognosis for the child and the family.

From 1985 to 1990 Davis conducted the most significant study for industrial countries on the incidence and aetiology of hearing loss in children aged 1–6 years, in a cohort of 366,480 children, in the Trent region in England, which has a population of 4.7 million (Table 10.1).

Concerning aetiology (Table 10.2), this study highlights that 43 per cent of congenital hearing losses are of genetic origin, whereas 4 per cent have prenatal and 7 per cent perinatal origin; a small percentage are due to craniofacial abnormalities and syndromic hearing losses. The high incidence of genetic hearing loss is evident. Genetic hearing loss is the only disease in 60 per cent of cases, while in the remaining 40 per cent of cases it is associated with other congenital anomalies in a syndrome. The most frequent mode of genetic transmission is Mendelian inheritance (monogenic hearing loss): autosomal recessive in about 75 per cent of cases, autosomal dominant in 25 per cent, X-linked in 5 per cent and mitochondrial in 1 per cent. Another, but rarer, mode of transmission is due to chromosomic mutations, as described by Dalla Piccola et al (1996).

Genetic research has recently highlighted that characteristic Cx26/GJB2 gene mutations are localized at chromosome 13q12 (DFNB1 and DFNA3) and cause non-syndromic

TABLE 10.1
Prevalence rate per 100,000 live births of permanent childhood hearing impairment in Trent region
PTA (0.5–2–4) ≥40 dBHL in 487 children (409 congenital; 78 acquired)

PTA dBHL	Total	Congenital	Acquired
≥ 40	100% (prev. 133)	100% (prev. 112)	100% (prev. 21)
≥ 50	83% (prev. 110)	81% (prev. 90)	92% (prev. 20)
40–50	17% (prev. 23)	19% (prev. 21)	8% (prev. 8)
51–69	38% (prev. 51)	38% (prev. 43)	36% (prev. 8)
70–94	22% (prev. 28)	20% (prev. 23)	24% (prev. 5)
≥95	23% (prev. 31)	22% (prev. 24)	32% (prev. 7)

dBHL = decibels hearing loss; prev. = prevalence; PTA = pure tone audiogram

Source: Trent, UK; birth cohort 1985–1990; number of live births 366,480 (Fortnum and Davis 1997).

TABLE 10.2
Classification of aetiology of hearing impairment

Aetiology	Total		Congenital (85%)		Acquired (15%)	
Genetic	259	(39.7%)	237	(42.6%)	22	(23.1%)
Prenatal	24	(3.7%)	23	(4.1%)	1	(1.0%)
Perinatal	44	(6.7%)	43	(7.7%)	1	(1.0%)
Postnatal acquired	40	(6.1%)	–		40	(41.2%)
Craniofacial anomalies	8	(1.2%)	8	(1.4%)	–	
Other	11	(1.7%)	8	(1.4%)	3	(3.0%)
Missing*	267	(40.9%)	237	(42.6%)	30	(30.9%)
Total	**653**		**556**		**97**	

* This refers to children lost during the study.

Source: Trent, UK; birth cohort 1985–1993; number of live births 552,558 (Fortnum and Davis 1997).

hearing losses (recessive or dominant) (Kelsell et al 1997, Denoyelle et al 1998, Estivill et al 1998).

The most frequent recessive genetic mutation of Cx26 is the deletion of a single base (35delG). Recently other genes of the connexin family have been associated with hearing loss: CX30, 31 and 32.

Improvement in neonatal intensive care and the introduction of universal immunization programmes have resulted in major changes in the epidemiology of hearing loss in children. In comparison with 25 years ago, when only 2 per cent of the child population with hearing loss was affected by hearing loss of perinatal origin, the incidence is now 27 per cent (Roizen 1999). In the UK, the prevalence of hearing impairment in children with a history of treatment in a neonatal intensive care unit has increased fourfold over a period of 15 years (Davis et al 1995), and is higher than in other European countries (Parving and Stephens 1997). A combination of neonatal intensive care unit status, family history of hearing loss and craniofacial abnormalities noticeable at birth may account for up to 64 per cent of all types of hearing loss.

It seems evident that the main aetiopathological factors have gradually changed in the last 30 years thanks to improved prevention programmes such as compulsory pre-menarche rubella vaccination, serological monitoring of pregnancy for TORCH-complex, Rh/AB0 histocompatibility monitoring, neonatal jaundice monitoring and therapy, careful use of ototoxic drugs, better control of pregnancy and birth, as well as prevention of genetic diseases.

With the spread of neonatal intensive care units (NICU) since 1960, infants born very preterm with complications due to severe preterm birth more often survive, and as a result the incidence of hearing loss has increased.

Hearing loss is normally classified in the following way:

1   Conductive hearing loss: an interference of any sort in the transmission of sound from the external auditory canal to the inner ear.
2   Sensorineural hearing loss: this occurs when damage has been sustained by the sensory organ or hair cells located within the cochlea.
3   Central auditory dysfunction: the vast majority of children with this diagnosis show communication disorders with normal hearing and no observable CNS pathologies (Stach 1998).

In the follow-up of high-risk newborns, the most important hearing loss is the 'sensorineural' with high threshold and low word perception. It is common practice to classify hearing loss in terms of pure tone threshold at 500–1000 and 2000 Hz in the best ear, and to consider four categories: mild, moderate, severe, and profound hearing impairment. Nowadays, we use the American National Standards Institute (1991) classification in which description of hearing loss is based on the reduced intelligibility of a speech message, the effects on speech perception and production, and learning abilities (Table 10.3).

The development of hearing and speech perception abilities in children occurs in the first two to three years of life. Recent studies have shown that children with hearing loss who are identified and receive early intervention prior to 6 months of age develop significantly better language abilities than children identified after 6 months.

The age at onset of hearing loss, together with the speech/language and cognitive skills of the child at that time, are the most important predictive factors for auditory development and central pathways organization. Early detection of the hearing loss, followed by early intervention (with use of appropriate hearing aids) and special education, is critical to speech/language, cognitive and social development.

In 1982 the Joint Committee on Infant Hearing (JCIH) developed a high-risk register for deafness to identify newborns at risk for severe to profound hearing impairment. The Joint Committee met again in 2000 to review and update new position statements, based on new knowledge and reviews of current literature. It recommended that all infants admitted to neonatal intensive care units for more than 24 hours should be screened for hearing loss before hospital discharge.

The high incidence of hearing loss in infants admitted to neonatal intensive care units (1–3 per cent of the infants admitted) is due to respiratory distress syndrome, hyper-bilirunemia, ototoxic medication, and complications during admission. They are all

TABLE 10.3

American National Standards Institute classification of hearing impairment as a function of average hearing threshold level of the better ear

Average threshold level at 500–2000 Hz (ANSI)	Description	Common causes	What can be heard without amplification	Degree of handicap if not treated in first (year of life)	Probable needs
0–15 dB	Normal range				
16–25 dB	Slight hearing loss	Serous otitis Perforation Monomeric membrane Sensorineural loss Timpanosclerosis	All speech sounds Vowel sounds heard clearly, may miss unvoiced consonant sounds	None Possible mild or transitory auditory dysfunction Difficulty in perceiving some speech sounds	None Consideration of need for hearing aid Lip reading Auditory training Speech therapy Preferential seating Appropriate surgery
26–40 dB	Mild hearing loss	Serous otitis Perforation Tympanosclerosis Monomeric membrane	Hears only some speech sounds – the louder voiced sounds	Auditory learning dysfunction Mild language retardation Mild speech problems Inattention	Hearing aid Lip reading Auditory training Speech therapy Appropriate surgery
41–65 dB	Moderate hearing loss	Sensorineural loss or mixed loss due to sensorineural loss plus middle ear disease	Misses most speech sounds at normal conversational level	Speech problems Language retardation Learning dysfunction Inattention	All of the above plus consideration of special classroom situation
66–95 dB	Severe hearing loss	Sensorineural loss or mixed loss due to sensorineural loss plus middle ear disease	Hears no speech sounds of normal conversation	Severe speech problems Language retardation Learning dysfunction Inattention	All of the above; probable assignment to special classes
96+ dB	Profound hearing loss	Sensorineural loss or mixed	Hears no speech or other sounds	Severe speech problems Language retardation Learning dysfunction Inattention	All of the above; probable assignment to special classes

considered as a single risk factor. In Tables 10.4 and 10.5 we report the position statement of the JCIH 2000 with the indicators that place an infant at risk for hearing loss at birth or for progressive or delayed onset of sensorineural and/or conductive hearing loss.

Early intervention in the first months of life is very important to avoid the consequences of late diagnosis which can seriously compromise language and learning skills as well as socio-emotional development. This diagnostic procedure (from the screening of at-risk children to the final diagnosis) has to be completed within the first year of life and, if possible, by 6–8 months. This can be achieved in two steps: identification of at-risk children (screening), and then, in positive cases, diagnostic and therapeutic evaluation. Only objective methods are used for both screening and diagnosis, since early infancy behavioural techniques cannot be precise enough for correct prosthetic and rehabilitative prescriptions.

At present, objective audiometric methodologies such as auditory evoked responses (AER) and oto-acoustic emissions (OAE) perform a fundamental screening role in the diagnosis. In the future it is likely that behavioural techniques, which allow a better definition

TABLE 10.4
Risk factors for hearing impairment from birth to 28 days (JCIH 2000)

(a) An illness or condition requiring admission of 48 hours or greater to a NICU.
(b) Stigmata or other findings associated with a syndrome known to include sensorineural and/or conductive hearing loss.
(c) Family history of permanent childhood sensorineural hearing loss.
(d) Craniofacial anomalies, including those with morphological abnormalities of the pinna and ear canal.
(e) *In utero* infections such as cytomegalovirus, herpes, toxoplasmosis or rubella (TORCH).

Source: JCIH 2000.

TABLE 10.5
Risk factors and indicators for rescreening infants from 29 days to 2 years

- Parental or caregiver concern regarding hearing, speech, language and/or developmental delay
- Family history of permanent childhood sensorineural hearing loss
- Stigmata or other findings associated with a syndrome known to include sensorineural and/or hearing loss or eustachian tube dysfunction
- Postnatal infections associated with sensorineural hearing loss including bacterial meningitis
- *In utero* infections such as cytomegalovirus, herpes, toxoplasmosis, rubella (TORCH) or syphilis
- Neonatal indicators specifically:

  – Hyperbilirubinemia at a serum level requiring exchange transfusion
  – Persistent pulmonary hypertension of the newborn associated with mechanical ventilation
  – Conditions requiring the use of ECMO

- Syndromes associated with progressive hearing loss such as neurofibromatosis, osteopetrosis and Usher's syndromes
- Neurodegenerative disorders, such as Hunter syndrome, or sensory-motor neuropathies, Friedreich's ataxia and Charcot-Marie-Tooth syndrome
- Head trauma
- Recurrent or persistent otitis media with effusion for at least three months

Source: JCIH 2000.

of hearing perception in terms of both audiometric threshold and acoustic disability (the child's verbal perceptual capacity with prosthetic aids), will become the basis of children's audiologic evaluation.

AUDITORY ASSESSMENT

Auditory screening is the process of applying unfailing, rapid and simple tests, examinations, or other procedures to a large number of people to identify those individuals with a high probability of having the disorder. Screening is not intended as a diagnostic procedure, but as the first step in the early identification of children with hearing loss.

Universal newborn hearing screening is based on a two-stage protocol using otoacoustic emissions, as the birth admission screening, followed by the auditory brainstem response (ABR) procedure. The cost and the positive predictive value of universal newborn hearing screening are closely comparable with the cost and predictive value of screening for other congenital conditions (Mehl and Thomson 1998).

The next diagnostic step is the application of objective procedures and particularly recording of the electrical activity of the auditory pathway, evoked by a loud sound. The auditory response may be near-field or far-field, depending on whether the electrodes are near or far from the bioelectrical potential generator. The near-field response is the electrocochleography performed with a trans-tympanic needle electrode on the promontory (the medial wall of the middle ear); and the far-field responses are the ABR, MLR, SVR and CNV recorded with electrodes on the vertex of the scalp (see below). Electrocochleography is an invasive procedure but with an improved signal/noise ratio and, consequently, with potentials of large magnitude.

Davis (1976) classified the evoked auditory responses in terms of their latencies:

- **Fast**: electrocochleography (ECochG) (Eggermont 1976) consists of more than one auditory electrical potential including the whole nerve action potential (AP), the cochlear microphonic (CM), and the summating potential (SP). The CM originates from the hair cells and from the auditory nerve. Latency is 0–5 ms.
- **Early**: ABRs (auditory brainstem responses) and FFR (frequency following responses) are electrical potentials originating from the brainstem and the auditory nerve. Latency is 1.5–15 ms. **Middle**: middle latency responses (MLRs) are generated from the thalamic region and the primary auditory cortex. Latency is 10–100 ms.
- **Slow**: slow vertex responses (SVRs) are generated from the auditory cortex. Latency is 100–300 ms.
- **Late**: cognitive negative variation (CNV), late positive component (P300) and slow wave (SW) are generated from the frontal cortex. Latency is 300–800 ms.

At present, only ABR and ECochG are used in routine clinical audiometric evaluation. Measuring ABR is straightforward and is thus considered the first-choice method for hearing assessment; it is now the cornerstone of all audiometric measurements in uncooperative children. Certain situations make the ECochG essential as a subsequent step to ensure a reliable audiological assessment in children.

The maturation of ABR is not complete until 12–18 months post-term; this confirms the importance of taking the chronological age of the infant into account when evaluating ABR latencies, and the importance of referring results to ABR normative standards in infants and young children (Gorga et al 1987).

The ABR is evoked with click stimuli, which have spectral energy between 1000 and 4000 Hz, and predominantly reflect the basal turn of the cochlea. When the stimulus intensity is near the auditory threshold, wave V is often the only remaining landmark in the response tracing (Moore 1983, Arslan and Conti 1994). The click-evoked ABR thresholds are closely related to behavioural audiometric thresholds at 2000–4000 Hz.

Any middle ear pathology can cause problems in detecting the true sensory peripheral hearing threshold, because of the overlapping conductive component. However, this easily recognizable pathology can only be responsible for a marginally worse threshold. By performing ABR testing and evaluating the latency of the fundamental components (the inter-peak intervals and the input–output functions), all the necessary information can be obtained for precise detection and subsequent assessment of any conductive hearing loss. In the case of mixed hearing loss, the conductive component can be suspected on the basis of otoscopic and tympanometric findings; in these cases ABR retesting and repeated follow-up measurements are needed after any medical and/or surgical treatment (Arslan et al 1997).

OUR EXPERIENCE

We have studied over 1300 children aged from 10 months to 13 years since 1974; most of the data have been obtained with ECochG (Arslan et al 1983, Conti et al 1984, Arslan et al 1997). ECochG was performed under general anaesthesia with a trans-tympanic needle electrode on the promontory. Each response was evoked by clicks, and the compound action potential (AP) (Kiang et al 1965, Dallos 1975) and cochlear microphonic (CM) were displayed separately.

ECochG has been largely replaced by widespread use of ABR for the objective assessment of hearing threshold. ABR methods are less invasive and are easier to perform because responses may be recorded in spontaneous sleep or conscious sedation. The clinical criteria for performing ECochG under general anaesthesia are the following:

1   A reliable threshold measure by ABR in spontaneous sleep or conscious sedation could not be obtained because of the child's restlessness.
2   ABR appeared unreliable as a threshold indicator for wave-latency functions not in accordance with normative data.
3   Presence of important morphological abnormalities which rendered ABR unreliable.
4   Suspected severe hearing loss associated with recurring otitis media with effusion.

Some differences of hearing thresholds between the two methods were found in individuals with central nervous system pathology or central maturation delay. In these cases ECochG may be the only reliable diagnostic tool for hearing assessment in uncooperative patients. ECochG is therefore a valid test after ABR for confirming the diagnosis. All infants and

175

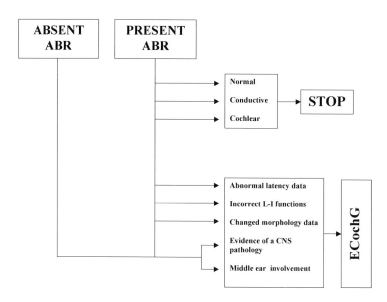

Fig. 10.1 Flowchart of electrophysiological procedures for the early diagnosis of hearing impairment.

children with significant hearing loss should be fitted with hearing aids. Appropriate amplification requires precise information concerning the function of the receptor.

The crucial point in the strategy for the early diagnosis of deafness is to establish when ABR testing alone is sufficient and when an ECochG is needed. A suitable diagnostic strategy can reduce the risks of error in objective threshold detection to a minimum (see Fig. 10.1).

It has been shown that a combination of these two methods attains a diagnostic sensitivity of about 100 per cent, thus allowing correct identification of all suspected hearing losses.

The absence of AP in the ECochG is indicative of profound neurosensorial hearing loss (nHL) due to cochlear lesions, with a threshold of about 90 dB nHL or more, for frequencies ranging from 2.0 to 4.0 KHz. Therefore, this finding does not exclude the presence of residual hearing on the low–middle frequencies which could be improved with hearing aids or a cochlear implant. This latter option could be evaluated during follow-up by assessing the child's perceptual and language skills after fitting hearing aids and appropriate rehabilitation. The presence of AP following a click of high intensity is indeed a favourable prognostic indicator for the acquisition of perceptual and language skills by means of a traditional hearing aid.

Development of language and communication in the first two years of life
Evaluation of language and communication in infants and toddlers is not an easy task. It requires both a comprehensive theoretical framework and clinical experience in the observation and description of young children's behaviour. From a theoretical point

of view, the so-called 'interactionist' model of language development assumes that readiness for or cognitive and communicative prerequisites to language acquisition are the foundations of development.

This perspective embraces Bloom and Lahey's (1978) three-dimensional view of normal and abnormal language acquisition, according to which precursors of language form, content and use are intimately linked and highly interdependent from the early stages of normal development, and dissociation between domains may result in clinically distinct types of disorder.

Infants perceive and produce sounds (form); they know about events in their immediate environment (content); and at the same time they interact with other persons and objects in the context (use). Data on development during the first year of life provide evidence of the infant's readiness in specific ways to acquire and use language. The behaviours that are hypothesized to be related to language acquisition appear to be a product of programmed structures and functions of the nervous system and of the maturational events that occur during development (biological, cognitive and social). Biological readiness refers to the uniqueness of the human infant's brain and the auditory vocal mechanisms which are pre-programmed to perceive and produce speech sounds.

Precursors of language content (or cognitive readiness) involve, among others, the ability to attend to only certain aspects of all sensory stimuli, which the infant manifests from birth. Processing abilities that seem to be especially designed for language acquisition include the ability to relate auditory and visual information, and the infant's very early imitative skills. According to Menyuk (1988), the newborn's 'attentional filter' and the developing ability to intermodally relate and recognize events, and recall them, are very important precursors to the development of language.

Moreover, since language is a communication system involving social interaction among participants, some forms of social readiness may also be an important prerequisite for the development of language. Social readiness also seems to be dependent on either innate structures and functions or predispositions, and refers to the infant's very early ability to attend to information that is crucial for comprehending the communication of others.

Before the beginning of language, infants show a wide repertoire of intentionally goal-directed actions, which are perceived by parents as intentional from birth, a construct that Reznick and Schwartz (2001) called 'parent perception of infant intentionality'.

SPEECH PERCEPTION AND PRODUCTION

Many years of experience with behavioural techniques, developed to determine the set of phonetic/phonemic contrasts that are perceived by preverbal infants, have clearly highlighted that human infants are capable of perceiving virtually all the speech contrasts used in natural languages, at birth and/or within the first few weeks of life. Acoustical perception of speech sounds seems to be already present during the last few weeks *in utero*. fMRI studies carried out on 3-month-old infants demonstrated an early left lateralization for language processing (Dehaene-Lambertz et al 2002). The selective loss or inhibition of non-native speech sounds is already under way by 10–12 months of age. This is precisely the point at which children begin to understand meaningful speech, start to recognize the intonational contours that are typical of their own language, and begin to produce the particular sounds of their native language in their own pre-speech babble.

In the first two months, the sounds produced by human infants are reflexive in nature, being linked to specific internal states (e.g. crying); between 2 and 6 months, vowel sounds (e.g. cooing and sound play) begin to be produced. So-called canonical or reduplicative babbling (babbling in short segments or in longer strings which are now punctuated by consonants, e.g. 'bababa') starts between 6 and 10 months in most children.

The development of speech production presupposes a well developed capacity to imitate (i.e. the ability to transform an auditory input into a motor output). The age between 8 and 10 months has been considered a 'turning point' (Bates et al 1992) at which several new skills emerge, in particular the ability to reproduce novel vocal and gestural patterns (including communicative gestures such as bye-bye), which document the child's growing attention to the characteristics of the input. Moreover, around 10 months of age, most children begin to produce 'word-like sounds', used in relatively consistent ways in particular contexts. Though there is considerable variability between infants in the particular speech sounds they prefer, there is a clear continuity from pre-speech babble to first words in an individual infant's 'favourite sounds' (Vihman et al 1985).

LANGUAGE MILESTONES

Language acquisition is an active process. Without a strong motivation to communicate with others and without understanding the relationship between sounds and meanings, the child will not develop an appropriate language. Infants do not take an active role in the establishment of joint reference until 8–9 months of age, when they begin to show, give and eventually point to objects as a form of social exchange.

Language development in the first two years is primarily reflected in the child's emerging ability to communicate via gestures and words, and in the acquisition of a lexicon.

Language comprehension

In normal development, language evolves in gradual stages from situational recognition, where all the perceptual clues are present, to a truly arbitrary representational system where the symbols have no perceptual similarity to their referents. Data drawn from experimental studies and from parental reports have extensively documented that children begin to show evidence of single-word comprehension between 8 and 10 months, during the so-called sensory-motor stage. At this stage, language comprehension manifests usually in response to specific, contextually supported sounds, and can be inferred when the child responds to linguistic commands with appropriate behaviours. Many children display a rapid spurt in comprehension after 10–12 months. Based on parental questionnaires (Fenson et al 1993, Caselli and Casadio 1995), the average receptive lexical repertoire appears to consist of about 58 words at 10 months, 128 at 13 months and 210 at 16 months.

During the second year, receptive language abilities progress from single-word to multi-word sentence comprehension. At about 20 months, the average child begins to understand predictable two-word utterances. Research has shown that at this stage children use a variety of non-linguistic strategies to decode verbal commands (Chapman 1978, Bridges 1980,

Miller et al 1980, Chilosi et al 2003), and that understanding of the relations among the words of a sentence relies on what the child knows about the world, rather than on true linguistic information.

Between 24 and 30 months children show a growing ability to carry out unpredictable (or unusual) instructions, two to three words long. When asked to perform unusual actions with dolls or toys (acting-out tests), the child will first act as the agent of the action and only later will be able to use objects as agents. During this period, an awareness of simple spatial relations starts to be acquired, but understanding of prepositions is still limited by the child's conceptualization of space. By 36 months most children have learnt to make use of some syntactic information (word order) as a cue for decoding simple active sentences (Chapman 1978). However, though crucial, this is but a first step in the acquisition of mature language processing strategies, as the process of learning complex grammar goes on well into the early school-age years (Bishop 1997).

Language production
True word production has usually been documented as occurring between 11 and 13 months. At this early stage a large gap exists between receptive and expressive language, with the latter lagging behind the former in normal development. However, as with comprehension, production is linked to specific situations and forms part of a well learnt sequence of events. It mainly consists of vocal routines, such as producing animal sounds in ritualized games, or using a specific sound when requesting an object or activity.

At the beginning, 'true' words are unstable, until the child has established a repertoire of about 10 consistently produced words. New words are gradually added until 50–75 words have been acquired. This stage has been considered crucial in development, as it generally coincides with a rapid acceleration in the rate at which new words are learned (Bates et al 1992). This so-called 'vocabulary burst' is accompanied by changes in vocabulary composition and use, with a qualitative shift from use for reference (single word meaning) to predication (relational meaning).

The onset of word combinations emerges around 18–20 months and it generally coincides with the acquisition of a cumulative vocabulary of about 50–100 words (Bates et al 1988, Fenson et al 1993). Interestingly, this is also the point at which children begin to produce verbs, adjectives and other predicative terms. Although there is a considerable variability from one language to another in the forms that children use to communicate, cross-linguistic studies (Slobin 1985) have shown that the same basic stock of relational meanings are encoded by 20-month-olds all around the world (e.g. appearance, dis-appearance and reappearance of interesting objects or events; refusal, denial and request; basic event relations).

After 20 months a rapid 'burst' of grammatical development occurs, but it is only around the age of 36–40 months that the average child acquires full control over the most complex grammatical and syntactic devices.

WHAT TO DO WHEN LANGUAGE DEVELOPMENT IS DELAYED

When a child is referred because he or she is supposedly delayed in speech development, clearly one of the initial tasks is to assess the level of language development. Because normal children vary considerably in the age at which they first use single words, as well as in the age at which they first string words together into phrases, there is a tendency among inexperienced clinicians to reassure parents without further assessment. However, before giving reassurance, it is necessary to check that all aspects of the child's development are proceeding normally (Rutter 1987). With respect to the milestones of language, it is crucial to be specific about what is being asked. Familial and personal histories must be collected, possibly by means of a structured interview. It is most productive to concentrate on key age periods that are easily remembered by parents.

Having obtained an outline history of the course of earlier language development, it is necessary to focus in some detail on the child's current level of language and language-related functioning. The following scheme, proposed by Rutter (1972, 1987), provides an outline of some of the chief aspects of speech and language which form the core of any basic clinical evaluation and must be covered by parental interview formats:

1   Imitation and imaginative play
2   Comprehension of spoken language and hearing behaviour: listening, attention and understanding
3   Vocalization and babble: amount, complexity, quality and social use
4   Language production: mode (gesture, speech, etc.), complexity (syntactical and semantic), amount, use for social communication
5   Word-sound production, phonation and rhythm of speech

It is also necessary to verify if the child was delayed in pre-linguistic development, and to look at the quantity and quality of social responses (facial expression and emotions, reciprocity and social interaction).

With a non-speaking child, 'hearing behaviour' deserves careful attention on the part of the observer. The term refers to *hearing oriented* behaviour, such as the child going to the door when the bell rings, *listening and attention* (by alerting when called, looking at the person who is speaking to them, and following the direction of mother's pointing), and the child's ability to follow instruction given without visual, contextual or gestural cues (understanding).

In general, this first informal assessment is sufficient for the clinician to determine the presence of any problems in speech and language development. Next, a series of 'decision-making' steps must be followed in order to determine whether the language delay is likely to reflect some clinically significant disorder.

Main tools for indirect and direct evaluation of language and communication in the first two years of life: an overview

The simplest means of language development quantification is provided by checklists and scales based on information given by parents about the child's skills in particular areas of functioning. Different checklists and early 'screening' tests have been developed, with the aim of both describing the early stages of lexical, gestural and grammatical acquisition in normal children and identifying children at risk for language delay.

Boyle et al (1996) have extensively analysed the particular suitability of tests of language production for screening in the 18–36 months age range, on account of their levels of predictive validity, especially when combined with parental report data.

According to the authors, 'multiphasic' screening tests (such as the Griffiths Mental Developmental Scales (Griffiths 1970), the Denver Developmental Screening Test (Frankenburg et al 1971) and the Bayley Scales of Infant Development (Bayley 1969)) are designed to assess several aspects of children's development (gross motor, fine motor, language, and social development) from an early age. These tests are basic to the assessment of any child referred for language delay. In fact, they allow the clinician to make a diagnostic distinction between *primary* (or specific) and *secondary* language delay. The latter term refers to an heterogeneous group of disorders that occur in association with other pathological conditions such as learning disability, pervasive developmental disorders, physical disability, hearing loss, etc. (ICD-10 and DSM-IV (ICD-10 1992, American Psychiatric Association 1994)). However, with regard to language and communication, generally these scales lack sensitivity, such that milder cases can be missed.

Parental report

In the last 15 years, the development of standardized parental reports and questionnaires on children's early communicative and linguistic abilities has highlighted the important role of parents as observers of their child's behaviour in a familiar context (Rescorla 1989, Fenson et al 1993). At present, the most widely used questionnaires among those available for the screening of early language development and delay (Table 10.6) are the MacArthur-Bates Communicative Development Inventories (MacArthur CDI; Fenson et al 1993).

The CDI use a checklist format and contain several different subscales designed to measure receptive and expressive vocabulary, use of communicative and symbolic gestures, and complexity of grammar; parents are instructed to complete them on their own. These inventories are suitable for children in the age range from 8 to 30 months. Standardized scores based on a normal distribution (percentiles) are available. The CDI have been adapted for many different languages (presently more than 35 languages) and their substantial reliability and validity have been largely demonstrated (Bates et al 1988, Fenson et al 1993; see website CDIs in other languages).

Despite cultural and linguistic differences, the results of cross-linguistic applications of these inventories resemble the American scales to a great degree. Moreover, several studies on English-, Japanese-, Spanish- and Hebrew-speaking children have shown

TABLE 10.6
Screening procedures for early language development (parental reports and questionnaires)

Checklists suitable for early communicative development	Checklists suitable for early language development
Checklist of Communicative Competence (Gerard 1986) From birth to 2 years. Detailed checklist dealing with comprehension, communicative development, cognitive development, social and motor development. Suggested age-norms are provided. Not fully standardized.	**Early Language Milestones Scale (ELM)** (Coplan 1987) Milestone-orientated developmental scale. Designed for use with children aged from birth to 3 years. Consists of parental report of milestones together with some direct elicitation of child's behaviour. The milestones are grouped into four quadrants: auditory expressive (AE), auditory receptive (AR), visual expressive (VE), visual receptive (VR).
Clinical Linguistic and Auditory Milestones (CLAMS) (Capute and Accardo 1978, Capute et al 1986) Milestone-orientated developmental scale. Designed for use with children aged from birth to 2 years. Parents are questioned about their child's age at attainment of 25 linguistic (both receptive and expressive) auditory milestones.	**Language Development Survey** (Rescorla 1989) Expressive vocabulary checklist designed for use with the parents of 2-year-old children. Parents indicate which words their children say.
Infant Intentionality Questionnaire (IIQ) Developed by Feldman and Reznick (1996) to assess parental attribution of infant intentionality, broadly defined as the capacity for deliberate action and an awareness of mental states.	**The MacArthur-Bates Communicative Development Inventories (MacArthur CDI)** (Fenson et al 1993) *Infant form* (I) for use with children aged from 0.8 to 1.4. It assesses vocabulary comprehension and expression, and use of gestures. *Toddler form* (II) for use with children aged 1.4–2.6 years. It assesses vocabulary expression and complexity of grammar.

that vocabulary is a more powerful predictor of grammatical development than age or gender.

Recently, short versions of the original CDI have been developed for several languages to be used in research and educational settings, where administration of the complete form is not feasible.

In spite of the validity of parental reports, in the case of children at high risk, or whenever a more precise assessment is required, information provided by parents must be supplemented by structured or semi-structured clinical procedures. In fact, direct observation and recording of the child's responses to a standard set of stimuli provide data which may not be readily seen in a natural setting, and also allow evaluation of children's language abilities out of their everyday context (which is a stronger predictor of subsequent language development) (Bates et al 1988). As outlined in the literature, the early identification of children at risk of language delay requires a valid and reliable diagnostic standard. No single source of information is adequate for assessment, whereas the combination of parental report and direct observation of the child's performance may increase predictive validity (Boyle et al 1996).

Standardized procedures
Standardized direct assessment procedures are therefore needed, though they are time-consuming and present several methodological problems, especially when very young children are being tested. One initial problem is related to the very wide individual variation in performance, and even discontinuities in development, which can be observed with any given language measure up to 24 months of age. A related issue, discussed by Tomblin et al (1996), strictly concerns measurement problems, in particular the type of norm-referenced scores to be employed and the size of the discrepancy between language achievement and chronological or mental age (the cut-off) necessary for determining specific developmental language delay.

More 'naturalistic' methods for the diagnosis of language delay employ quasi-standardized measures of spontaneous speech. These are 'criterion-referenced' procedures using experimental data derived from studies in developmental psycholinguistics, as thoroughly described by Miller (1981). According to several authors, informal but guided observation of the child in a natural communication setting is most appropriate, though standardized interpretative schemes and referenced norms are at present limited.

In Table 10.7 we have selected some standardized scales suitable for the assessment of language in English- and Italian-speaking children.

Receptive language assessment
The aim of this section is not to give a comprehensive review of language tests, but rather to provide some guidelines for the assessment of young children, given the paucity of standardized instruments suitable for children under 3-4 years of age.

It is well known that the assessment of receptive language skills is important, because it is through the detection, discrimination and identification of speech sounds and words, and the interpretation of connected speech (sentences), that the very young child gets access to the language code. Evaluation must therefore be performed according to the following separate (but complementary) developmental steps:

1　Speech perception and attention to acoustic stimuli in a shared highly interactive social context
2　Understanding the meaning of unfamiliar and familiar words (including body parts, onomatopoeia, verbal routines and social games)
3　Understanding the meaning of sentences uttered in a highly familiar context
4　Understanding words and sentences out of context, including semantically implausible utterances
5　Understanding the meanings encoded by relational terms (space and time words) and decoding semantically and syntactically complex structures, relying solely on linguistic-driven (grammatical) information

TABLE 10.7
Some suggested standardized procedures for early language assessment

Tests	Areas of language assessed (language: E = English, I = Italian)	Age range	Description
Peabody Picture Vocabulary Test (PPVT-III) (Dunn and Dunn 1997)	Receptive vocabulary (E)	2.5–18 years	Children are presented with a four-choice picture array and they are required to point to the picture representing the noun or verb spoken by the examiner
Reynell Developmental Language Scales (RDLS-III), Comprehension Scale (Edwards et al 1997)	Receptive vocabulary (E)	1–7 years	The earliest items involve asking parents about the kinds of words the child responds to
RDLS-III, Comprehension Scale (Edwards et al 1997)	Sentence comprehension (E)	1–7 years	In later stages, the child is asked to first pick out a named item from an array, and then to act out commands of increasing complexity
Test of Early Comprehension (TCP) (Chilosi et al 2003)	Sentence comprehension (I)		
RDLS-III, Expressive Scale (Edwards et al 1997)	Expressive vocabulary (E)	1–7 years	The child is asked to name objects and pictures, and to define simple words
Expressive One-Word Picture Vocabulary Test –revised (EOWPVT) (Gardner 1990)	Expressive vocabulary (E)	2–12 years	The child must label black and white line drawings
RDLS-III, Expressive Scale (Edwards et al 1997)	Expressive grammar (E)	1–7 years	Throughout the testing session, the examiner notes down all the spontaneous and provoked language produced by the child. This is analysed for its complexity and structures. The child is also asked to look at pictures, and to tell short stories about pictures
Analysis of free speech samples (CHILDES) (Mac Whinney 1991, Bortolini and Pizzuto 1997)	Expressive grammar (E/I)		

For children below the age of 30 months only the first three stages are consistently attained and must be covered by formal and/or informal testing.

The typical method used for assessing receptive vocabulary is the multiple-choice picture-pointing format, according to which the child is required to select a picture to match a word spoken by the tester (such as the Peabody Picture Vocabulary Test). This method may not give reliable results for normally developing children below the age of 30 months, and its use is often problematic with older children with poor concentration and attention problems (Bishop 1997). In very young or inattentive children receptive vocabulary may be more adequately evaluated by means of parental report such as the CDI. However, the language comprehension inventory is only suitable in the age range from 8 to 18 months of age, because after 18 months parents can no longer keep track of all the words their children know, due to the acceleration of vocabulary growth (lexical burst).

As outlined earlier, language comprehension undergoes significant changes from 18 to 24 months, such that evaluation of the child's understanding of connected speech becomes critical at that stage. Standardized tests are, however, limited and are generally too coarsely grained for describing and analysing the quality of processing strategies children can make use of for decoding syntax. Clinical applications of experimental procedures, as suggested by Miller (1981), are similarly scarce. For English-speaking children one can refer to the study by Miller et al (1980) and to the research on early language development in full-term and preterm infants published by Menyuk et al in 1995.

For Italian-speaking children we have devised an acting-out test similar (with modification) to the one used by Miller et al (1980). The test (called the Test of Early Comprehension (TCP; Chilosi et al 2003)) has been standardized on Italian children aged from 16 to 36 months. It includes 56 items of increasing complexity and the child is required to act-out simple verbal commands in the presence of a set of toys or familiar objects. Complexity varies with respect to sentence length (from one to two and three words), semantic complexity (predictable vs unpredictable or anomalous sentences), agency (child vs object as agent of the action). Normative data are available for five age groups and are expressed in percentiles and standard scores. The test is currently being used in our clinic as part of an assessment protocol suitable for children with language delay and other developmental disorders. It has also been used for research purposes to study language acquisition in focal brain-injured (Chilosi et al 2005) and late talking children (Cipriani et al 2002) and in children who have undergone early cochlear implant.

Alternative methods for testing early comprehension are based on behavioural techniques and experimental paradigms originally developed to study attention and perception in pre-verbal infants. One such method involves the recording of cortical event-related potentials (ERP) and has been used to evaluate word comprehension as well as sentence processing (Molfese 1990, Mills et al 1997).

Another technique, the *preferential looking paradigm*, is based on the evidence that very young children (as young as 14–16 months) will prefer to watch a picture that matches a spoken utterance more than one that does not. To date, the method has been used in a series of experiments which have shed new light on the organizational principles that young

185

children use to interpret their language input (see Hirsh-Pasek and Michnik-Golinkoff 1991 for a review). However, its clinical application is not yet clearly established.

According to Bates et al (1988), before 28 months production tasks which tap into the vocabulary burst (typically occurring between 18 and 24 months) may themselves tap into processes which also involve aspects of comprehension. This assumption supports the idea that reliable and valid measures of expressive language would detect not only children with expressive delay but also the vast majority of those with comprehension problems (Whitehurst and Fischel 1994). The above assumption and the difficulty of testing young children would also explain why few clinical standardized tests of early language comprehension have been developed. However, in children who are delayed in language acquisition, evaluation of comprehension is more informative than evaluation of production, given their limited repertoire of expressive skills. Moreover, follow-up studies of late talking children with language delay persisting beyond 36 months of age indicate that early receptive language skills are one of the most significant predictors of subsequent language outcome.

Assessment of speech and language production

Speech
The assessment of speech development should include observation of the child's speech and articulation skills, examination of the oral speech mechanism for oro-facial abnormalities of the vocal apparatus, and informal testing of oral motor skills by asking the child to imitate simple oral motor gestures (Cantwell and Baker 1987). The absence of any vocalization or spontaneous imitation of sounds by the age of 6 months, and the absence of any babbling involving consonant sounds by the age of 1 year, must be considered as abnormal and warrants fuller investigation.

In order to measure phonological development, Paul and Jennings (1992) suggested computing the number of different consonant types produced during a 10-minute parent–child videotaped interaction. According to the authors the resulting indices (phonetic inventory and consonants to words ratio) are highly informative and allow identification of toddlers with slow expressive language development. The average number of different consonants produced by normal children is about 14 between 18 and 24 months, and about 18 between 24 and 34 months, whereas it is significantly lower in children with language delay.

Vocabulary and grammar
Evaluation of expressive vocabulary and grammar may be performed by means of both informal and formal testing. As outlined by Yule (1987), standardized scales such as the grammatical complexity score of the CDI and the Expressive Scales of the Reynell test are useful for measuring language level, but do not provide any detailed description of grammatical development in terms of syntactic 'stage' (or level).

Spontaneous language sampling in a semi-structured context (play situation) and in the presence of a familiar adult allows evaluation of not only the level of grammatical organization (language form), but also the child's pragmatic, interactive and symbolic skills (language content and use).

The analysis of transcripts can take a number of different directions, depending upon the assessment goals set for the child. After transcribing the adult/child conversation, the clinician usually has a good notion of the child's general productive abilities. Specific analytic procedures should be selected to quantify and document the child's language organization. For English-speaking children, referenced norms are provided by Miller (1981) for both the measurement of mean length of utterances (MLU) and Brown's stage-assignment (Brown 1973). A number of different computational tools have been developed for automatically analysing the transcripts. For cross-linguistic comparisons, the extensive language production databases in the Child Language Data Exchange System (MacWhinney 1991, Bortolini and Pizzuto 1997) are now available.

For Italian children we have developed a system for the coding of free speech samples based on data drawn from a longitudinal study of language acquisition by six normally developing children (Cipriani et al 1993). For each child a level of language development (grammatical score) can be derived from the transcripts according to a six-level rating system ranging from level 0 (pre-linguistic) to level 5 (complex grammar).

According to Edwards et al (1999), 'no test can fully assess every aspect of language; essentially a test must be practical in terms of design and, for screening purposes, sufficiently comprehensive' to be used with children referred for early language delay. In addition, any assessment procedures must also provide some diagnostic indicators of the main areas of difficulty and decision-making criteria for clinical management and follow-up (see Fig. 10.2).

Disorders of communication: early signs of autism

BACKGROUND

Aetiological hypotheses in infantile autism suggest a strong genetic component, as well as possible environmental risks linked to early fetal development; in particular, intrauterine and neonatal factors related to deviant intrauterine growth or fetal distress seem important in the pathogenesis of autism. Moreover several studies have investigated the correlation between pre-, peri- and neonatal factors and autism, suggesting a consistent association with unfavourable events in pregnancy, delivery and the neonatal phase. These include uterine bleeding, prolonged labour and emergency caesarean section, preterm birth (<36 weeks), low birth weight (<2500 g), oxygen requirement and respiratory distress syndrome, rhesus incompatibility, hemolytic anemia, and hyperbilirubinemia (Juul-Dam et al 2001) (see Table 10.8).

However, other studies point out that autism is unlikely to be caused by a single obstetric factor. The increased prevalence of obstetric complications among autism cases is most likely due to the underlying genetic factors or an interaction of these factors with the environment (Glasson et al 2004).

To summarize, children who are at greatly increased risk of cerebral damage have been noted to have a high rate of autistic symptoms, as well as increased chances of

TABLE 10.8

Incidence of pre-, peri- and neonatal factors in autism, PDD-NOS (pervasive developmental disorder not otherwise specified), and general population groups: percentage of affected children

Factor	Authors and groups studied					
	Study 1 (Finegan and Quarrington 1979)		Study 2 (Deykin and MacMahon 1980)		Study 3 (Gillberg and Gillberg 1983)	
	Autistic (*n* = 15)	Siblings (*n* = 15)	Autistic (*n* = 118)	Siblings (*n* = 246)	Autistic (*n* = 25)	Controls (*n* = 25)
Prenatal						
Bleeding	20	7	13	9	44	8
Infection/illness	7	0	16	15	27	8
Oedema			18	18	48	24
Preeclampsia			3	4	12	12
Accident/injury	7	0	4	1		
Use of medication	20	0	44	37	40	16
Weeks' gestation <37 wks	20	13				
<36 wks					48	12
>42 wks					12	0
Perinatal						
Malposition	13	0	13	9	4	8
General anaesthesia	67	40				
Forceps/vacuum extraction	40	53	60	59	12	16
Caesarean section	7	7	8	2		
Cord complications	7	7	18	14	12	16
Amniotic fluid (clear)	27	0			24	4
Prolonged labour	7	0	15	9		
Neonatal						
Low birthweight/small for gestational age	20	7	7	3	12	0
Respiratory distress	20	0			4	4
Oxygen treatment	13	0	20	15	4	0
Low Apgar score/poor condition	20	7	14	8	24	4
Jaundice	20	0	8	9	4	0
Clinical dysmaturity					50	2

Source: Juul-Dam et al 2001.

developing general problems in social communication or cognitive development. Therefore, screening for early signs of autism should be included as part of the follow-up of the developmental trajectory of these high-risk profile infants.

EARLY DIAGNOSIS OF AUTISM

The majority of children with autism spectrum disorders (ASD) are usually identified by 24 months of age. Several factors have contributed to the decrease in the age of referral and diagnosis of autism. First, there has been an increase in recognition of the early features of autism amongst primary healthcare practitioners, and this has led to earlier referral to paediatric and child development specialists. Second, attempts have been made to prospectively identify cases of autism using screening instruments. These have been applied both to general populations (Checklist for Autism in Toddlers – CHAT) and to referred populations (Modified-CHAT; Pervasive Developmental Disorders Screening Test – PDDST). These studies have demonstrated that it is possible to identify some cases of autism by the age of 18 months. Third, there is increasing evidence that appropriately targeted intervention improves outcome in children with ASD in terms of IQ gains and reduction in symptom severity.

Further, it is possible that early intervention might ameliorate the negative secondary consequences of the primary social orienting and communication deficits that characterize ASD. Finally, another impetus for the promotion of earlier identification is the fact that the risk of having a subsequent child with autism is 5 per cent, many times greater than even the highest reported prevalence rate.

TOOLS FOR DETECTION

Most studies have confirmed great stability of symptoms from the second year of life (Gillberg et al 1990, Baron-Cohen et al 1992, Lord 1995) or even from the 20th month (Cox et al 1999). But these studies have also confirmed the difficulties in detecting autism during the first 18 months of life. So we can consider as 'early' the period before 18 months, when autism, in most cases, is considered present but is still not clearly evident.

Specific knowledge on this topic mostly comes from three main sources: retrospective studies based on parental report, home video recordings, and longitudinal studies based on large population-based samples.

Parental report

Retrospective studies based on parental recall report a variety of symptoms in the social and communicative areas under 2 years of age. Consistent with Kanner's early reports (1943), several studies have noted that parents report a pervasive lack of responsiveness at some point in their child's development. Overall interpersonal engagement is diminished such that the child displays less frequency and intensity of eye contact; and he/she uses eye contact less often for referential communication. Moreover, the child is not very cuddly and lacks the range of affective expression, particularly around positive interactions with familiar persons. In some cases, these deficits are reported by parents from early in infancy, and in other cases they are reported to be 'lost' following some period of normal development.

Interestingly, other parental reports converge on a variety of unusual reactivity patterns in their infants, such as hypersensitivities to sound (covers ears to loud noises), lack of response to pain, problems regulating sleep cycles, and perseverative play behaviours. For instance, based on the Early Development Interview which consists of questions about the child's behaviour from birth to 2 years of age, children with autism were reported by Werner et al (2005) to have elevated symptoms in the regulatory domain (difficult to hold/cuddle; exceptionally fussy or easy baby; sleeping and feeding problems; overly sensitive to noise and/or touch) by 3–6 months.

189

However, the most serious factor related to parental concern is the length of the interval between the time when the parents begin to suspect that something is wrong in their young child and the time when they decide to refer the child for a psychiatric consultation. This gap has necessitated a conceptual distinction between age of onset and age of recognition of the symptoms.

Home videos

The retrospective analysis of home videos provides another potential research resource which has confirmed the early emergence of developmental impairments in infants with autism. These are videos taken by parents of their children – later diagnosed as having autism – at an early age, before the child's problems are diagnosed. They are considered as an excellent opportunity for direct observation of the earliest stages of autism development. Up to now they have been the only instrument available to study the actual course of onset of the disorder in infants with autism. Recent research, based on this methodology, has pointed out that diagnosis at 8–12 months is feasible (Baranek 1999, Maestro et al 2001, 2002, 2005), and that consideration of behaviours not previously thought to be diagnostic, such as motor behaviours or basic social skills, may enhance autism identification (Teitelbaum et al 1998). Retrospective video analysis can be considered a valid and eco-logical tool for the identification of early ASD signs (Massie 1977, Losche 1990, Adrien et al 1991, 1993, Grimes and Walker 1994, Osterling and Dawson 1994, Baranek 1999, Maestro et al 1999, Osterling and Dawson 1999, 2000, Osterling et al 2002).

Different studies developed through this methodology have pointed out that young children, later diagnosed as ASD, can be distinguished from typical children with respect to interaction and attachment, social attention, communication, motility and attention, intentional communication and imitative ability. In some of these studies the Behavioral Summarized Evaluation (BSE) scale was used to quantify symptom severity. This scale was developed by Adrien et al (1992) to evaluate the severity of behavioural problems in children with autism. The scale consists of 20 items on a single sheet, easy to handle, and accessible to professionals involved in the assessment of ASD. A total score is obtained in order to have information on the clinical state of the child at the time of observation. The glossary of the scale has been integrated with examples and descriptions from the Infant form of the BSE because of the very young age of infants observed in the home videos. Each infant's behaviour is rated on a 5-point scale, where 0 corresponds to never observed; 1 corresponds to sometimes; 2 corresponds to often; 3 corresponds to very often; and 4 represents a behaviour that is always observed.

The findings from retrospective video analysis allow a more accurate recognition of symptoms compared to retrospective interviews, even if the results seem to confirm parents' concern. In fact most of the infants display signs in the first year of life: some of them from the very beginning (very early onset), others in the second semester of life (early onset). Only a very low percentage are completely symptom-free in the first year of life and become symptomatic in the second year. Moreover most of the studies report a group of more frequently rated items, which constitute a typical symptom constellation charac-terized by item 2 (ignores people), item 3 (poor social interaction), item 4 (difficulties in eye contact), item 5 (does not make effort to communicate with mimic expression and with gestures), item 8 (lack of initiative and hypoactivity), and item 17 (lack of emotional modulation); this constellation suggests a mood disorder. However, a step forward was achieved when research moved from the detection of specific signs of autism towards the search for typically developing behaviours (such as pointing, joint attention, and responding to name).

Table 10.9 summarizes the results of this body of research, focused both on the domain of the specific autistic symptoms and on the domain of the typical behaviours. In particular the table shows the more frequently rated items, which discriminate children with ASD from typical children in the first 18 months of life.

Longitudinal studies
A new approach to early identification is to assess, observe and follow the infant siblings of children with autism and compare their development with that of the siblings of typical and developmentally delayed (but not autistic) children. Because the siblings of children with autism are at greater risk, for genetic reasons, than the siblings of children without

TABLE 10.9
Checklist of signs of autism and social competence which
discriminate autistic infants from typical infants

Symptoms	0–6 months	6–12 months	12–18 months
Is eager for aloneness		x	x
Ignores people		x	x
Poor social interaction	x	x	x
Abnormal eye contact	x	x	x
Does not make an effort to communicate using voice and/or words		x	x
Lack of appropriate facial expressions and gestures	x	x	x
Lack of initiative, hypoactivity	x	x	x
Mood difficulties	x	x	x
Competence			
Syntony	x		
Contact with objects		x	
Orienting to name		x	
Smiling at people			x
Maintaining social engagement		x	x
Simple vocalizing		x	x
Accepting invitation		x	x
Enjoying physical or visual contact with people			x
Pointing		x	
Soliciting social interaction			x
Meaningful vocalization			x
Referential gaze			x

Note: The symbol 'x' indicates the age range in which it is possible to observe the presence of the symptoms and/or the absence of the developmental competence autism, the assumption behind this methodology is that some of the siblings of children with autism will develop either autism or the broader autism phenotype later in childhood. If that occurs, the early behaviours of the children who develop autism can be contrasted with behaviours of infants who show typical development.

Preliminary results of a study using this new methodology (Zwaigenbaum et al 2005) indicate that by 12 months of age, siblings who are later diagnosed with autism may be distinguished from other siblings and low-risk controls on the basis of: (1) several specific behavioural markers, including atypicalities in eye contact and visual tracking, disengagement of visual attention, orienting to name, imitation, social smiling, reactivity, social interest and affect, and sensory-oriented behaviours; (2) prolonged latency to disengage visual attention; (3) a characteristic pattern of early temperament, with marked passivity and decreased activity level at 6 months, a tendency to fixate on particular objects in the environment, and decreased expression of positive affect by 12 months; and (4) delayed expressive and receptive language.

Studies of infants siblings of children with autism may have the most potential for teaching us about early deficiencies in autism, even if they are very difficult to conduct.

Conclusions

As already pointed out, language and communication are the foundations of human relations and of cognitive development; they are biologically constrained but need strong social support. They are early-onset functions but have a rather protracted course, with age-dependent variable degrees of plasticity but also vulnerability to many different adverse conditions. This may explain why possible language delay is the concern most commonly raised by parents in the 18 to 36 months age period. It always warrants careful diagnostic investigation, because at that age language is one of the most sensitive indicators and the commonest 'surface' manifestation of quite diverse paraphysiological or frankly pathological conditions. Therefore:

- Assessment of high-risk newborns in the first two years of life must be multi-dimensional.
- It requires information from multiple sources.
- One single diagnostic observation may be poorly informative, given the wide inter-individual variability in the pace and style of acquisition; this means that repeated evaluations during the most 'critical' stages of development are needed.
- Hearing defects and possible communication disorders due to autism must be ruled out.

Fig. 10.2 shows a decision tree based on an outline of the diagnosis and follow-up of children with language delay from the perspective of reducing long-term risks.

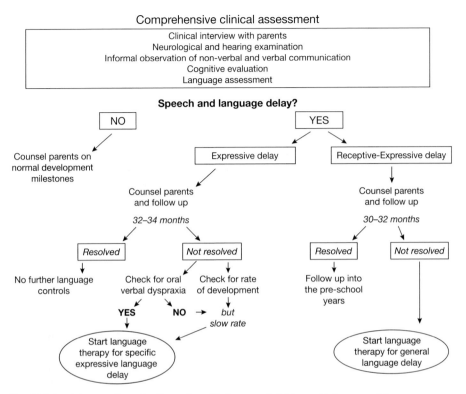

Fig. 10.2 Decision tree for early diagnosis and follow-up of children with language delay.

REFERENCES

Adrien JL, Faure M, Perrot A, Haumery L, Garreau B, Barthelemy C, Sauvage D (1991) Autism and family HM: preliminary findings. *J Autism Dev Disabil* 21: 43–49.

Adrien JL, Barthelemy C, Perrot A (1992) Validity and reliability of the infant behavioral summarized evaluation (IBSE): a rating scale for the assessment of young children with autism and developmental disorders. *J Autism Dev Disord* 22: 375–394.

Adrien JL, Lenoir P, Martineau J, Perot A, Hameury L, Larmande C, Sauvage D (1993) Blind ratings of early symptoms of autism based upon family HM. *J Am Acad Child Adolesc Psychiatry* 33: 617–625.

American National Standards Institute (1991) Hearing handicap as a function of average hearing threshold level of the better ear. In: Northern JL, Downs MP, editors. *Hearing in Children*. Baltimore, MD: Williams & Wilkins, pp 98–99.

American Psychiatric Association (1994) *Diagnostic and Statistical Manual of Mental Disorders, 4th edition* (DSM-IV). Washington, DC: APA.

Arslan E, Conti G (1994) I potenziali evocati troncoencefalici (ABR) nella diagnosi delle ipoacusie infantili. *Audiologia Italiana* 11: 210–223.

Arslan E, Prosse S, Conti G, Michelini S (1983) Electrocochleography and brainstem potentials in the diagnosis of the deaf child. *Int J Otorhinolaryngol* 5: 251–259.

Arslan E, Turrini M, Lupi G, Genovese E, Orzan E (1997) Hearing threshold assessment with auditory brainstem response (ABR) and electrocochleography (EcochG) in uncooperative children. *Scand Audiol* 26: 32–37.

Baranek GT (1999), Autism during infancy: a retrospective video analysis of sensory-motor and social behaviours at 9–12 months of age. *J Autism Dev Disord* 29: 213–224.

Baron-Cohen S, Allen J, Gillberg C (1992) Can autism be detected at 18 months? The needle, the haystack, and the CHAT. *Br J Psychiatry* 138: 839–843.

Bates E, Bretherton I, Snyder L (1988) *From First Words to Grammar*. Cambridge: Cambridge University Press.

Bates E, Thal D, Janowsky J (1992) Early language development and its neural correlates. In: Rapin I, Segalowitz S, editors. *Handbook of Neuropsychology. Vol 7 Child Neuropsychology*. Amsterdam: Elsevier, pp 69–110.

Bayley N (1969) *Bayley Scales of Infant Development*. New York: The Psychological Corporation..

Bishop DVM (1997) *Uncommon Understanding. Development and Disorders of Language Comprehension in Children*. Hove, UK: Psychology Press, pp 86–87.

Bloom L, Lahey E (1978) *Language Development and Language Disorders*. New York: John Wiley & Sons, pp 67–97.

Bortolini U, Pizzuto E, editors (1997) *Il Progetto CHILDES Italia*. Tirrenia (Pisa): Edizioni del Cerro.

Boyle J, Gillham B, Smith N (1996) Screening for early language delay in the 18–36 month age-range: the predictive validity of tests of production, and implications for practice. *Child Lang Teach Ther* 12: 113–127.

Bridges A (1980) SVO comprehension strategies reconsidered – the evidence of individual patterns of response. *J Child Lang* 7: 89–104.

Brown R (1973) *A First Language*. Cambridge, MA: Harvard University Press.

Cantwell DP, Baker L (1987) *Developmental Speech and Language Disorders*. London: Guilford Press, pp 40–45.

Capute AJ, Accardo PJ (1978) Linguistic and auditory milestones during the first two years of life. *Clin Pediatr* 17: 847–853.

Capute AJ, Palmer FB, Shapiro BK, Wachtel RC, Schmidt S, Ross A (1986) Clinical Linguistic and Auditory Milestone Scale: prediction of cognition in infancy. *Dev Med Child Neurol* 28: 762–771.

Caselli MC, Casadio P (1995) *Il primo vocabolario del bambino: guida all'uso del questionario MacArthur per la valutazione della comunicazione e del linguaggio nei primi anni di vita* [The child's first words: guide for the use of the MacArthur questionnaire for assessing communication and language in the first years of life]. Milan: Franco Angeli.

Chapman RS (1978) Comprehension strategies in children: a discussion of Bransford and Nitsch's paper. In: Kavanagh J, Strange W, editors. *Speech and Language in the Laboratory, School and Clinic*. Cambridge, MA: MIT Press, pp 308–327.

Chilosi AM, Cipriani P, Villani S, Pfanner L (2003) Capire giocando: uno strumento per la valutazione verbale precoce (TCVP). Technical Report, Italian National Research Council, CNR002D39-004.

Chilosi AM, Pecini C, Cipriani P, Brovedani P, Brizzolara D, Ferretti G, Pfanner L, Cioni G (2005) Atypical language lateralization and early linguistic development in children with focal brain lesions. *Dev Med Child Neurol* 47: 725–730.

Cipriani P, Chilosi AM, Bottari P, Pfanner L (1993) *L'acquisizione della morfosintassi in Italiano: fasi e processi*. Padova: Unipress.

Cipriani P, Chilosi AM, Pfanner L, Villani S, Bottari P (2002) Il ritardo del linguaggio in età precoce: profili evolutivi ed indici di rischio. In: Caselli MC, Capirci O, editors. *Indici di rischio nel primo sviluppo del linguaggio: ricerca, clinica, educazione*. Milano: Franco Angeli, pp 95–108.

Conti G, Arslan E, Camurri L, Prosser S (1984) Elettrocochleografia e ABR in audiologia infantile. Comparazione dei risultati nelle determinazioni di soglia. *Acta Otorhinol Ital* 4: 655.

Coplan J (1987) *The Early Language Milestones Scale*. Austin, TX: Pro-Ed.

Cox A, Klein K, Charman T, Baird G, Baron-Cohen S, Swettenham J, Drew A, Wheelwright S (1999) Autism spectrum disorders at 20 and 42 months of age: stability of clinical and ADI-R diagnosis. *J Child Psychol Psychiatry* 40(5): 719–732.

Dalla Piccola B, Mingarelli R, Gennarelli M (1996) Aspetti genetici della sordità. *Acta Otorhinol Ital* 16: 79–90.

Dallos P (1975) Electrical correlates of mechanical events in the cochlea. *Audiology* 14: 408.

Davidovitch M, Glick L, Holtzman G, Tirosh E, Safir MP (2000) Developmental regression in autism: maternal perception. *J Aut Dev Disord* 30: 113–119.

Davis A (1976). Brainstem and other responses in electric response audiometry. *Ann Otol* 85: 3–13.

Davis A, Wood S, Healy R, Webb H, Rowe S (1995) Risk factors for hearing disorders: epidemiologic evidence of change over time in the UK. *J Am Acad Audiol* 6: 365–370.

Dehaene-Lambertz G, Dehaene S, Hertz Pannier L (2002) Functional neuroimaging of speech perception in infants. *Science* 298: 2013–2016.

194

Denoyelle F, Lina-Granade G, Plauchu H, Bruzzone R, Chaib H, Levi-Acobas F, Weil D, Petit C (1998) Cx 26 gene linked to a dominant deafness. *Nature* 393: 319–320.

Deykin EY, MacMahon B (1980) Pregnancy, delivery, and neonatal complications among autistic children. *Am J Disabled Child* 134: 860–864.

Dunn LM, Dunn LM (1997) *Peabody Picture Vocabulary Test – PPVT, 3rd edition.* Circle Pines, MN: American Guidance Service Inc.

Edwards S, Garman M, Hughes A, Letts C, Sinka I (1997) *Reynell Developmental Language Scales 3.* University of Reading edition. Windsor: NFER-Nelson.

Edwards S, Garman M, Hughes A, Letts C, Sinka I (1999) Assessing the comprehension and production of language in young children: an account of the Reynell Developmental Language Scales 3. *Int J Lang Commun Disord* 34: 151–171.

Eggermont JJ (1976) Electrocochleography. In: Keidel WD, Neff WD, editors. *Handbook of Sensory Physiology: Auditory System.* Berlin: Springer Verlag, pp 625–705.

Estivill X, Fortin P, Surrey S, Rabionet R, Melchionda S, D'Agruma L, Mansfield E, Rappaport E (1998) Cx-26 mutations in sporadic and inherited sensorineural deafness. *Lancet* 351: 394–398.

Feldman R, Reznick JS (1996) Maternal perception of infant intentionality at 4 and 8 months. *Infant Behav Dev* 19: 483–496.

Fenson L, Dale PS, Reznick JS, Thal D, Bates E, Hartung JP, Pethick S, Reilly JS (1993) *Mac Arthur Communicative Development Inventories: User's Guide and Technical Manual.* San Diego: Singular Publishing Group.

Finegan JA, Quarrington B (1979) Pre, peri and neonatal factors and infantile autism. *J Child Psychol Psychiatry* 20: 119–128.

Fortnum H, Davis A (1997) Epidemiology of permanent childhood hearing impairment in Trent region, 1985–1993. *Br J Audiol* 31: 409–446.

Frankenburg WK, Goldstein AD, Camp B (1971) The revised Denver Developmental Screening Test: its accuracy as a screening instrument. *J Pediatr* 79: 988.

Gardner MF (1990) *Expressive One-Word Picture Vocabulary Test – Revised (EOWPVT).* Novato, CA: Academic Therapy Publications.

Gerard K (1986) The Checklist of Communicative Competence. Available from the author (3 Perry Mansions, 113 Catford Hill, London SE6).

Gillberg C, Gillberg IC (1983) Infantile autism: a total population study of reduced optimality in the pre, peri and neonatal period. *J Autism Dev Disord*.13: 153–166.

Gillberg C, Ehlers S, Schaumann H, Jakibsson G, Dahlgren SO, Lindblom R, Bagenholm A, Tjuus T, Bloinder E (1990) Autism under age 3 years: a clinical study of 28 cases referred for autistic symptoms in infancy. *J Child Psychol Psychiatry* 31: 921–934.

Glasson EJ, Bower C, Petterson B, de Klerk N, Chaney G, Hallmayer JF (2004) Perinatal factors and the development of autism: a population study. *Arch Gen Psychiatry* 61: 618–627.

Gorga MP, Reiland JK, Beauchaine KA, Worthington DW, Jesteadt W (1987) Auditory brainstem response from graduates of an intensive care nursery: normal patterns of response. *J Speech Hear Res* 30: 311–318.

Griffiths R (1970) *The Abilities of Babies.* London: University of London Press.

Grimes K, Walker EF (1994) Childhood emotional expressions, educational attainment, and age at onset of illness in schizophrenia. *J Abnorm Psychol* 103: 784–790.

Hirsh-Pasek K, Michnik-Golinkoff R (1991) Language comprehension: a new look at some old themes. In: Krasnegor N, Rumbaugh D, Studdert-Kennedy M, Schiefelbusch R, editors. *Biological and Behavioural Aspects of Language Acquisition.* Hillsdale, NJ: Lawrence Erlbaum Associates, pp 301–320.

ICD-10 (1992) ICD-10 Classification of Mental and Behavioural Disorders: Conversion tables between ICD-8, ICD-9 and ICD-10. Geneva: World Health Organization.

Joint Committee on Infant Hearing (1982) Position statement. *Pediatrics* 70: 496–497.

Joint Committee on Infant Hearing (2000) High risk register. Principles and guidelines for early intervention programs: Year 2000 position statement.

Juul-Dam N, Townsend J, Courchesne E (2001) Prenatal, perinatal, and neonatal factors in autism, pervasive developmental disorder – not otherwise specified, and the general population. *Pediatrics* 107: 63.

Kanner L (1943) Autistic disturbances of affective contact. *Nerv Child* 2: 217–250.

Kelsell DP, Dunlop J, Stevens HP, Lench HJ, Liang JN, Parry G, Mueller RF, Leigh IM (1997) Cx 26 mutations in hereditary non-syndromic sensorineural deafness. *Nature* 387: 80–83.

Kiang NYS, Watanabe T, Thomas EC, Clarck LF (1965) *Discharge Patterns of Single Fibres in the Cat's Auditory Nerve.* Cambridge, MA: MIT Press.

195

Lelord G, Barthélémy C, Adrien JL, Lancrenons S, Sauvage D (1987) L'échelle ERC (Evaluation Résumée du Comportement). Problèmes techniques, psychopathologiques et sociologiques suscités par la publication française d'une échelle d'évaluation quantitative des symptomes autistiques chez l'enfant. In: Grémy F, Tomkiewicz S, Ferrari P, Lelord G, editors. *Autisme infantile*. Paris: INSERM, 147, pp 311–316.

Lord C (1995) Follow-up of two-year-olds referred for possible autism. *J Child Psychol Psychiatry* 36: 1365–1382.

Losche G (1990) Sensorimotor and action development in autistic children from infancy to early childhood. *J Child Psychol Psychiatry* 31: 749–761.

MacWhinney B (1991) *The CHILDES Project: Tools for Analyzing Talk*. Hillsdale, NJ: Lawrence Erlbaum Associates.

MacWhinney B (1997) *The CHILDES Project: Tools for Analyzing Talk* (in Italian). Pizzuto E, Bortolini U, editors. Tirrenia: Edizioni Il Cerro.

Maestro S, Casella C, Milone A, Muratori F, Palacio-Espasa F (1999) Study of the onset of autism through home-movies. *Psychopathology* 32: 292–300.

Maestro S, Muratori F, Barbieri F, Casella C, Cattaneo V, Cavallaro MC, Cesari C, Milone A, Rizzo L, Viglione V, Stern D, Palacio-Espasa F (2001) Early behavioural development in autistic children: the first 2 years of life through HM. *Psychopathology* 34: 147–152.

Maestro S, Muratori F, Cavallaro MC, Pei F, Stern D, Golse B, Palacio-Espasa F (2002) Attentional skills during the first 6 months of age in autism spectrum disorders. *J Am Acad Child Adolesc Psychiatry* 41: 1239–1245.

Maestro S, Muratori F, Cesari A, Cavallaro MC, Paziente A, Pecini C, Grassi C, Manfredi A, Sommario C (2005) Course of autism signs in the first year of life. *Psychopathology* 38: 26–31.

Massie HN (1977) Patterns of mother–infant interaction in home-movies of psychotic and normal infants. *Am J Psychiatry* 135: 1371–1374.

Mehl A, Thomson V (1998) Newborn hearing screening: the great omission. *Pediatrics* 101: E4–.

Menyuk P (1988) *Language Development: Knowledge and Use*. New York: HarperCollins.

Menyuk P, Liebergott JW, Schulz MC (1995) *Early Language Development in Full-term and Premature Infants*. Hillsdale, NJ: Lawrence Erlbaum Associates.

Miller JF (1981) *Assessing Language Production in Children*. Austin, TX: Pro-Ed.

Miller JF, Chapman RS, Branston M, Reichle I (1980) Comprehension development in sensorimotor stages 5 and 6. *J Speech Hear Res* 23: 284–311.

Mills DL, Coffey-Corina SA, Neville HJ (1997) Language comprehension and cerebral specialization from 13 to 20 months. *Dev Neuropsychol* 13: 397–445.

Molfese D (1990) Auditory evoked responses recorded from 16-month-old human infants to words they did not know. *Brain Lang* 38: 345–363.

Moore EJ (1983) *Bases of Auditory Brain-stem Auditory Evoked Responses*. New York: Grune and Stratton.

Osterling J, Dawson G (1994) Early recognition of children with autism: a study of first birthday home videotapes. *J Autism Dev Disord* 24: 247–257.

Osterling J, Dawson G (1999) Early identification of one-year-old with autism versus mental retardation. Poster presented at the 1999 meeting of the Society of Research in Child Development, Albuquerque, NM.

Osterling J, Dawson G (2000) Brief report: Recognition of autism spectrum disorder before one year of age: a retrospective study based on home-videotapes. *J Autism Dev Disord* 30: 157–162.

Osterling JA, Dawson G, Munson JA (2002) Early recognition of 1-year-old infants with autism spectrum disorder versus mental retardation. *Dev Psychopathol* 14: 239–251.

Pabla HS, McCormick B, Gibbin KP (1991) Retrospective study of the prevalence of bilateral sensorineural deafness in childhood. *Int J Pediatr Otorhinolaryngol* 22: 161–165.

Parving A, Stephens D (1997) Profound hearing impairment in childhood: causative factors in two European countries. *Acta Otolaryngol* 117: 158–160.

Paul R, Jennings P (1992) Phonological behaviour in toddlers with slow expressive language development. *J Speech Hear Res* 35: 99–107.

Rescorla L (1989) The Language Development Survey: a screening tool for delayed language in toddlers. *J Speech Hear Disord* 54: 587–599.

Reznick JS, Schwartz BB (2001) When is an assessment an intervention? Parent perception of infant intentionality and language. *J Am Acad Child Adolesc Psychiatry* 40: 11–18.

Roizen NJ (1999) Etiology of hearing loss in children. Nongenetic causes. *Paediatr Clin North Am* 46: 49–64.

Rutter M (1972) Clinical assessment of language disorders in the young child. In: Rutter M, Martin JAM. *The Child with Delayed Speech*. London: William Heinemann Medical Books Ltd, pp 33–47.

Rutter M (1987) Assessment of language disorders. In: Jule W, Rutter M, editors. *Language Development and Disorders*. London: Mac Keith Press, pp 295–311.

Slobin DI (1985) Introduction: why study language crosslinguistically? In: Slobin DI, editor. *The Crosslinguistic Study of Language Acquisition. Vol 1. The Data Mahwah*. Hillsdale, NJ: Lawrence Erlbaum Associates, pp 3–24.

Stach B (1998) Central auditory disorders. In: Lalwani A, Grundfast K, editors. *Pediatric Otology and Neurotology*. Philadelphia: Lippincott-Raven, pp 378–396.

Teitelbaum P, Teitelbaum O, Nye J, Fryman J, Maurer RG (1998) Movement analysis in infancy may be useful for early diagnosis in autism. *Proc Natl Acad Sci USA* 95: 1392–1397.

Tomblin JB, Records NL, Zhang X (1996) A system for diagnosis of Specific Language Impairment in kindergarten children. *J Speech Hear Res* 39: 1284–1294.

Vartainien E, Kemppinen P, Karjalainen S (1997) Prevalence of bilateral sensorineural hearing impairment in a Finnish childhood population. *Int J Pediatr Otorhinolaryngol* 41: 175–185.

Vihman MM, Macken MA, Miller R, Simmons H, Miller J (1985) From babbling to speech: a reassessment of the continuity issue. *Language* 61: 395–443.

Werner E, Dawson G, Munson J, Osterling J, (2005) Variation in early developmental course in autism and its relation with behavioral outcome at 3–4 years of age. *J Autism Dev Disord* 35: 337–350.

Whitehurst GJ, Fischel JE (1994) Practitioner review: Early developmental language delay: what, if anything, should the clinician do about it? *J Child Psychol Psychiatry* 35: 613–648.

Yule W (1987) Psychological assessment. In: Jule W, Rutter M, editors. *Language Development and Disorders*. London: Mac Keith Press, pp 317–320.

Zwaigenbaum L, Bryson S, Rogers T, Roberts W, Brian J, Szatmari P (2005) Behavioral manifestations of autism in the first year of life. *Int J Dev Neurosci* 23(2–3): 143–152.

11
DEVELOPMENT OF VISION AND VISUAL ATTENTION

Anthony Norcia and Francesca Pei

Introduction

The visual system of the human infant is highly immature at birth and undergoes an extensive period of postnatal development. As the retina and visual cortex mature, so too does infant cognition and it is sometimes difficult to separate the development of one from the other. The goal of this chapter is to review, in a succinct fashion, the major developmental trends in vision and visual attention during infancy, and to consider their possible interaction. Recent reviews of each of these fields considered separately are already available (Atkinson 2000, Colombo 2001, Hopkins and Johnson 2003, Norcia and Manny 2003, Richards, 2003b).

Methodology plays a central role in all discussions of visual development. Because infants cannot be instructed and can give no direct report of their perceptual experience, researchers in this area must rely on specialized behavioural testing procedures or on oculomotor, psychophysiological and electrophysiological techniques. In this review, we focus on electrophysiological studies of early and mid-level visual processing mechanisms and the development of low-level forms of visual attention, such as arousal and orienting. It is inevitable that the distinction between vision and attention is somewhat blurred as we discuss higher-level visual processing. The hierarchy of processing stages which organizes this chapter is shown in Fig. 11.1.

The hierarchy of visual processing

We divide visual processing into three stages – early, middle and late – which correspond roughly with both anatomical distance from the retina and complexity of visual processing. Early vision mechanisms extract image contrast and temporal change, producing local estimates of orientation, direction of motion, spatial scale and disparity. Refined estimates of these quantities are first available in striate cortex, but rough tuning for orientation and direction of motion exists at lower levels (Xu et al 2002). As early vision gives way to middle vision, local measurements of image features such as line orientation are integrated across space into more extended representations of borders and surfaces. The content of the representation at the level of middle vision includes information regarding the shape of extended contours, figure/ground relationships, the symmetry of objects, surface depths, but not the identity of the objects in the scene.

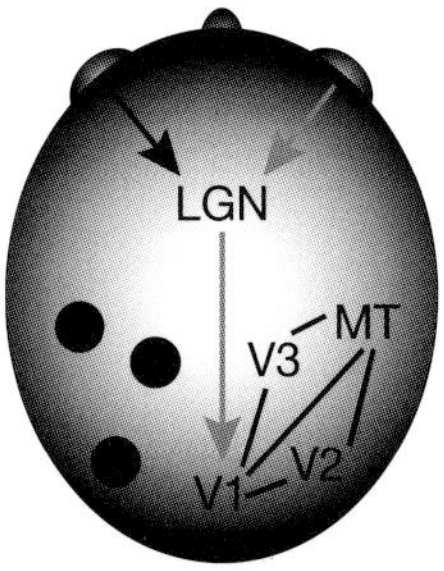

Visual Hierarchy

	Early	Middle	Late
Attributes	Contrast Color Disparity Direction Speed Orientation	Collinearity Symmetry Figure/Ground Occlusion Texture Depth Shape	Object category Object recognition Visual memory
Where	Retina, LGN, V1	V1-Vn	Fusiform Face Area Lateral Occipital Complex Temporal Lobe
When	Up to 100 msec	100 to 200 msec	After 150 msec

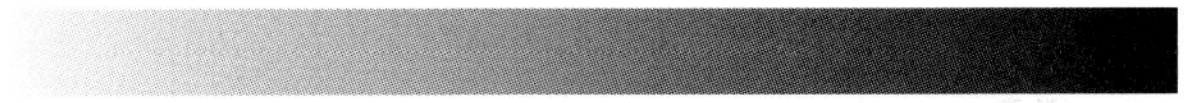

Attentional Modulation Strength

Fig. 11.1 The visual processing hierarchy. The left section of the figure shows a schematic diagram of the visual system. Information originating in the retina is fed to the lateral geniculate nucleus (LGN) and then on to the striate cortex (V1). V1 is shown to project to extra-striate cortical areas V2, V3 and MT. Lines with arrows indicate feed-forward connections, lines without arrows indicate reciprocal connections between areas. The VEP monitors activity in the different areas which is passively conducted through the brain, skull and scalp where it is measured with surface electrodes. The right section shows a conceptual hierarchy of visual processing broken down into early, middle and late processing stages. Each stage is largely responsible for certain stimulus attributes, has an anatomical locus and a largely sequential timing relationship to the onset of a stimulus. The shaded bar indicates the degree to which attention can modulate activity, with darker shading indicating greater modulation.

Middle vision is thought to begin in striate cortex and extend into both first-tier (V2, V3, V4, MT) and second-tier extra-striate visual areas such as V3a (see Allbright and Stoner 2002 for review). The identification of objects (object recognition) involves not only visual perception, but memory and category specificity (e.g. identification of faces and various types of objects) and is conceptualized as occurring in higher-order visual and visual association areas functionally associated with 'late vision' (see Grill-Spector et al 2001).

The effects of visual attention on simple stimuli such as checkerboards can be seen as early as striate cortex, but appear to be stronger at progressively higher levels of the visual hierarchy (Schwartz et al 2005). More complex stimuli which are processed outside of striate cortex, such as coherent motion (Rees et al 1997), show strong effects of attention. This increasing gradient of attentional modulation is schematized by the shaded bar in Fig. 11.1. The study of attention in infancy is particularly difficult since only limited means are available for cueing attention to specific aspects of a visual task. We will therefore concentrate on lower-level forms of visual attention which are 'reflexive' or involuntary to a substantial degree.

199

The development of early vision

Of all the levels of processing, early vision has received the most attention. Within early vision, the development of sensitivity to visual contrast as a function of spatial frequency (image element size) has been the most thoroughly studied. Across all techniques, contrast sensitivity improves during infancy and the improvement is greatest for high spatial frequencies (Norcia et al 1990, Peterzell et al 1993, 1995, Hainline and Abramov 1997).

Fig. 11.2 plots the development of contrast sensitivity at several spatial frequencies determined by the swept-parameter VEP (Norcia et al 1990). Sensitivity is highest at low spatial frequencies at all ages due to the use of gratings that were reversing in contrast at 6 Hz. Development is most marked for the highest spatial frequencies, with low spatial frequency sensitivity showing little additional development beyond 10–12 weeks. High spatial frequency sensitivity can also be studied by measuring grating acuity – the highest resolvable spatial frequency.

Fig. 11.3 plots results of six studies of grating acuity development which have used the spatial frequency sweep VEP (Norcia and Tyler 1985, Norcia et al 1990, Sokol et al 1992, Allen et al 1996, Auestad et al 1997, Birch et al 1998). Grating acuity develops linearly as a function of age, up to around 8 months of age, in each of the studies. By this age, grating acuity is about a factor of two lower than that of the adult. The development of grating acuity can be approximately modelled by developmental changes in cone density and the size of receptive fields in V1 (Jacobs and Blakemore 1988, Wilson 1993).

Resolving image features is a critical first step in visual processing. An essential second step is encoding the relative position and orientation of different features. The

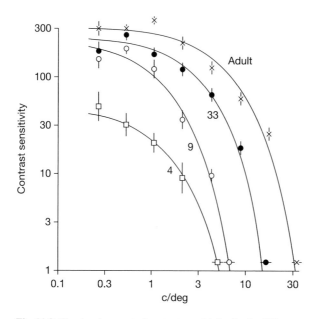

Fig. 11.2 The development of contrast sensitivity for the 6 Hz pattern reversal VEP (Norcia et al 1990).

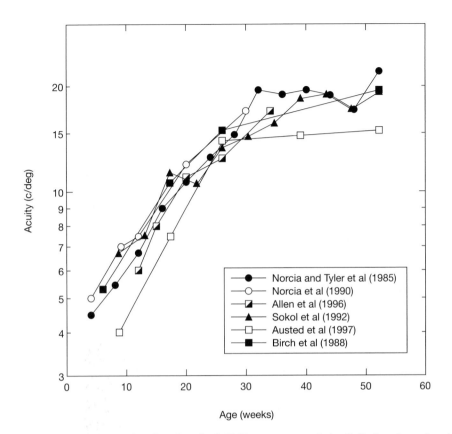

Fig. 11.3 Grating acuity as a function of age for 5–10 Hz pattern reversal stimuli. Each study employed the swept spatial frequency technique. Acuity growth functions are similar across studies, with acuity increasing from 4–6 cpd in 1-month-olds to around 15–20 cpd around 8 months of age. Data are re-plotted from Norcia and Tyler (1985) – filled circles; Norcia et al (1990) – open circles; Allen et al (1996) – half-filled squares; Sokol et al (1992) – triangles; Auestad et al (1997) – open squares; Birch et al (1988) – filled squares.

Source: Norcia and Manny 2003.

development of relative position sensitivity has been most extensively studied using vernier offset targets.

Vernier acuity measures the ability to discriminate the relative position of different components of a visual pattern (Westheimer 1975). In this task the individual is required to discriminate lines that are perfectly aligned, from lines that are offset. During normal development, vernier acuity develops significantly later than grating acuity, suggesting that the two functions are limited by different visual mechanisms. Vernier offset sensitivity (i.e. vernier acuity) shows a more prolonged developmental sequence than does grating acuity, as can be seen in Fig. 11.4 which plots VEP vernier acuity and grating acuity development through adulthood for VEP (Skoczenski and Norcia 2002) and behavioural measures (Zanker et al 1992, Carkeet et al 1997).

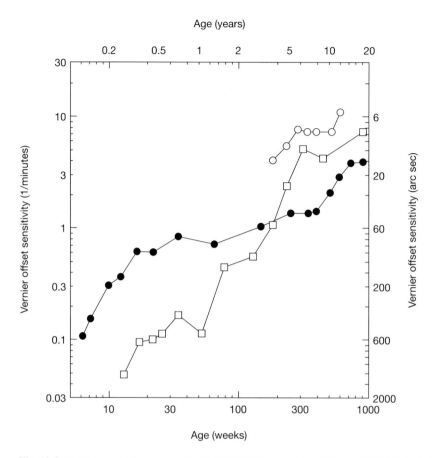

Fig. 11.4 Development of vernier acuity. Both VEP (Skoczenski and Norcia 2002, filled circles) and behavioural data (Carkeet et al 1997, open circles; Zanker et al 1992, open squares) show development into adolescence. Vernier sensitivity is plotted in inverse minutes.

Vernier offsets are one of the primary cues used to segment objects from their backgrounds, and studies of vernier offset sensitivity provide the gateway to understanding the first stages of object processing. Object processing begins with segmentation of the object from its background. Cells in macaque monkey occipital areas V1 and V2 are highly sensitive to vernier breaks (Grosof et al 1993, Marcus and Van Essen 2002) and appear capable of at least crude forms of figure/ground segmentation. Figure/ground-related activity in V1 appears to be the result of feedback from higher-level visual areas (Lamme et al 1999, Lee and Mumford 2003), suggesting that vernier offset detection may engage both early and middle-level mechanisms. The involvement of higher-level visual areas may contribute to the relatively late development of vernier acuity, since it is thought that cortical development proceeds forward from the occipital pole (Landing et al 2002).

The development of middle vision

Mid-level or 'middle' vision centres on the processes by which local measurements of orientation, motion, colour, spatial frequency and disparity are integrated over larger areas of the visual field. At this level of processing, the perceptual organization of the visual image begins to emerge: representations of borders and surface relationships have emerged, along with depth relationships and estimates of shape.

The development of texture processing

The most studied mid-level visual function in the adult VEP literature is texture segmentation (Bach and Meigen 1992, Lamme et al 1992, Bach and Meigen 1998, Caputo and Casco 1999). Textures are spatially homogeneous patterns which typically contain repeated structures, often with some random variation (e.g. random positions, orientations or colours). Textures are deformed systematically by the volumetric shape of an object or by the layout of a surface. These deformations thus provide powerful cues for segmenting objects from their backgrounds and for shape recognition.

The perception of texture-defined forms is limited by the ability to extract the appropriate image statistics, to integrate these statistics across scales and to resolve or segment the shape that is represented. Two behavioural studies of texture discrimination in infants (Sireteanu and Rieth 1992, Rieth and Sireteanu 1994) found that texture segmentation based on line-orientation emerges at 9 to 12 months of age, becoming adult-like around school age. In contrast, another study (Atkinson and Braddick 1992) found discrimination of orientation-defined forms as early as 14–18 weeks.

We studied the ability of very young infants to encode the difference between organized textures and random stimuli using the VEP (Norcia et al 2005). We chose to not study figure/ground segmentation in the hope of being able to tap the most primitive level of global sensitivity – the extraction of a difference in the orientation statistics between patterns. To do this we used simple textures comprised of Gabor patches. Gabor patches are small, localized patches of sine wave luminance gratings (see Fig. 11.5). They are both local in space (location) and in spatial frequency (a single spatial scale) and have a definite orientation. By varying the overall orientation of the Gabor patches we could test, using the VEP, whether differences in the orientation statistics of different Gabor-defined textures were encoded by the infant visual system.

In a first experiment, we alternated a texture comprised of vertically oriented Gabor patches with a second texture comprised of the same number of randomly oriented patches (see Fig. 11.5). Responses in this condition were compared to those from a matched sequence of random-image updates. Fig. 11.6 shows response waveforms for 2- to 4-month-olds and 5- to 9-month-olds. Both infant groups showed bifid positivities at Oz after each image update (latencies of 100–200 ms). For the random/random sequence, the major negativity was at nearly 300 ms for the younger group. The responses in the organized/random condition contained a slow component superimposed on the basic waveform of the control condition. The difference potential between the text and control conditions consisted almost entirely of a sinusoid with a period equal to that of the full image sequence. The significant difference potentials in this first experiment suggested that the infant's

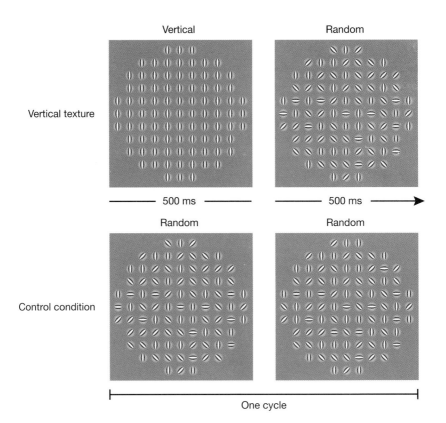

Fig. 11.5 Stimuli used to elicit texture VEPs (Norcia et al 2005). In the test condition (top), a set of vertically aligned Gabor patches was alternated with the same number of randomly oriented patches. These responses were compared to a control condition consisting of alternations between two randomly oriented sets of patches.

visual system can encode the difference in orientation statistics between the organized and random Gabor fields. There was, however, the possibility that local, orientation-specific adaptation could underlie the difference potential, since the vertical texture is presented over half of the duration of the stimulus.

In a second experiment (Norcia et al 2005), we again measured responses to an organized texture comprised of many Gabor patches of the same orientation, alternated with images containing the same number of patches, but all of random orientation. In the test condition, a pattern in which the Gabor patches all had the same orientation was alternated with a pattern in which the orientations were randomized but, unlike the first experiment, the global orientation of the single orientation images was changed each time a new alternation occurred. Responses in the test condition were compared with a control condition consisting of alternation between two independently random configurations. Locally both test and control conditions comprised a random sequence of orientation changes.

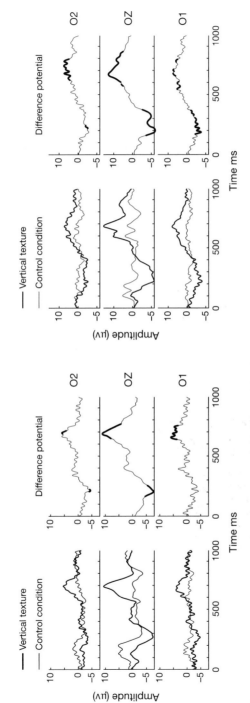
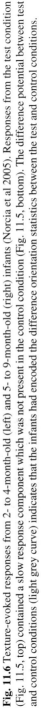

Fig. 11.6 Texture-evoked responses from 2- to 4-month-old (left) and 5- to 9-month-old (right) infants (Norcia et al 2005). Responses from the test condition (Fig. 11.5, top) contained a slow response component which was not present in the control condition (Fig. 11.5, bottom). The difference potential between test and control conditions (light grey curve) indicates that the infants had encoded the difference orientation statistics between the test and control conditions.

We found significant differences between test and control waveforms at 8.8 to 18.4 and 25.4 to 30.7 weeks old, although the difference between test and control conditions was smaller than in the first experiment. We thus concluded that infants can encode a difference in orientation statistics no later than 8 weeks of age. This age of onset agrees with other VEP estimates of the onset of orientation selectivity (Braddick et al 1986, Manny 1992).

The development of contour integration

The pattern of orientation changes along the borders of objects provides a strong cue for shape. Orientation changes relatively slowly along the borders of objects and the detection of orientation changes is thus critical for determining the shape of objects (Geisler et al 2001, Elder and Goldberg 2002). This process is often referred to as 'contour integration'.

Contour integration has been extensively studied in adults using a variety of psychophysical tasks (Field et al 1993, Kovacs and Julesz 1993, Kovacs et al 1999, 2000, Geisler et al 2001). One of the most widely used approaches to the study of contour integration is the use of artificial contours comprised of strings of Gabor patches (see Fig. 11.7). The visibility of a Gabor-defined contour can be systematically degraded by the addition of randomly-oriented Gabor patches. The Gabor-defined contour is undetectable once a

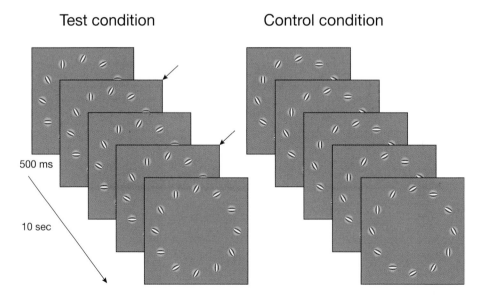

Fig. 11.7 Stimuli used to elicit contour VEPs (Norcia et al 2005). In the test condition, Gabor patches were aligned to be tangent to an imaginary circle in one phase of the alternation, and consistently offset from the circle by 60 degrees in the other phase. In the control condition, the display alternated between two mirror symmetric patterns, each consisting of patches with a 30 degree orientation offset with respect to the imaginary circle. In both test and control conditions, the Gabor patches each rotated through 60 degrees.

critical level of background 'noise' Gabor patches have been added (Kovacs et al 2000). Children as young as age 3 can point to contours embedded in noise (Pennefather et al 1999), but adult performance is achieved only in late childhood (Kovacs et al 1999).

We recently studied the development of contour integration using visual evoked potentials in infants aged between 8 and 56 weeks (Norcia et al 2005). Gabor patches were organized as 'circles' (all patches present were organized in tangent to an imaginary circular path) and as a 'pinwheel' configuration (all patches having a fixed orientation offset from the path), and responses were measured. Each contour contained 12 Gabor patches and there were a total of 11 contours present on the screen. In the test condition a 'circle' configuration alternated with a 'pinwheel' configuration every 500 ms, while in the control condition two different 'pinwheel' configurations were used. Local rotations of single patches were thus always 60 degrees in both the circle/pinwheel condition and the pinwheel/pinwheel control condition.

In the infant group we studied (24 to 56 weeks of age), the response in the pinwheel/pinwheel control condition was similar in amplitude and waveform to that measured in the texture control condition (compare Fig. 11.8 with Fig. 11.6). In contrast to the texture case, the infant difference potential did not reach statistical significance. Spectrum analysis, however, indicated the presence of a small, but significant first harmonic in the pinwheel/circle condition (Norcia et al 2005). The contour integration response was thus substantially less well developed than the texture integration response in infants.

Contour integration may require more specific spatial integration – e.g. integration specifically along the orientation axis. Adults have specialized integration mechanisms

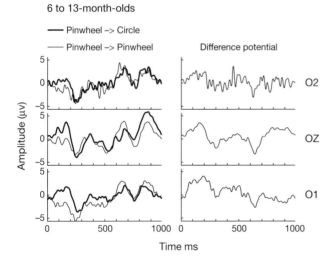

Fig. 11.8 Responses of 6- to 13-month-old infants to contour (Fig. 11.7, left) and control stimuli (Fig. 11.7, right; Norcia et al 2005). Responses in the test and control conditions are similar and the difference potential is not significantly different from zero. Spectrum analysis was able to detect a small, but significant difference between conditions.

for such collinear information (Hou et al 2003). In infants, integration appears to be less specific: stimuli of the same orientation are integrated equally well if they are collinear (end-to-end) or not (side-to-side; Hou et al 2003). The relatively poor vernier acuity of infants (Zanker et al 1992, Carkeet et al 1997, Skoczenski and Norcia 1999, Skoczenski and Norcia 2002) is also a sign of an immature specialization for collinear information. In spite of the quantitative differences in the texture and contour responses of infants, rudimentary sensitivity is present: differential responses to our texture and contour stimuli and their controls could only have been generated by mechanisms that are capable of comparing the relative orientation of two or more patches, as no local information at a single patch distinguished the random and organized textures or the circle and pinwheel configurations.

The development of visual attention

Attention mechanisms are the inevitable main actors of behavioural development, as perception and action as well as higher cognitive function require attention to work. Attentional processes rely on multiple neuro-cognitive processes and it is therefore difficult to separate attention from the complex of visually driven behaviours, especially in non-communicative infants.

In this part of the chapter, we will review event-related potential (ERP) and VEP studies of the development of visual attention. We will mainly focus on low-level properties of attention such as general arousal and alertness and spatial orienting since these are most probably the first attentional functions to emerge in the postnatal period.

During the earliest postnatal period, attention can best be considered as the activation of very basic arousal mechanisms in response to exogenous events occurring in the central visual field. During this period of development, orientation to external visual stimuli is strongly limited by sensory immaturities caused by the lack of development of foveal photoreceptors (Hendrickson and Yuodelis 1984) and general immaturities of cortical development. In spite of the immaturity of the fovea, grating acuity still appears to be highest in the central visual field (Spinelli et al 1983, Allen et al 1996). The development of orienting behaviour thus involves a complex interplay between developing sensory capabilities and the development of attentional mechanisms *per se*.

Arousal effects on brain responsiveness

The state of arousal is a general physiological activation increasing behavioural performance when attention is engaged. The arousal, which originates from brainstem structures, is not system specific, but affects all perceptual modalities and cognitive activities (see Richards 2003a). By 3 months the distinction between sleep, alertness and wakefulness is sharp and the infant shows sustained periods of alertness (see Mirmiran et al 2003 for review). Alertness can be considered as a state where the participant is receptive to the presentation of the stimuli.

The effect of behavioural state on neural functioning and responsivity has been studied in infants by showing changes in the waveform, latency and amplitude of the evoked response during different arousal states and during sleep. Apkarian et al (1991) found remarkable alterations of the EEG and of the VEP response to a transient luminance stimulus across four different sleep–wake cycles (quiet sleep, active sleep, quiet wakefulness, active wakefulness). Sleep state was found to affect all factors of the response (amplitude, latency and waveform). The background EEG showed higher power in the low-frequency band during quiet sleep than in the other three states. During wakefulness, low EEG voltages and irregularity were predominant. The usual P3 component present in the VEP flash response was affected by state and present only during wakefulness. The study also showed that when the VEP is recorded under carefully controlled state conditions, the within and between participant variability reduced considerably (see also Shepherd et al 1999 and Roy et al 2004 for additional results and review). The degree of arousal strongly affected visual performance as measured by the critical flicker frequency, e.g. the highest frequency of flicker capable of eliciting a time-locked response (Apkarian 1993).

The development of spatial orienting

Shifts of attention to different parts of the visual field are often accompanied by fixational saccades. Attention can also be shifted to different spatial locations during central fixation. These shifts of attention are referred to as 'covert attention' shifts. Covert attention was first discovered by showing that saccadic reaction times were faster to a peripheral location that had been previously cued (Posner 1980).

Infants also show effects of spatial cueing on saccadic reaction times (Hood 1993, 1995, Johnson and Tucker 1996). It is generally assumed that reaction time is facilitated due to an increase in response to peripheral targets that have been cued. That is, attention to a location increases responsiveness to stimuli presented at that location (see Reynolds and Chelazzi 2004 for review). A recent event-related potential (ERP) study (Richards 2000) showed that the P1 ERP component elicited by a grating pattern presented in the periphery was larger when that location had been previously cued compared to when the cue was in the opposite hemi-field. The pattern of response observed was adult-like at 20 and 26 weeks, but not at 14 weeks.

The development of non-spatial orienting

The most frequently used electrophysiological approach to study visual attention in infants is to compare responses to novel and familiar stimuli. In the first infant study of this type, infants were presented with a series of two faces, one of which was presented frequently and the other infrequently (Courchesne et al 1981). The faces were matched in size and a number of low-level visual features; one was male and the other female. The infrequently presented stimuli, called 'novel stimuli' or 'odd-balls', were presently randomly along with the more frequent stimuli, called 'standards'. This task elicited a long latency negative component on central and frontal leads (referred to as the Nc component) which was larger for the novel stimuli. It was initially hypothesized that the Nc component reflected selective attention to novel or discrepant stimuli (Courchesne et al 1981). Successful performance on this task requires that the infant encode the two stimuli and retain a visual memory that can be used to compare novel to familiar stimuli, and there has been considerable debate over which aspect(s) of the task are most important (see Ackles and Cook 1998, Nelson ?' Webb 2003, Richards 2003a).

More recently, John Richards has made the most direct connection between Nc and attention. In his study (Richards 2003a), Nc components were measured during states of attentiveness and inattentiveness as determined by simultaneously and independently measured heart-rate patterns. The heart-rate data were used to classify the evoked responses as having occurred during a period of orienting (the period before a heart-rate deceleration occurred), a period of sustained attention (a period of time during which the inter-beat interval was longer than the pre-stimulus baseline), and a period of inattentiveness (the period after a deceleration when the heart-rate returned to baseline; see Richards 2003b for a review of the heart-rate measure and attention). The Nc component was larger during periods of attention than during non-attention and Richards has argued that it may thus reflect a general orienting reflex.

Future directions for infant visual electrophysiology

While much is known about basic sensitivity to image contrast, we are only beginning to understand the neural development of the mechanisms responsible for the perceptual organization of low-level features into objects such as faces (see de Haan et al 2003, Halit et al 2003, 2004 for reviews of infant face-related ERPs). As one ascends the visual hierarchy, it is clear that controlling for the attentional state of the infant will become increasingly important, so as not to confuse lack of attention with lack of visual sensitivity. Even low-level responses such as the pattern reversal (Di Russo et al 2001, Di Russo and Spinelli 2002, Chen et al 2003) or motion VEPs (Valdes-Sosa et al 1998, Torriente et al 1999, Pei et al 2002) are subject to attentional modulation. It would be of considerable interest to determine the extent to which infant acuity and contrast sensitivity depend on the state of visual attention.

Attentional control is likely to be critical to understanding the development of mid-level responses, since it appears that responses to only moderately complex motion stimuli are strongly modulated by attention (Rees et al 1997), as are the responses of higher visual areas to simple stimuli (Schwartz et al 2005). Combining mid-level visual tasks with strong attentional controls would bring together two traditions that have remained largely separate – infant visual development and infant cognitive development. It is hoped that this review provides a stimulus to workers in both fields to begin this new endeavour.

REFERENCES

Ackles PK, Cook KG (1998) Stimulus probability and event-related potentials of the brain in 6-month-old human infants: a parametric study. *Int J Psychophysiol* 29(2): 115–143.

Albright TD, Stoner GR (2002) Contextual influences on visual processing. *Annu Rev Neurosci* 25: 339–379.

Allen D, Tyler CW, Norcia AM (1996) Development of grating acuity and contrast sensitivity in the central and peripheral visual field of the human infant. *Vision Res* 36(13): 1945–1953.

Apkarian P (1993) Temporal frequency responsivity shows multiple maturational phases: state-dependent visual evoked potential luminance flicker fusion from birth to 9 months. *Vis Neurosci* 10(6): 1007–1018.

Apkarian P, Mirmiran M, Tijssen R (1991) Effects of behavioural state on visual processing in neonates. *Neuropediatrics* 22(2): 85–91.

Atkinson J (2000) *The Developing Visual Brain*. Oxford: Oxford University Press.

Atkinson J, Braddick O (1992) Visual segmentation of oriented textures by infants. *Behav Brain Res* 49(1): 123–131.

Auestad N, Montalto MB, Hall RT, Fitzgerald KM, Wheeler RE, Connor WE, Neuringer M, Connor SL, Taylor JA, Hartmann EE (1997) Visual acuity, erythrocyte fatty acid composition, and growth in term infants fed formulas with long chain polyunsaturated fatty acids for one year. Ross Pediatric Lipid Study. *Pediatr Res* 41(1): 1–10.

Bach M, Meigen T (1992) Electrophysiological correlates of texture segregation in the human visual evoked potential. *Vision Res* 32(3): 417–424.

Bach M, Meigen T (1998) Electrophysiological correlates of human texture segregation, an overview. *Doc Ophthalmol* 95(3–4): 335–347.

Birch EE, Hoffman DR, Uauy R, Birch DG, Prestidge C (1998) Visual acuity and the essentiality of docosahexaenoic acid and arachidonic acid in the diet of term infants. *Pediatr Res* 44(2): 201–209.

Braddick OJ, Wattam-Bell J, Atkinson J (1986) Orientation-specific cortical responses develop in early infancy. *Nature* 320(6063): 617–619.

Caputo G, Casco C (1999) A visual evoked potential correlate of global figure-ground segmentation. *Vision Res* 39(9): 1597–1610.

Carkeet A, Levi DM, Manny RE (1997) Development of Vernier acuity in childhood. *Optom Vis Sci* 74(9): 741–750.

Chen Y, Seth AK, Gally JA, Edelman GM (2003) The power of human brain magnetoencephalographic signals can be modulated up or down by changes in an attentive visual task. *Proc Natl Acad Sci USA* 100(6): 3501–3506.

Colombo J (2001) The development of visual attention in infancy. *Annu Rev Psychol* 52: 337–367.

Courchesne E, Ganz L, Norcia AM (1981) Event-related brain potentials to human faces in infants. *Child Dev* 52(3): 804–811.

de Haan M, Johnson MH, Halit H (2003) Development of face-sensitive event-related potentials during infancy: a review. *Int J Psychophysiol* 51(1): 45–58.

Di Russo F, Spinelli D (2002) Effects of sustained, voluntary attention on amplitude and latency of steady-state visual evoked potential: a costs and benefits analysis. *Clin Neurophysiol* 113(11): 1771–1777.

Di Russo F, Spinelli D, Morrone MC (2001) Automatic gain control contrast mechanisms are modulated by attention in humans: evidence from visual evoked potentials. *Vision Res* 41(19): 2435–2447.

Elder JH, Goldberg RM (2002) Ecological statistics of Gestalt laws for the perceptual organization of contours. *J Vis* 2(4): 324–353.

Field DJ, Hayes A, Hess RF (1993) Contour integration by the human visual system: evidence for a local 'association field'. *Vision Res* 33(2): 173–193.

Geisler WS, Perry JS, Super BJ, Gallogly DP (2001) Edge co-occurrence in natural images predicts contour grouping performance. *Vision Res* 41(6): 711–724.

Grill-Spector K, Kourtzi Z, Kanwisher N (2001) The lateral occipital complex and its role in object recognition. *Vision Res* 41(10–11): 1409–1422.

Grosof DH, Shapley RM, Hawken MJ (1993) Macaque V1 neurons can signal 'illusory' contours. *Nature* 365(6446): 550–552.

Hainline L, Abramov I (1997) Eye movement-based measures of development of spatial contrast sensitivity in infants. *Optom Vis Sci* 74(10): 790–799.

Halit H, de Haan M, Johnson MH (2003) Cortical specialisation for face processing: face-sensitive event-related potential components in 3- and 12-month-old infants. *Neuroimage* 19(3): 1180–1193.

Halit H, Csibra G, Volein A, Johnson MH (2004) Face-sensitive cortical processing in early infancy. *J Child Psychol Psychiatry* 45(7): 1228–1234.

Hendrickson AE, Yuodelis C (1984) The morphological development of the human fovea. *Ophthalmology* 91(6): 603–612.

Hood BM (1993) Inhibition of return produced by covert shifts of visual attention in 6-month-old infants. *Infant Behav Dev* 16: 245–254.

Hood BM (1995) Shifts of visual attention in the human infant: a neuroscientific approach. *Adv Infancy Res* 10: 163–216.

Hopkins B, Johnson SP (2003) *Neurobiology of Infant Vision.* Westport, CT: Praeger Publishers.

Hou C, Pettet MW, Sampath V, Candy TR, Norcia AM (2003) Development of the spatial organization and dynamics of lateral interactions in the human visual system. *J Neurosci* 23(25): 8630–8640.

Jacobs DS, Blakemore C (1988) Factors limiting the postnatal development of visual acuity in the monkey. *Vision Res* 28(8): 947–958.

Johnson MH, Tucker LA (1996) The development and temporal dynamics of spatial orienting in infants. *J Exp Child Psychol* 63(1): 171–188.

211

Kovacs I, Julesz B (1993) A closed curve is much more than an incomplete one: effect of closure in figure-ground segmentation. *Proc Natl Acad Sci USA* 90(16): 7495–7497.

Kovacs I, Kozma P, Feher A, Benedek G (1999) Late maturation of visual spatial integration in humans. *Proc Natl Acad Sci USA* 96(21): 12204–12209.

Kovacs I, Polat U, Pennefather PM, Chandna A, Norcia AM (2000) A new test of contour integration deficits in patients with a history of disrupted binocular experience during visual development. *Vision Res* 40(13): 1775–1783.

Lamme VA, Van Dijk BW, Spekreijse H (1992) Texture segregation is processed by primary visual cortex in man and monkey. Evidence from VEP experiments. *Vision Res* 32(5): 797–807.

Lamme VA, Rodriguez-Rodriguez V, Spekreijse H (1999) Separate processing dynamics for texture elements, boundaries and surfaces in primary visual cortex of the macaque monkey. *Cereb Cortex* 9(4): 406–413.

Landing BH, Shankle WR, Hara J, Brannock J, Fallon JH (2002) The development of structure and function in the postnatal human cerebral cortex from birth to 72 months: changes in thickness of layers II and III co-relate to the onset of new age-specific behaviors. *Pediatr Pathol Mol Med* 21(3): 321–342.

Lee TS, Mumford D (2003) Hierarchical Bayesian inference in the visual cortex. *J Opt Soc Am A Opt Image Sci Vis* 20(7): 1434–1448.

Manny RE (1992) Orientation selectivity of 3-month-old infants. *Vision Res* 32(10): 1817–1828.

Marcus DS, Van Essen DC (2002) Scene segmentation and attention in primate cortical areas V1 and V2. *J Neurophysiol* 88(5): 2648–2658.

Mirmiran M, Maas YG, Ariagno RL (2003) Development of fetal and neonatal sleep and circadian rhythms. *Sleep Med Rev* 7(4): 321–334.

Nelson CA, Webb S (2003) A cognitive neuroscience perspective on early memory development. In: de Haan M, Johnson MH, editors. *The Cognitive Neuroscience of Development*. Hove, UK: Psychology Press.

Norcia AM, Manny RE (2003) Development of vision in infants. In: Kaufman PL, Alm A, editors. *Adler's Physiology of the Eye*. St Louis, MO: Mosby, pp 531–551.

Norcia AM, Tyler CW (1985) Spatial frequency sweep VEP: visual acuity during the first year of life. *Vision Res* 25(10): 1399–1408.

Norcia AM, Tyler CW, Hamer RD (1990) Development of contrast sensitivity in the human infant. *Vision Res* 30(10): 1475–1486.

Norcia AM, Pei F, Bonneh Y, Hou C, Sampath V, Pettet MW (2005) Development of sensitivity to texture and contour information in the human infant. *J Cogn Neurosci* 17(4): 569–579.

Pei F, Pettet MW, Norcia AM (2002) Neural correlates of object-based attention. *J Vis* 2(9): 588–596.

Pennefather PM, Chandna A, Kovacs I, Polat U, Norcia AM (1999) Contour detection threshold: repeatability and learning with 'contour cards'. *Spat Vis* 12(3): 257–266.

Peterzell DH, Werner JS, Kaplan PS (1993) Individual differences in contrast sensitivity functions: the first four months of life in humans. *Vision Res* 33(3): 381–396.

Peterzell DH, Werner JS, Kaplan PS (1995) Individual differences in contrast sensitivity functions: longitudinal study of 4-, 6- and 8-month-old human infants. *Vision Res* 35(7): 961–979.

Posner MI (1980) Orienting of attention. *Q J Exp Psychol* 32(1): 3–25.

Rees G, Frith CD, Lavie N (1997) Modulating irrelevant motion perception by varying attentional load in an unrelated task. *Science* 278(5343): 1616–1619.

Reynolds JH, Chelazzi L (2004) Attentional modulation of visual processing. *Annu Rev Neurosci* 27: 611–647.

Richards JE (2000) Localizing the development of covert attention in infants with scalp event-related potentials. *Dev Psychol* 36(1): 91–108.

Richards JE (2003a) Attention affects the recognition of briefly presented visual stimuli in infants: an ERP study. *Dev Sci* 6(3): 312–328.

Richards JE (2003b) The development of visual attention and the brain. In: de Haan M, Johnson MH, editors. *The Cognitive Neuroscience of Development*. Hove, UK: Psychology Press, pp 321–338.

Rieth C, Sireteanu R (1994) Texture segmentation and 'pop-out' in infants and children: the effect of test field size. *Spat Vis* 8(2): 173–191.

Roy MS, Gosselin J, Hanna N, Orquin J, Chemtob S (2004) Influence of the state of alertness on the pattern visual evoked potentials (PVEP) in very young infant. *Brain Dev* 26(3): 197–202.

Schwartz S, Vuilleumier P, Hutton C, Maravita A, Dolan RJ, Driver J (2005) Attentional load and sensory competition in human vision: modulation of fMRI responses by load at fixation during task-irrelevant stimulation in the peripheral visual field. *Cereb Cortex* 15(6): 770–786.

Shepherd A, Saunders K, McCulloch D (1999) Effect of sleep state on the flash visual evoked potential. A case study. *Doc Ophthalmol* 98(3): 247–256.

Sireteanu R, Rieth C (1992) Texture segregation in infants and children. *Behav Brain Res* 49(1): 133–139.

Skoczenski AM, Norcia AM (1999) Development of VEP Vernier acuity and grating acuity in human infants. *Invest Ophthalmol Vis Sci* 40(10): 2411–2417.

Skoczenski AM, Norcia AM (2002) Late maturation of visual hyperacuity. *Psychol Sci* 13(6): 537–541.

Sokol S, Moskowitz A, McCormack G (1992) Infant VEP and preferential looking acuity measured with phase alternating gratings. *Invest Ophthalmol Vis Sci* 33(11): 3156–3161.

Spinelli D, Pirchio M, Sandini G (1983) Visual acuity in the young infant is highest in a small retinal area. *Vision Res* 23(10): 1133–1136.

Torriente I, Valdes-Sosa M, Ramirez D, Bobes MA (1999) Visual evoked potentials related to motion-onset are modulated by attention. *Vision Res* 39(24): 4122–4139.

Valdes-Sosa M, Bobes MA, Rodriguez V, Pinilla T (1998) Switching attention without shifting the spotlight object-based attentional modulation of brain potentials. *J Cogn Neurosci* 10(1): 137–151.

Westheimer G. (1975) Visual acuity and hyperacuity. *Invest Ophthalmol* 14: 570–572.

Wilson HR (1993) Theories of infant visual development. In: Simons K, editor. *Early Visual Development: Normal and Abnormal.* New York: Oxford, pp 560–572.

Xu X, Ichida J, Shostak Y, Bonds AB, Casagrande VA (2002) Are primate lateral geniculate nucleus (LGN) cells really sensitive to orientation or direction? *Vis Neurosci* 19(1): 97–108.

Zanker J, Mohn G, Weber U, Zeitler-Driess K, Fahle M (1992) The development of vernier acuity in human infants. *Vision Res* 32(8): 1557–1564

12
VISUAL FUNCTION IN CHILDREN WITH NEONATAL BRAIN LESIONS

Eugenio Mercuri, Andrea Guzzetta, Francesca Tinelli, Daniela Ricci and Giovanni Cioni

Introduction

Disorders of visual function are a common finding in children with neonatal brain lesions of antenatal and perinatal onset. In some cases they are secondary to ophthalmological abnormalities such as cataract or retinopathy, but more often they are related to damage of the central visual pathway, known as cerebral visual impairment (CVI). While most of the early studies only reported retrospectively the prevalence of abnormal visual function in children with cerebral palsy, in the last few years increasing attention has been devoted to the development of visual function in infants with brain lesions. This has been due to a dramatic improvement in both neonatal imaging and the ability to assess visual function in the first years.

As reviewed in Chapter 6, in the last two decades neonatal MRI and serial imaging have increasingly been applied in infants with risk factors such as severe preterm birth or birth asphyxia with ultrasound abnormalities. This has made it possible to achieve much more precise information on the type and extent of the lesion and on the involvement of the various cortical and subcortical areas related to visual function, providing a better understanding of the correlation between structure and function. These studies have provided evidence that the normal development of vision depends on the integrity of a complex network which includes optic radiations and primary visual cortex but also other cortical and subcortical areas, such as the frontal or the temporal lobes or the basal ganglia, which are known to be associated with visual attention and other aspects of visual function. These findings are in agreement with animal studies and functional studies in adults and children, which have significantly improved our knowledge of the neurophysiological bases of vision.

It is now well established that the process of vision involves different brain areas and multiple levels of increasing complexity, from mechanisms of local perception of image features, which are partially of subcortical origin, up to complete object recognition and localization, based on complex interactions between striate cortex and associative areas (see also Chapter 11). Brain lesions are therefore often associated with an impairment of one or more aspects of visual function, which may involve different levels of visual processing according to the neurophysiological role of the damaged areas. This general picture is further complicated by the interaction between lesion and development, or, in other words, by the complex mechanisms of plasticity and reorganization that invariably follow early brain damage.

The possibility of testing various aspects of visual function from the first weeks of life has significantly improved our understanding of the correlation between visual function and neonatal brain lesions and of the effect of a neonatal lesion on the developing brain. Various tests specifically designed to assess aspects of visual function such as acuity, visual fields and visual attention, from the early postnatal period, are now available even in preterm infants, and this has made it possible to follow the onset and maturation of all those aspects of visual function and to provide age-dependent normative data.

In this chapter we will report: (a) brief details on the assessment of visual function to be used in infants with brain lesions, in relation to the maturation of the various aspects of visual development; and (b) the patterns of visual function observed in the first years of life in infants with neonatal brain lesions.

Assessment of visual function in the first years of life
The assessment of visual function in young infants includes behavioural and electro-physiological techniques. Application of these tests should be preceded by a standard ophthalmological examination to ascertain the presence of eye abnormalities such as retinopathy, cataract or optic atrophy.

BEHAVIOURAL TECHNIQUES
Behavioural techniques are based on the observation and assessment of spontaneous or elicited behaviours of the infant. A number of methods are presented here which have been specifically designed or modified for the assessment of very young infants and uncooperative patients.

Oculomotor behaviour can be assessed by testing fixation, following reactions and saccadic movements, i.e. the rapid eye movement to shift fixation from one stimulus to another. A short period of fixation on a target can be observed by 30 weeks post-menstrual age (PMA). Following reactions are better observed from 34 weeks PMA. At term age, newborns are generally able to follow a target, such as a red ball, in a full arc. Saccadic movements can be elicited from birth for short distances, but they have high latency and little accuracy. A more mature pattern is reached at around 3 months post-term.

Roving eye movements are common in young preterm infants. The presence of abnormal eye movements, such as spontaneous nystagmus, can also be noted. Strabismus and eye alignment can be tested by commonly used orthoptic techniques, such as the cover test. *The blink reflex* (threatening response) can already be observed in infants born at 26 weeks gestation (Hacke et al 1981).

Acuity can be tested by using forced-choice preferential looking (FCPL). The target is presented to the infant at eye level on one side of the midline; it consists of black and white stripes, paired with a uniform grey background on the other side. The level of acuity is measured as the finest grating (i.e. width of black and white stripes) for which the infant shows a consistent preference (in cycles/degree), and compared to age-specific normative data (Teller et al 1986). As a rule of thumb, visual acuity shows a maturation of 1 cycle/

degree per month in the first year of life. The acuity cards commercially available are a simplified adaptation of the FCPL technique (Fig. 12.1). Other measures of acuity can be obtained by means of visual evoked potentials (see below).

Contrast sensitivity is tested with grating patterns in which the stripes are not sharp but have a sine-wave distribution of light intensity. Contrast is defined as the intensity difference between the brightest and the darkest points of the grating, divided by the sum of these intensities, and it can vary from 0 to 100 per cent. A rapid increment in contrast sensitivity has been found over the first two to three months of life (Banks et al 1975, Atkinson 1979). In particular, at 4 weeks post-term, peak contrast sensitivity is a factor of about 5 to 6 lower than that of adults (Norcia et al 1990). By 33 weeks post-term, adult levels are reached. The contrast sensitivity function as a whole has proved useful in showing pathological visual losses (e.g. amblyopia, glaucoma, and demyelinating diseases) which are not adequately revealed by acuity measures alone.

Visual fields can be assessed using kinetic perimetry. The apparatus consists of two perpendicular black metal strips bent to form two arcs, each with a radius of 40 cm (Fig. 12.2). The infant is held in the centre of the arc perimeter. During central fixation of a white ball, an identical target is moved from the periphery towards the fixation point along

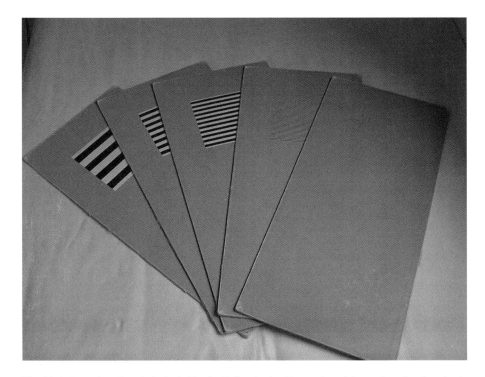

Fig. 12.1 Examples of cards included in the Teller Acuity Test and used for testing visual acuity in infants.

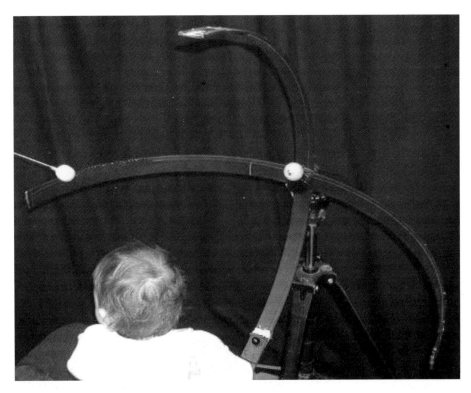

Fig. 12.2 Example of testing visual fields by means of the kinetic perimeter.

one of the arcs of the perimeter. Eye and head movements towards the peripheral ball are used to estimate the outline of the visual fields. Normative data for full-term and preterm infants are available (Mohn and van Hof-van Duin 1986, van Hof-van Duin et al 1992). The fields are quite narrow in the first months of life (approximately 30 degrees) and become progressively wider (approximately 60 degrees at 6 months and 80–90 degrees at 1 year of age).

Optokinetic nystagmus (OKN) can be elicited by using a large piece of paper or a computer-generated random dot pattern in front of the infant's face. The examiner observes the infant's eye movements, recording the presence and the symmetry of the OKN in response to the movement of the pattern in either direction. Normally, binocular OKN is symmetrical from birth onwards, whereas monocular OKN shows a better response to stimulation in a temporo-nasal direction up to about 3 to 6 months corrected age (Atkinson and Braddick 1981).

Fixation shift is a test of visual attention evaluating the direction and the latency of saccadic eye movements in response to a peripheral target in the lateral field (Fig. 12.3). A central target is used as a fixation stimulus before the appearance of the peripheral target. While in some trials the central target disappears simultaneously with the appearance of the peripheral target (non-competition), in others the central target remains visible,

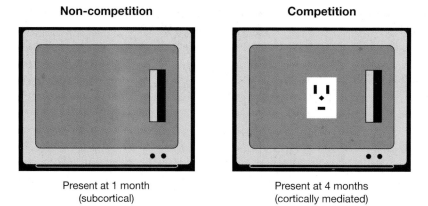

Non-competition　　　　　　　**Competition**

Present at 1 month　　　　　　　Present at 4 months
(subcortical)　　　　　　　　　　(cortically mediated)

Fig. 12.3 Stimuli used for testing fixation shift in infants.

generating a situation of competition between the two stimuli. Normal children can reliably shift their attention in a situation of non-competition during the first weeks after birth, but prompt refixation in a situation of competition is only found after 6–8 weeks post-term and reliably by 12–18 weeks post-term. Absent or delayed (a latency of more than 1.2 sec) refixation at 5 months of age is considered abnormal (Atkinson et al 1992).

A final group of behavioural tests related to visual processing which are usable in the first two years of life are intelligence tests based on the theory of *information processing*. As reported in Chapter 11 of this book, these tests aim to evaluate the information processing efficiency of the child, mainly by testing her/his visual recognition memory. It has been shown that these abilities can be evaluated even in very young infants or in those whose severe motor dysfunction does not permit a response to traditional tests of sensorimotor intelligence (Drotar et al 1989).

Some instruments are now available for the assessment of visual information processing in infancy even in clinical situations; one of these is the Fagan Test for Infant Intelligence (FTII), standardized for infants at ages 6, 9 and 12 months. This test measures recognition memory on the basis of novelty preference. It consists of a set of pictures showing human faces: after a familiarization phase, a familiar stimulus and a novel face, different for sex, orientation or other features, are simultaneously presented to the child (Fig. 12.4). The time spent by the child looking at each stimulus is registered. After several trials a novelty score can be computed, and compared to standardized values; such a score allows us to identify infants as having a low, suspect or high risk level for developmental delay. Several studies of high-risk infants have been performed to investigate the predictive value of the FTII in relation to later cognitive level, with controversial but promising results (for reviews see Fagan and Singer 1983, Bornstein and Sigman 1986, McCall and Carriger 1993). On the whole, novelty preference during early infancy appears to provide a promising measure for assessing an infant's mental faculties and for predicting intelligence later in life, perhaps more predictive than other psychometric tests.

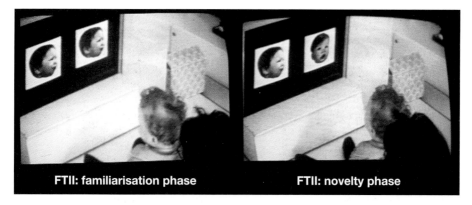

FTII: familiarisation phase   **FTII: novelty phase**

Fig. 12.4 Example, taken from a video, of the administration of the Fagan Test of Infant Intelligence (FTII) to a young infant with brain lesions.

ELECTROPHYSIOLOGICAL TECHNIQUES

Different types of visual evoked potentials (VEPs) can be used for the early assessment of visual functions (see also Chapter 11).

Flash VEPs can be used to follow the normal or abnormal maturation of the visual pathway (Hrbek et al 1973, Taylor et al 1987, Eken et al 1996, Tsuneishi and Casaer 1997, 2000), although their contribution to the assessment of infants at risk of CVI is quite limited.

Steady-state VEPs can be recorded by using orientation-reversal and phase-reversal stimuli, and are used to assess the maturation of visual cortical processing (Mercuri et al 1995). For phase-reversal VEPs the orientation of the black and white stripes is fixed but the contrast reversed periodically. For orientation-reversal VEPs, stimuli periodically change orientation between 45 and 135 degrees. The phase-reversal response is already present at term, while the orientation-reversal response is only consistently elicited at 10 weeks post-term for slow changes (4 rev/sec) and after 12 weeks for faster changes (8 rev/sec) (Braddick et al 1986).

VEPs can also be used to assess *vernier acuity*, which measures the ability to discriminate the relative position of different components of a visual pattern (Westheimer 1975). In this task, the infant is required to discriminate lines that are perfectly aligned, from lines that are offset. The ability to identify fine offsets exceeds the visual resolution predicted by photoreceptor cell spacing. During normal development, vernier acuity develops significantly later than grating acuity. Some studies (Shimojo and Held 1987, Skoczenski and Norcia 2002) show that vernier acuity is a 'hypo-acuity' (inferior to grating acuity) during early infancy in children with normal visual experience, while it is a 'hyper-acuity' (superior to grating acuity) in adults with normal vision.

Sweep VEPs are a new technique for the assessment of grating acuity. In the steady-state sweep VEP, the spatial frequency of a high-contrast grating is systematically varied, and acuity is measured by extrapolating the VEP amplitude versus the spatial frequency. Grating acuity measured by this technique develops from around 5 c/deg at 1 month to around 15 to 20 c/deg by 8 months (Allen et al 1996, Auestad et al 1997, Birch et al 1998).

219

Other aspects of visual function, both of higher and lower levels of processing, are obviously present from the first months of life, but we have limited our review to the functions that can be assessed by standardized tests, available for the clinical setting. Other tools are available for older children.

In the first years of life, the combined use of behavioural and electrophysiological techniques allows a detailed assessment of many different aspects of visual function and their maturation from birth (Fig. 12.5). Moreover, the availability of precise normative data for each one of the tests is useful for the longitudinal follow-up of single aspects of vision in infants at risk for cerebral visual impairment, and for a better understanding of the mechanisms of cerebral reorganization following brain lesion.

Visual disorders in children with brain lesions

The significant improvement in neonatal intensive care and in the early assessment of brain lesions by means of neuroimaging has allowed a detailed evaluation of the type and extent of brain damage immediately after birth (see also Chapter 6). This new scenario has made it possible to explore at an early stage the correlation between development of visual functions and brain damage, significantly improving our understanding of the pathogenic mechanisms of visual disorders of central origin. Due to the previously under-lined complexity of the visual system, most of the more common types of brain disorder are associated with a significant risk of impairment of different aspects of visual function,

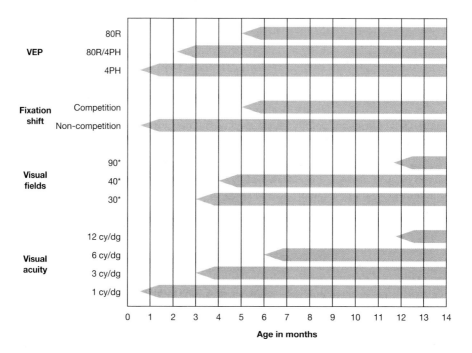

Fig. 12.5 Graph illustrating the maturation of some visual functions in the first year of life.

in relation to the brain areas involved. The main types of congenital brain lesions and the associated disorders of visual function will now be analysed.

PERIVENTRICULAR LEUKOMALACIA

Periventricular leukomalacia (PVL) is the most common cause of cerebral palsy (Shevell et al 2003). Recent studies have reported that approximately 10 per cent of very low birthweight infants develop cerebral palsy, which is caused by periventricular leukomalacia in nearly 90 per cent of cases. The original description of the pathology of PVL by Banker and Larroche (1962) highlighted that the lesion often involves the axons in the optic radiations and that the individual is therefore at high risk of abnormal visual function.

While a few studies in the 1980s had already reported the association of PVL, cerebral palsy and visual impairment (Brozynski et al 1985, de Vries and Dubowitz 1985, de Vries et al 1987), visual function in infants with PVL was more systematically investigated in the 1990s. Several studies using a combined clinical and imaging approach have shown that the presence and the severity of visual abnormalities are related to the severity and the extent of the lesion.

In our own series published in 1997, infants with 'prolonged flares', persisting for more than seven days (PVL type 1 according to the classification proposed by de Vries et al 1990) or evolving into small localized frontoparietal cysts (PVL type 2), generally had normal acuity (Eken et al 1995, Cioni et al 1997). Isolated abnormalities of ocular movements, usually strabismus (squint; 50 per cent), or of other aspects of visual function, such as visual fields (22 per cent) or OKN (35 per cent), could, however, occasionally be found in infants with such lesions (Eken et al 1995, Uggetti et al 1996, Cioni et al 1997). In contrast, infants with PVL grades 3 and 4 show almost invariably severe visual abnormalities with impairment of multiple aspects of visual function (Scher et al 1989, Gibson et al 1990, Eken et al 1994, Cioni et al 1997, Lanzi et al 1998). In our series only 20 per cent of infants with grade 3 and 4 PVL had normal visual function, while the remaining 80 per cent had abnormalities on several aspects of visual function, including strabismus (70 per cent), acuity (57 per cent), visual fields (62 per cent) and OKN (45 per cent). Other studies have also reported abnormal acuity in 44 to 75 per cent of infants (Eken et al 1995, Uggetti et al 1996).

The presence of abnormal acuity, and abnormal visual function more generally, has been related to lesions in the peritrigonal white matter and in the optic radiations, as well as to the extent of occipital cortex involvement (Eken et al 1995, Uggetti et al 1996, Cioni et al 1997). Accordingly, Eken et al (1994) have reported that in infants with cystic PVL visual abnormalities are more frequent in infants with gestational ages of 35 to 37 weeks than in those with gestational ages below 32 weeks, possibly as a consequence of the distribution of the lesion, which in more mature infants extends further into the subcortical white matter.

Although the association between the involvement of optic radiations/occipital cortex and abnormal visual findings is statistically significant, the correlation does not hold true in all cases, suggesting that other factors may play a role in determining visual impairment. We have recently reviewed the MRI scans performed in 13 infants with cystic PVL assessed for ocular movements, acuity, and visual fields and fixation shift. In agreement with previous studies we found that visual abnormalities were more frequent in infants with severely abnormal optic radiations, but we were also able to demonstrate that the severity of visual impairment was correlated to the involvement of other cortical and subcortical areas, and, more specifically, to the involvement of the thalami.

The early diagnosis of visual impairment in infants with PVL is also important because of the relation between visual function and neurodevelopment in these children. It has been previously reported that infants with more severe and diffuse abnormalities of visual functions also have a low DQ (Eken et al 1995, Cioni et al 2000). In particular, we have shown in our series, by means of a multivariate analysis, that visual impairment is the most important variable in determining the neurodevelopmental scores in these infants – more important than the severity of motor disability or the extent of lesions on MRI (Cioni et al 2000).

Several other aspects of vision, in particular the higher levels of visual processing, can be impaired in children with PVL, although their detection is usually not possible in the first years of life. Disorders of global form recognition have been consistently reported by Stiers and co-workers (1998, 1999, 2001, 2002). They have shown significant visual perceptual abnormalities in children with PVL in a series of studies in children with congenital brain lesions tested around 5 years of age. Some of these difficulties have been interpreted in relation to the reported impairment of ocular motility in these infants which may lead to significant abnormalities of visual scanning (Fedrizzi et al 1998, Jacobson et al 2002).

More recently, we have also investigated motion perception in children with brain lesions, by means of behavioural, electrophysiological and functional MRI measures (Guzzetta et al 2004). A significant impairment of motion perception was present in children with PVL, but similar results were found in children with other types of brain lesion, suggesting a more general vulnerability of this function.

Intraventricular Haemorrhage

Abnormalities of visual function are frequent among preterm infants with intraventricular haemorrhages (IVH) but they are less common and generally less severe than in infants with periventricular leucomalacia. A recent study investigated visual function in a large cohort of 171 infants with different degrees of IVH, reporting deficit of visual acuity and visual fields. While the visual fields defects were usually transient and only persisted until 1 year of age, the reduction of visual acuity did persist until the fourth year (Harvey et al 1997). Interestingly, in this study visual impairment did not correlate to the severity of the haemorrhage (Papile et al 1983) but was more often observed in infants who subsequently developed cerebral palsy. These results are in partial agreement with previous studies which showed a reduction of visual acuity in infants with IVH during the neonatal period (Morante et al 1982, Dubowitz et al 1983), which tended, however, to recover during the first months of life (Eken et al 1994). In this last study, a correlation with the degree of IVH was also found.

Transient anomalies of visual function may be due to the effect of intraventricular haemorrhage on the thalamus or inferior colliculi, or to haemorrhage of the germinal matrix at the origin of the optic radiations and the posterior thalami. On the other hand, permanent effects may be present in case of deeper tissue involvement, as demonstrated by the positive association between visual deficit and neuromotor impairment. It has to be noted, however, that not all infants with parenchymal involvement (grade IV lesions) show a deficit of visual function, as the lesion is more often located in the mid-anterior parietal lobe and therefore not in sites affecting the primary visual pathway, i.e. posterior parietal and occipital lobes.

NEONATAL CEREBRAL INFARCTION

Several studies have reported abnormalities of visual function in adults who suffered ischaemic brain stroke and in children with stroke acquired after the neonatal period. In these patients, lesions affecting the striate occipital cortex and the optic radiations were almost invariably associated with contralateral hemianopia, while lesions affecting the parietal lobe generally resulted in abnormal visual attention and, in the most severe cases, contralateral visual neglect.

Little has been reported on possible visual impairment in infants with neonatal stroke, an entity which has become increasingly recognized since neonatal imaging has become more widely available. Arterial infarcts are the most frequent strokes in full-term infants, and in the great majority of cases involve the left middle cerebral artery.

In 1996 we reported a short-term visual follow-up in a cohort of 12 infants with neonatal infarction (Mercuri et al 1996b). Using a battery of tests specifically designed to evaluate visual function in the first years of life, we demonstrated that while acuity and ocular movements were always normal, other aspects of visual function were impaired. These were visual fields and visual attention, as tested by fixation shift, which were abnormal in 58 per cent of cases. The correlation of neurobehavioural visual tests with neonatal MRI did not show the same association previously reported in adults and in children with post-natal acquired stroke. More specifically, although 50 per cent of the children showed unilateral involvement of optic radiations and/or the visual areas in the occipital cortex, only half of them had contralateral visual fields abnormalities. Similarly, although in all the 12 patients the infarcted area involved the parietal lobe, only 50 per cent had abnormal fixation shift in the first year of life.

These preliminary results have been subsequently confirmed in a larger cohort of 30 infants. These findings suggested that early lesions affecting the visual pathway were, to some extent, compensated for by the immature brain, but we were unable to identify any other marker which could help to identify infants with normal visual function and those with visual abnormalities.

When the same infants were tested at school age, when more mature aspects of visual function, such as stereopsis and crowding acuity, could be studied, the proportion of children with visual abnormalities was even lower than on the assessment performed in the neonatal period. Crowding acuity refers to the ability of an individual to identify target stimuli if these are surrounded by nearby contours. Crowding effect is more pronounced in eccentric vision, compared with central vision; whereas crowding in central vision is caused chiefly by contour interaction, crowding in eccentric vision is caused by both attentional and contour interaction effects.

Crowding acuity gives an equivalent measure in children to that in adults, testing with standard Snellen linear charts. In our study, at school age only 28 per cent of children with neonatal focal infarction had some abnormalities of visual function, compared to 58 per cent of the same children who were found to have some abnormalities in the first year after birth. One of the main differences is that a proportion of the children (12.5 per cent) who had normal results on preferential looking in the first year had developed abnormal crowding acuity. This discrepancy probably reflects the sensitivity of the assessment at school age rather than a deterioration of acuity with age.

The test of crowding acuity reflects visual functioning in everyday life rather than monocular or single letter acuity. In this test letters are presented on cards, either alone (single optotype), or surrounded by four other letters which are half a letter-width away (crowded optotype). The results of the single and crowded optotypes are compared and if the child fails to identify the letter surrounded by others, but can easily see the single letter, this is a measure of cortical visual impairment rather than a refractive error.

Only a small proportion of the children who had abnormal fields in infancy still had abnormal results at school age. These findings suggest that caution should be used when interpreting the results of assessment of visual fields in infants, and that visual outcome in infants with neonatal infarction is normal in the great majority of cases.

In our experience (Mercuri et al 1996a) the risk of developing visual abnormalities is higher in children who develop hemiplegia (33 per cent) than in those with normal outcome. This reflects the extent of the lesion as demonstrated by the fact that visual abnormalities are significantly more frequently associated with lesions involving the main branch of the middle cerebral artery than with those localized in the territory of one of the cortical branches of the middle cerebral artery (75 vs 32 per cent). This information is important when counselling in the neonatal period, when the extent of the lesion is fully appreciated on MRI but clinical signs of hemiplegia are not yet present.

These findings suggest that abnormality of acuity, visual fields and stereopsis are not common in children who had neonatal infarction. The relatively low prevalence of abnormal visual findings cannot only be explained by the type and the extent of the lesions, which are usually in the territory of the middle cerebral artery and show little or no involvement of the optic radiations and sparing of the primary visual cortex. Normal visual function can also be found in children with involvement of optic radiations and occipital cortex. This is also confirmed by the low association of abnormal visual findings with border-zone lesions which are always associated with involvement of the optic radiations.

The low incidence of abnormal visual function following cortical infarction, in comparison with adults with similar lesions, may be related to the existence of effective mechanisms of plasticity of the visual structures, as also shown by the presence of normal vision in children with damaged optic radiations and visual cortex.

However, these children may show more subtle visual deficits which are difficult to detect early in life. Preliminary results of visual recognition memory testing in infants with brain infarct, using the FTII, indicate a high percentage of abnormal results (Cioni et al 1998, Guzzetta et al 2006). It has also been noted that other subtle defects of visual function can be identified in children with focal lesions at school age. An abnormal perception of motion stimuli has recently been found, for instance, in children with congenital hemiplegia, possibly due to a higher vulnerability of the function of the *dorsal stream*, i.e. the occipito-parietal visual pathway which has a role in action control, in these patients (Gunn et al 2002). The use of functional MRI or fibre tracking analysis in relation to the reorganization of visual structures may be of extreme help in the future for understanding the plasticity of the brain after early lesion.

NEONATAL ENCEPHALOPATHY/HYPOXIC-ISCHAEMIC ENCEPHALOPATHY

Neonatal encephalopathy is characterized by an abnormal neurological state, with or without seizures, and affects 2–8 in 1000 term infants (Badawi et al 2005, Pierrat et al 2005). The majority of studies in the literature have focused on infants who had neonatal encephalopathy due to perinatal hypoxic-ischaemic events, and have used the definition of hypoxic-ischaemic encephalopathy (HIE).

A few studies in the early 1990s, including both preterm and full-term infants with hypoxic-ischaemic lesions, reported that visual abnormalities are very common in infants with such lesions (de Vries and Dubowitz 1985, Groenendaal et al 1989, Cioni et al 1996). More recent studies have correlated the presence and the severity of abnormalities of various aspects of visual function to the severity of HIE at birth, graded according to Sarnat and Sarnat (1976), and to the pattern of brain lesions on neonatal brain MRI in full-term infants with HIE. The severity of HIE at birth cannot always predict the severity of visual impairment (Mercuri et al 1997a, 1997b). Although all the infants with stage I HIE (Sarnat and Sarnat 1976) have normal visual function, and those with stage III HIE who survive the neonatal period always have severe visual impairment, visual outcome in stage II HIE is less predictable as both normal and abnormal visual outcome can be found in these infants.

The presence and the severity of visual impairment, in contrast, appear to be related to the pattern of lesions seen on brain MRI and particularly to the involvement of the basal ganglia and thalami. When basal ganglia and thalami are not involved, not all lesions involving the occipital lobes are associated with impaired visual function, suggesting a possible plasticity of the brain. The involvement of basal ganglia and thalami is, in contrast, more often associated with visual impairment. More specifically, children with severe basal ganglia lesions are very severely visually impaired from the first months of life and do not show any improvement with age, generally only showing a response to light. Children with moderate basal ganglia lesions also have abnormal results on various aspects of visual function, such as acuity, fields and fixation shift, but they have much better residual vision which they can use in everyday life. When tested at school age these infants still show a similar degree of impairment even when more mature aspects of visual function, such as crowding acuity or stereopsis, are tested.

The only infants who show different results on the assessments performed in the first year and at school age are those with minimal basal ganglia lesions. A proportion of infants with minimal basal ganglia lesions may also have visual abnormalities in the first months after birth but these tend to recover by the end of the first year (Mercuri et al 1997c). These infants are described as having 'delayed visual maturation' (DVM), a term used to describe

225

infants with reduced vision at birth, which improves by the end of the first year of life (Tresidder et al 1990).

The role played by basal ganglia and thalami in visual maturation is still not fully understood, but several studies have reported extensive reciprocal connections between visual cortical areas and basal ganglia (Ungerleider et al 1984, Updyke 1993, Serizawa et al 1994). One hypothesis is that the integrity of these connections is essential not only for the normal development of visual function but also for an exchange of information within the brain when damage to the developing brain occurs. An interruption to these connections may preclude the possibility of functional reorganization, reducing the possibility that other cortical areas may take over functions from a damaged occipital region.

Conclusions

In recent decades major transformations have occurred in the clinical management of infants with early brain lesions, and in the diagnosis of visual disorders. On the one hand, early detailed neuroimaging can give important information from birth concerning the specific risk of visual problems of central origin. On the other hand, reliable new methods can be applied in early infancy for the assessment and monitoring of visual disorders in newborns at risk. This is particularly relevant in relation to the essential role of early visual function in cognitive development (Mercuri et al 1999, Cioni et al 2000), and the important therapeutic function of early planning of specific rehabilitation. Recognition of visual impairment should lead to enrolment in early intervention programmes, which have been shown to have a favourable influence on the visual outcome of these infants (Sonksen et al 1991).

REFERENCES

Allen D, Tyler CW, Norcia AM (1996) Development of grating acuity and contrast sensitivity on the central and peripheral visual field of the human infant. *Vision Res* 36: 1945–1953.
Atkinson J (1979) Development of optokinetic nystagmus in the human infant and monkey infant: an analogue to development in kittens. In: Freeman RD, editor. *Developmental Neurobiology of Vision*. New York: Plenum Pless.
Atkinson J, Braddick OJ (1981) Development of optokinetic nystagmus in infants: an indicator of cortical binocularity. In: Fisher DF, Monty RA, Sender JW, editors. *Eye Movements: Cognition and Visual Perception*. Hillsdale, NJ: Lawrence Erlbaum Associates, pp 53–64.
Atkinson J, Hood B, Wattam-Bell J, Braddick O (1992) Changes in infants' ability to switch visual attention in the first three months of life. *Perception* 21: 643–653.
Auestad N, Montalto BM, Hall RT, Fitzgerald KM, Wheeler RE, Connor E, Neuringer M, Connor SL, Taylor JA, Hartmann EE (1997) Visual acuity, erythrocyte fatty acid composition, and growth in term infants fed formulas with long chain polyunsaturated fatty acids for one year. *Pediatr Res* 41: 1–10.
Badawi N, Felix JF, Kurinczuk JJ, Dixon G, Watson L, Keogh LM, Valentine J, Stanley FJ (2005) Cerebral palsy following term newborn encephalopathy: a population-based study. *Dev Med Child Neurol* 47: 293–298.
Banker BQ, Larroche JC (1962) Periventricular leukomalacia of infancy. A form of neonatal anoxic encephalopathy. *Arch Neurol* 7: 386–410.
Banks MS, Aslin RN, Letson RD (1975) Sensitive period for the development of human binocular vision. *Science* 190: 675–677.
Birch EE, Hoffman DR, Uauy R, Birch DG, Prestidge C (1998) Visual acuity and the essentiality of docosahexaenoic acid and arachidonic acid in diet of term infants. *Pediatr Res* 44: 201–209.
Bornstein MH, Sigman MD (1986) Continuity in mental development from infancy. *Child Dev* 57, 251–274.

Braddick OJ, Wattam-Bell J, Atkinson J (1986) Orientation-specific cortical responses develop in early infancy. *Nature* 320: 617–619.

Brozynski ME, Nelson MN, Matalon TA, Genaze DR, Rosati-Skertich C, Naughton PM, Meier WA (1985) Cavitary periventricular leukomalacia: incidence and short-term outcome in infants weighing less than or equal to 1200 grams at birth. *Dev Med Child Neurol* 27: 572–577.

Cioni G, Fazzi B, Ipata AE, Canapicchi R, van Hof-van Duin J (1996) Correlation between cerebral visual impairment and magnetic resonance imaging in children with neonatal encephalopathy. *Dev Med Child Neurol* 38: 120–132.

Cioni G, Fazzi B, Coluccini M, Bartalena L, Boldrini A, van Hof-van Duin J (1997) Cerebral visual impairment in preterm infants with periventricular leukomalacia. *Pediatr Neurol* 17: 331–338.

Cioni G, Brizzolara D, Ferretti G, Bertuccelli B, Fazzi B (1998) Visual information processing in infants with focal brain lesions. *Exp Brain Res* 123, 95–101.

Cioni G, Bertuccelli B, Boldrini A, Canapicchi R, Fazzi B, Guzzetta A, Mercuri E (2000) Correlation between visual function, neurodevelopmental outcome, and magnetic resonance imaging findings in infants with periventricular leucomalacia. *Arch Dis Child Fetal Neonatal Ed* 82: F134–F140.

de Vries LS, Dubowitz LMS (1985) Cystic leukomalacia in the preterm infant: site of lesion in relation to prognosis. *Lancet* 2: 1075–1076.

de Vries LS, Connel JA, Dubowitz LMS, Oozeer RC, Dubowitz V, Pennock JM (1987) Neurological, electrophysiological and MRI abnormalities in infants with extensive cystic leukomalacia. *Neuropediatrics* 18: 61–66.

de Vries LS, Dubowitz LMS, Pennock JM, Dubowitz V (1990) *Brain Disorder in the Newborn*. London: Wolfe Medical Publications.

Drotar D, Mortimer J, Shepherd PA, Fagan JF (1989) Recognition memory as a method of assessing intelligence of an infant with quadriplegia. *Dev Med Child Neurol* 31: 391–394.

Dubowitz LMS, Mushin J, Morante A, Placzek M (1983) The maturation of visual acuity in neurologically normal and abnormal newborn infants. *Behav Brain Res* 10: 39–45.

Eken P, van Nieuwenhuizen O, van der Graaf Y, Schalij-Delfos NE, de Vries L (1994) Relation between neonatal cranial ultrasound abnormalities and cerebral visual impairment in infancy. *Dev Med Child Neurol* 36: 3–15.

Eken P, de Vries L, van der Graaf Y, Meiners LC, van Nieuwenhuizen O (1995) Haemorrhagic-ischaemic lesions of the neonatal brain: correlation between cerebral visual impairment, neurodevelopmental outcome and MRI in infancy. *Dev Med Child Neurol* 37: 41–55.

Eken P, de Vries LS, van Nieuwenhuizen O, Schalij-Delfos NE, Reits D, Spekreijse H (1996) Early predictors of cerebral visual impairment in infants with cystic leukomalacia. *Neuropediatrics* 27: 16–25.

Fagan JF, Singer LT (1983) Infant recognition memory as a measure of intelligence. In: Lisitt L, editor. *Advances in Infancy Research*, Vol 2. Norwood, NJ: Ablex, pp 31–78.

Fedrizzi E, Anderloni A, Bono R, Bova S, Farinotti M, Inverno M, Savoiardo S (1998) Eye-movement disorders and visual-perceptual impairment in diplegic children born preterm: a clinical evaluation. *Dev Med Child Neurol* 40: 682–688.

Gibson NA, Fielder AR, Trounce JQ, Levine MI (1990) Ophthalmic findings in infants of very low birthweight. *Dev Med Child Neurol* 32: 7–13.

Groenendaal F, van Hof-van Duin J, Baerts W, Fetter WP (1989) Effects of perinatal hypoxia on visual development during the first year of (corrected) age. *Early Hum Dev* 20: 267–279.

Gunn A, Cory E, Atkinson J, Braddick O, Wattam-Bell J, Guzzetta A, Cioni G (2002) Dorsal and ventral stream sensitivity in normal development and hemiplegia. *NeuroReport* 13(6): 843–847.

Guzzetta A, Morrone MC, Del Viva M, Montanaro D, Tosetti M, Tinelli F, Cioni G (2004) Perceiving the opposite direction of motion in children with congenital brain lesions. *Dev Med Child Neurol* 46: 17.

Guzzetta A, Mazzotti S, Tinelli F, Bancale A, Ferretti G, Battini R, Bartalena L, Boldrini A, Cioni G (2006) Early assessment of visual information processing and neurological outcome in preterm infants. *Neuropediatrics* 37: 278–285.

Hacke W, Schaar B, Schafer C (1981) Comparison of the blink-reflex obtained using needle electrodes and surface electrodes (author's transl). *EG EMG Z Elektroenzephalogr Elektromyogr Verwandte Geb* 12: 190–194.

Harvey EM, Dobson V, Luna B, Scher MS (1997) Grating acuity and visual-field development in children with intraventricular hemorrhage. *Dev Med Child Neurol* 39: 305–312.

Hrbek A, Karlberg P, Olsson T (1973) Development of visual and somatosensory evoked responses in pre-term newborn infants. *Electroencephalogr Clin Neurophysiol* 34: 225–232.

Jacobson L, Ygge J, Flodmark O, Ek U (2002) Visual and perceptual characteristics, ocular motility and strabismus in children with periventricular leukomalacia. *Strabismus* 10: 179–183.

Lanzi G, Fazzi E, Uggetti C (1998) Cerebral visual impairment in periventricular leukomalacia. *Neuropediatrics* 29: 145–150.

McCall RB, Carriger MS (1993) A meta-analysis of infant habituation and recognition memory performance as predictors of later IQ. *Child Dev* 64: 57–79.

Mercuri E, von Siebenthal K, Tutuncuoglu S, Guzzetta F, Casaer P (1995) The effect of behavioural states on visual evoked responses in preterm and full-term newborns. *Neuropediatrics* 26: 211–213.

Mercuri E, Atkinson J, Braddick O, Anker S, Nokes L, Cowan F, Rutherford M, Pennock J, Dubowitz L (1996a) Visual function and perinatal focal cerebral infarction. *Arch Dis Child Fetal Neonatal Ed* 75: F76–F81.

Mercuri E, Spanò M, Bruccini G, Frisone MF, Trombetta JC, Blandino A, Longo M, Guzzetta F (1996b) Visual outcome in children with congenital hemiplegia: correlation with MRI findings. *Neuropediatrics* 27: 184–188.

Mercuri E, Atkinson J, Braddick O, Anker S, Cowan F, Rutherford M, Pennock J, Dubowitz L (1997a) Visual function in full-term infants with hypoxic-ischaemic encephalopathy. *Neuropediatrics* 28: 155–161.

Mercuri E, Atkinson J, Braddick O, Anker S, Cowan F, Rutherford M, Pennock J, Dubowitz L (1997b) Basal ganglia damage and impaired visual function in the newborn infant. *Arch Dis Child Fetal Neonatal Ed* 77: F111–F114.

Mercuri E, Atkinson J, Braddick O Anker S, Cowan F, Pennock J, Rutherford MA, Dubowitz LM (1997c) The aetiology of delayed visual maturation: short review and personal findings in relation to magnetic resonance imaging. *Eur J Paed Neurol* 1: 31–34.

Mercuri E, Haataja L, Guzzetta A, et al (1999) Visual function in full term infants with brain lesions: correlation with neurologic and developmental status at 2 years of age. *Arch Dis Child Fetal Neonatal Ed* 80: F99–F104.

Mohn G, van Hof-van Duin J (1986) Development of the binocular and monocular visual field during the first year of life. *Clin Vis Sci* 1: 51–64.

Morante A, Dubowitz LMS, Levene MI, Dubowitz V (1982) The development of visual function in normal and neurologically abnormal preterm and fulllterm infants. *Dev Med Child Neurol* 24: 771–784.

Norcia AM, Tyler CW, Hamer RD (1990) Development of contrast sensitivity in the human infant. *Vision Res* 30: 1475–1486.

Papile LA, Munsick-Bruno G, Schaefer A (1983) Relationship of cerebral intraventricular hemorrhage and early childhood neurologic handicaps. *J Pediatr* 103: 273–277.

Pierrat V, Haouari N, Liska A, Thomas D, Subtil D, Truffert P, Groupe d'Etudes en Epidemiologie Perinatale (2005) Prevalence, causes, and outcome at 2 years of age of newborn encephalopathy: population based study. *Arch Dis Child Fetal Neonatal Ed* 90: F257–F261.

Sarnat HB, Sarnat MS (1976) Neonatal encephalopathy following neonatal distress. A clinical and electroencephalographic study. *Arch Neurol* 33: 696–705.

Scher MS, Dobson V, Carpenter NA, Guthrie RD (1989) Visual and neurological outcome of infants with periventricular leukomalacia. *Dev Med Child Neurol* 31: 353–365.

Serizawa M, Mc Haffie JG, Hoshino K, Norita M (1994) Corticostriatal and corticotectal projections from visual cortical areas 17, 18 and 18a in the pigmented rat. *Arch Histol Cytol* 57: 493–507.

Shevell MI, Majnemer A, Morin I (2003) Etiologic yield of cerebral palsy: a contemporary case series. *Pediatr Neurol* 28: 352–359.

Shimojo S, Held R (1987) Vernier acuity is less than grating acuity in 2- and 3-month-olds. *Vision Res* 27: 77–86.

Skoczenski AM, Norcia AM (2002) Late maturation of visual hyperacuity. *Psychol Sci* 13: 537–541.

Sonksen PM, Petrie A, Drew KJ (1991) Promotion of visual development of severally visual impaired babies: evaluation of a developmentally based program. *Dev Med Child Neurol* 22: 320–335.

Stiers P, De Cock P, Vandenbussche E (1998) Impaired visual perceptual performance on an object recognition task in children with cerebral visual impairment. *Neuropediatrics* 29(2): 80–88.

Stiers P, De Cock P, Vandenbussche E (1999) Separating visual perception and non-verbal intelligence in children with early brain injury. *Brain Dev* 21(6): 397–406.

Stiers P, van den Hout BM, Haers M, Vanderkelen R, de Vries LS, van Nieuwenhuizen O, Vandenbussche E (2001) The variety of visual perceptual impairments in pre-school children with perinatal brain damage. *Brain Dev* 23(5): 333–348.

Stiers P, Vanderkelen R, Vanneste G, Coene S, De Rammelaere M, Vandenbussche E (2002) Visual-perceptual impairment in a random sample of children with cerebral palsy. *Dev Med Child Neurol* 44(6): 370–382.

Taylor MJ, Keenan NK, Gallant T, Skarf B, Freedman MH, Logan WJ (1987) Subclinical VEP abnormalities in patients on chronic deferoxamine therapy: longitudinal studies. *Electroencephalogr Clin Neurophysiol* 68: 81–87.

Teller DY, McDonald MA, Preston K, Sebris SL, Dobson V (1986) Assessment of visual acuity in infants and children: the acuity card procedure. *Dev Med Child Neurol* 26: 779–789.

Tresidder J, Fielder AR, Nicholson J (1990) Delayed visual maturation: ophthalmic and neurodevelopmental aspects. *Dev Med Child Neurol* 32: 872–881.

Tsuneishi S, Casaer P (1997) Stepwise decrease in VEP latencies and the process of myelination in the human visual pathway. *Brain Dev* 19: 547–551.

Tsuneishi S, Casaer P (2000) Effects of preterm extrauterine visual experience on the development of the human visual system: a flash VEP study. *Dev Med Child Neurol* 42: 663–668.

Uggetti C, Egitto MG, Fazzi E, Bianchi PE, Bergamaschi R, Zappoli F, Sibilla L, Martelli A, Lanzi G (1996) Cerebral visual impairment in periventricular leukomalacia: MR correlation. *Am J Neuroradiol* 17: 979–985.

Ungerleider LG, Desimone R, Galwin TW, Mishkin M (1984) Subcortical projections of area MT in the macaque. *J Comp Neurol* 223: 368–386.

Updyke BV (1993) Organisation of visual corticostriatal projections in the cat, with observations on visual projections to claustrum and amygdala. *J Comp Neurol* 327: 159–193.

van Hof-van Duin J, Heersema DJ, Groenendaal F, Baerts W, Fetter WPF (1992) Visual field and grating acuity development in low-risk preterm infants during the first 2½ years after term. *Behav Brain Res* 49: 115–122.

Westheimer G (1975) Visual acuity and hyperacuity. *Invest Ophthalmol* 14: 570–572.

13
FROM OBSERVATION TO REHABILITATION

Laura Zawacki and Suzann Campbell

The development of postural control is the foundation for functional movement in infancy, and observations of quality of movement and postural alignment in infants at risk for poor developmental outcome have long formed the basis of examination of motor development by physical therapists. Diagnosis of delayed development for the purpose of qualifying children for rehabilitation services, however, requires the additional use of observations from standardized tests for comparison of infant performance to age-related norms. Two commonly used tests for this purpose are the Test of Infant Motor Performance (TIMP; Campbell 2001) and the Alberta Infant Motor Scale (AIMS; Piper and Darrah 1994). The purpose of this chapter is to describe how results of the TIMP and the AIMS can be used to (1) establish a diagnosis of delayed motor development in infants under 12 months of age (age adjusted for preterm birth when necessary); (2) identify profiles of individual item performance which suggest risk for cerebral palsy (CP) versus delayed development without neurological signs; (3) plan intervention based on test performance profiles; and (4) measure outcomes of intervention programmes.

The practice of physical and occupational therapy in neonatal intensive care units (NICUs) and in developmental follow-up clinics is highly variable. A recent multi-centre study involved 13 different clinical sites across the United States, each with a level II or level III NICU and some form of follow-up for their NICU graduates. The therapy practice patterns both in the NICUs and in the follow-up clinics were highly inconsistent. Some NICUs had a blanket referral for therapists to evaluate and treat all infants in the nursery. Others relied more on medical diagnoses likely to lead to motor impairments to prompt a referral for service. Still others used a symptom-driven approach whereby infants who demonstrated abnormal movement, abnormal muscle tone or difficulty with feeding or behavioural organization were referred for therapy. Across the board, however, therapists practising in these NICUs did not utilize any form of standardized testing that would yield a score to compare performance to that of a peer group. As a result, the outcome of the assessment is highly dependent on the level of experience or expertise of the therapist.

The variability in the provision of follow-up services was equally as broad. The 13 sites had no consistent age or schedule for follow-up testing, nor was the type of assessment utilized consistent. Some sites offered a therapist's descriptive evaluation of the infant's motor performance, which again would vary depending on the therapist's level of experience. Other sites did offer standardized testing using the Peabody Developmental

Motor Scales, the Bayley Scales of Infant Development or the AIMS. Still other sites had no therapists actively involved in their follow-up clinics at all.

It is the belief of these authors that some form of standardized testing should be a part of the assessment process both in the NICU and in the follow-up clinics. Furthermore, the decision of whether or not to treat these infants should be based on performance falling below that of their peers. Utilization of a standardized assessment provides some degree of consistency across different facilities. Some of the available assessment tools to determine the need for intervention are the TIMP, the AIMS, the Bayley Scales of Infant Development – 2nd edition (BSID-II; Bayley 1993), and the Peabody Developmental Motor Scales – 2nd edition (PDMS-2; Folio and Fewell 2000). (These assessment tools are described in detail in Chapter 8.)

The motor assessments most commonly used by physical therapists are the PDMS-2 and the BSID-II, despite recent peer-reviewed citations refuting their utility (Darrah et al 1998a, Provost et al 2000). These assessments do not cover the age range of infants in the NICU, and their clinical utility is quite limited for infants younger than 6 months of age. The TIMP and the AIMS, however, were both created by therapists and are intended for use by therapists to diagnose delayed gross motor development in infancy. As such they yield the kind of clinical information of particular interest to physical therapists and occupational therapists. Specifically, the items in these tests assess postural control and quality of movement rather than only gross motor skill acquisition. These authors believe that the TIMP and the AIMS are superior assessment options to the traditionally used Peabody and Bayley scales. This chapter will review the evidence-based use of the TIMP and the AIMS, and clinical decision making based on these tests, demonstrated through case examples.

Review of the literature on the Test of Infant Motor Performance (TIMP)

The TIMP is a norm-referenced assessment of the postural control and alignment needed for functional activity in early infancy (Campbell 2001). The TIMP can be used with infants from 34 weeks postconceptional age (PCA) to 4 months adjusted age (AA) post-term (Campbell et al 1995). Thirteen Observed Items record presence or absence of a variety of spontaneous movements such as centring the head along the midline axis of the body, flexing the lower extremities against gravity, reciprocal kicking, and isolated finger and ankle movements. There are 29 Elicited Items which present movement problems for infants to solve, in a variety of positions, such as righting the head in supported sitting, turning the head to visually track a bright red ball, or lifting the head in prone. The Observed Items are scored as either 0 for absent or 1 for present, and the Elicited Items are scored on a 4- to 7-level scale, depending on the item.

The TIMP thus yields a total raw score which is then compared to the age standards published in the Test User's Manual (Campbell 2005). Raw scores can be used to calculate standard or Z-scores, percentile rankings, age equivalent scores and percentages of delay, depending on the local agency requirements for qualification for services. Psychometricians caution against the use of age equivalent scores and percentages of delay, but some government agencies continue to require these scores to determine eligibility for services.

Typically developing infants change significantly on the TIMP every two weeks, and age standards are available for each two-week interval from 34–35 weeks PCA to 16–17 weeks AA post-term, based on the performance of a national sample of 990 US infants of all races and ethnicities (Campbell et al 2006). The items in the test have demonstrated ecologic validity, i.e. demands for movement placed on infants during TIMP testing by clinicians have been shown to be similar to those placed on babies by their mothers during dressing, bathing and play (Murney and Campbell 1998).

The TIMP has also been shown to have predictive validity based on infant performance scores at 3 months AA that fall below -0.5 SD from the mean (Campbell et al 2002, Kolobe et al 2004). Prediction of delayed motor development on the AIMS (Piper and Darrah 1994) at 12 months of age is achieved with a sensitivity of 92 per cent and specificity of 76 per cent. The relatively low specificity means that some infants who perform poorly on the TIMP at 3 months AA can be expected to recover to achieve scores above the 5th percentile on the AIMS at 12 months AA.

TIMP scores in infancy are correlated with Bruininks-Oseretsky Test of Motor Proficiency scores at school age (partial correlation = .36; Flegel and Kolobe 2002). Furthermore, prediction of motor outcomes more then 2 SD below the mean on the Peabody Developmental Motor Scales (PDMS; Folio and Fewell 2000) at preschool age has a sensitivity of 72 per cent and a specificity of 91 per cent, with a positive predictive validity of 75 per cent, suggesting that the apparent early recovery at 12 months AA from the effects of medical complications may not persist in some infants (Kolobe et al 2004). Finally, a longitudinal study of 10 infants who were later diagnosed as having CP showed that motor development on the TIMP was delayed in six (60 per cent) of the infants as early as 7 days AA post-term, and that eight (80 per cent) of the infants showed delayed development by 3 months AA (Barbosa et al 2003). Two of the 10 children did not show delayed development until tested with the AIMS at 6 months AA.

Two controlled clinical trials have demonstrated that the TIMP is sensitive to the effects of physical therapy in the form of Neuro-Developmental Treatment in the special care nursery (Girolami and Campbell 1994), and in the form of a home programme following nursery discharge (Lekskulchai and Cole 2001). The latter study also documented the usefulness of the TIMP in identifying children at hospital discharge who showed delayed development that could be improved through physical therapy.

In summary, the TIMP is sensitive to biweekly change in motor performance of infants born preterm and other infants at risk for impaired motor outcome, it can be used to identify those with motor developmental delay, and it is sensitive to the effects of physical therapy on rate of functional motor development.

Review of the literature on the Alberta Infant Motor Scale
The Alberta Infant Motor Scale (AIMS) is a norm-referenced gross motor assessment comprised of items which assess quality and components of movement rather than motor skill acquisition in isolation (Piper and Darrah 1994). It is appropriate for use from birth or term equivalent age up to 18 months of age. The infant is observed in the prone, supine, sitting and standing positions, and the clinician determines the infant's current motor

repertoire or window of skills in these positions. Because the AIMS is observational, stranger anxiety is lessened. The clinician simply watches the mother play with her infant in various positions and notes the skills that are present.

The AIMS emphasizes quality of movement, such that an infant who lifts his head in prone using excessive neck extension and scapular retraction would receive a lower score than an infant who executes this skill with a chin tuck and the ability to bring the arms forward and align the elbows in front of the shoulders. There are 58 possible items which are scored dichotomously as either Observed or Not Observed, and the raw scores can be compared to normative tables to yield a percentile ranking compared to same-age peers. The reporting of test results as a percentile ranking is a method that parents can easily understand, as they are used to hearing this for their infant's height, weight and head circumference.

The intended purposes of the AIMS are to identify infants with gross motor delay, to evaluate change in motor performance over time, to assist clinicians with treatment planning, and to educate parents about infant motor development (Piper and Darrah 1994). The AIMS was normed on a representative sample of 2202 infants from the province of Alberta, Canada. Concurrent validity with the motor scale of the Bayley Scales of Infant Development (BSID; Bayley 1969) and the gross motor scale of the Peabody Developmental Motor Scales (PDMS; Folio and Fewell 1983) was .99 and .97, respectively, for typically developing infants. When used to assess at-risk and atypically developing infants, the concurrent validity between the AIMS and the BSID was .93, and with the PDMS it was .95 (Piper et al 1992, Piper and Darrah 1994). Concurrent validity with the TIMP at 3 months AA is .64 (Campbell and Kolobe 2000).

When the AIMS manual (Piper and Darrah 1994) was published, the predictive capabilities of the tool had not yet been studied. Since that time, however, two studies have been published reporting the predictive capability of the AIMS. The test developers compared the predictive capabilities of the AIMS with those of the Movement Assessment of Infants (MAI; Chandler et al 1980) and the gross motor scale of the PDMS (Darrah et al 1998a). There were 164 infants in the study, tested at 4 and 8 months AA with all three assessments, and rated at 18 months by a physician as normal, suspicious or abnormal for gross motor development.

Based on the results of this study, the authors revised the recommended cut-off scores for clinicians using the AIMS, based on which cut-offs yielded the best combination of sensitivity and specificity for predicting later outcome. The recommended cut-off on the AIMS at 4 months is the 10th percentile, which carries a sensitivity value of 77 per cent and a specificity of 82 per cent. At 8 months, however, the recommended cut-off is the 5th percentile, with a sensitivity of 86 per cent and a specificity value of 93 per cent. The authors recommend the use of the MAI at 4 months due to better specificity values, but conclude that the AIMS is a superior tool at 8 months. Furthermore, the authors offer an excellent discussion about the selection of cut-off scores to use for discriminating low performance, based on the intent of the programme and the availability of resources.

A second group of researchers reported lower sensitivity and specificity values for the AIMS at 4 and 7 months in a group of cocaine-exposed infants, and concluded that the 2nd percentile at 7 months was the cut-off score yielding the best combination of sensitivity and specificity for prediction of motor performance at 15 months, as measured by the gross motor scale of the PDMS (Fetters and Tronick 2000). In this study, while the AIMS did a better job of identifying typically developing infants, it tended to miss more infants with delays.

Similarly, in a study reviewing AIMS performance in 10 infants later diagnosed as having CP, seven of the 10 infants were not identified by the AIMS at 3 months AA because they were able to achieve a score above the 20th percentile (Barbosa et al 2003). By 6 months of age, however, all but one of the infants with CP was correctly labelled as delayed by the AIMS. Clinicians using the AIMS should also be aware that in an analysis of the intra-individual stability of AIMS scores over time, 31 per cent of typically developing infants tested repeatedly on the AIMS had at least one score that fell below the 10th percentile (Darrah et al 1998b).

Although the test developers state that the age range for the AIMS is from birth to 18 months, two different authors have reported a ceiling effect on the AIMS. Rasch analysis of the AIMS items revealed that there are too few items below 3 months of age as well as too few beyond the stage of lowering from standing, so that the AIMS offers the best precision of measurement from 3 to 9 months of age (Liao and Campbell 2004). Additionally, a group of infants who scored poorly on the AIMS at 10 months were assessed again at 15 months with the AIMS and the PDMS and compared to a group that scored well on the AIMS at 10 months (Bartlett 2000). Both groups scored in the normal range on the AIMS at 15 months, but the study group (low-scoring 10-month-old infants) scored lower on the locomotor section of the gross motor scale of the PDMS. The author concludes that the AIMS alone at 15 months is not an adequate assessment of motor function, as most infants will ceiling out by then.

In this chapter we present information from our experience of using test results on the TIMP and the AIMS for making clinical decisions and planning and evaluating results of intervention for children who are (1) delayed in motor performance, (2) within the average range for overall motor performance but demonstrating atypical quality of movement, and (3) at high risk for CP because of a profile of item performance combining 'advanced' performance in items using extension patterns and slow development or regression in items requiring anti-gravity activity and balanced use of flexion-extension patterns of muscle activity.

Infant QA: diagnosis of delayed functional motor performance

MEDICAL HISTORY

QA was born via normal spontaneous vaginal delivery (NSVD) to a schizophrenic mother with a history of alcohol abuse and no prenatal care. He was born in a hotel room and was taken to the hospital emergency room (ER) several hours later. Upon presentation to the ER, he was hypothermic and hypoglycemic. He weighed 1519 grams at birth, and his estimated gestational age (EGA) at birth by physical examination was 33–35 weeks. His neonatal course included bilateral grade IV intraventricular hemorrhage (IVH), hydrocephalus, gastroesophageal reflux disease (GERD), as well as orthopedic deformities of his hands and feet (bilateral club feet and PIP and DIP flexion contractures as well as hyper-extension of the MP joint). Hydrocephalus was managed with a ventriculoperitoneal (VP) shunt which subsequently became infected resulting in meningitis. He repeatedly aspirated during oral feeding and required a gastrostomy tube for enteral feedings. For his multiple and complex problems, QA was followed by a variety of medical specialists. He received physical therapy, occupational therapy and speech therapy services while in the neonatal intensive care unit (NICU), and he was referred for early intervention (EI) services upon discharge to a foster home.

DEVELOPMENTAL EXAMINATION RESULTS

In the USA, eligibility for provision of EI services is determined by each state operating under overall federal guidelines. In the state of Illinois, developmental diagnosis must be based on use of approved tests with documented reliability and validity. QA was assessed with both the TIMP and the AIMS. Calculated via the TIMP age correction calculation wheel (www.thetimp.com), QA's AA on the day of testing was 14 weeks. He received a raw score of 62 on the TIMP (the range of possible scores is 0–142), placing him in the far below average performance range compared to age-matched peers (Fig. 13.1; Campbell 2001). His age equivalent score was that of an infant at 38–39 weeks PCA, and his standard score or Z-score was -2.3, far below the cut-off of -.5 SD for prediction of poor motor outcome. In this case the TIMP allowed the therapist to objectively quantify QA's paucity of self-generated movement and lack of postural control as well as document his lack of gross motor skill acquisition compared to similar-age peers.

On the AIMS, QA obtained a raw score of 8 (Fig. 13.2; the maximum possible score on the AIMS is 58 but for this age the maximum is approximately 19). Using the traditional subtraction method to calculate AA, referenced by many authors, including the developers of the AIMS, QA's AA on the day of testing was 3 months 4 days. Based on their research findings, the AIMS developers recommend using a cut-off of <10th percentile at 4 months as indicative of motor delay (Darrah et al 1998a). QA's raw score of 8 on the AIMS placed him in the 10th percentile for gross motor development compared to same-age peers (Fig. 13.3) and, contrary to the TIMP results, did not identify him as delayed. Conversely, if his AIMS raw score of 8 was plotted on the percentile graph as a 14-week AA infant as

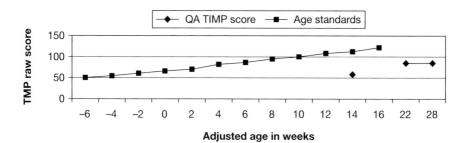

Fig. 13.1 Infant QA's TIMP raw scores compared to age standards.

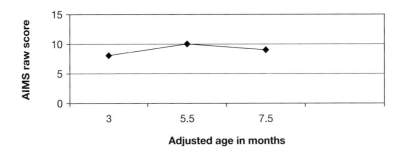

Fig. 13.2 Infant QA's AIMS raw scores.

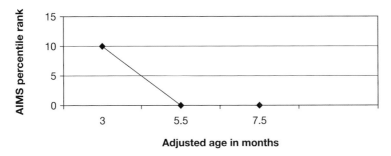

Fig. 13.3 Infant QA's AIMS percentile rank.

calculated via the more accurate TIMP age correction calculation wheel, then he would have been labelled as delayed. The age wheel is the more accurate method to calculate AA, and its use may qualify children who are near the cut-off for service eligibility.

Although both the TIMP and the AIMS assess postural control, quality of movement, and motor skill acquisition, and the tests have been shown to have some commonalities (concurrent validity = .64 at 3 months AA; Campbell and Kolobe 2000), the test results were remarkably different in this case. It is the authors' belief that the TIMP should be the examination tool of choice for clinicians working with infants under 4 months AA. The AIMS does a good job of identifying motor delay in infants above 5–6 months of age, but there are too few items for the lower age range of the test to have a high degree of precision at ages under 4 months AA (Liao and Campbell 2004). The primary motor skill required to receive credit for the few available AIMS items in the younger age ranges of the test is neck extension. As a result, infants who eventually present with developmental disabilities are able to score well on the AIMS at the younger ages if they use excessive neck extension to perform anti-gravity activities of the head (Barbosa et al 2005).

This discussion is included as a potential explanation for why QA was able to 'pass' the AIMS yet he 'failed' the TIMP. Additionally, QA's performance on the AIMS was determined by only 8 items, versus 42 items on the TIMP, a more sensitive test in the early months of life. By approximately 5–6 months of age, however, the AIMS does an excellent job of identifying children with poor motor performance (Barbosa et al 2003).

236

QA was reassessed two additional times with the AIMS at approximately 5½ and 7½ months AA and showed minor improvements in raw scores (Fig. 13.2). Plotting these AIMS results in terms of percentile ranks compared to same-age peers yields clinically useful information. QA's scores plummeted from the low end of the typical range at 3 months AA to far below average with repeated testing (Fig. 13.3).

INTERVENTION AND OUTCOME

In QA's case the TIMP was used to diagnose his delayed gross motor development and thus qualify him for intervention. Exercise prescription, parent education and treatment planning were also guided by the TIMP results. QA scored poorly on TIMP items requiring anterior neck muscle strength, lateral head righting and lower extremity strength. He presented with marked imbalance between flexion and extension of his neck, with extension being his preferred movement pattern. His foster mother received a copy of the pictorial version of the TIMP score sheet with items 17 (Head Control – Anterior Neck Muscles), 18 (Head Control – Lowered from Sitting) and 32 (Pull to Sit) circled as exercises to improve anterior neck muscle strength. Items 28/29 (Rolling: Elicited from Legs) and 40 (Standing) were also prescribed as part of his home programme to improve head righting and lower extremity weight bearing. All exercises were demonstrated and discussed with his foster mother in detail.

The TIMP was also used to evaluate change in QA's motor performance over time. Over a six-week interval QA showed no improvement in his TIMP score; in fact, his performance worsened slightly (Fig. 13.1). We know from research that there is a linear relationship between age and TIMP scores, such that as age increases, TIMP scores improve, with a correlation of .89 (Campbell et al 1995). Although the rate of change in TIMP scores is slower for children with neonatal brain insult, their scores have also been shown to improve over time (Campbell and Hedeker 2001).

The therapist was alarmed by QA's lack of improvement on the TIMP. She recommended to his foster mother that they return to the neurology clinic for further work-up of his condition. Over time QA began to lose motor milestones that he had previously achieved, and he eventually died of respiratory compromise shortly after his first birthday. In this case, lack of progress and TIMP performance regression over time served as an early warning sign for what may have been a progressive neuromuscular condition.

Infant SG: average functional motor performance with asymmetry

MEDICAL HISTORY

SG was born at 28 weeks EGA via emergency cesarean section to a 34-year-old mother. His birth weight was 488 grams, evidence of severe intrauterine growth retardation (IUGR). His Apgar scores were 6, 7 and 7 at 1, 5 and 10 minutes, respectively. Other neonatal history included respiratory distress syndrome (RDS), sepsis ruled out, multiple blood transfusions for anaemia, apnea and bradycardia, osteopenia of preterm birth, and difficulty with oral feeding. His primary medical diagnosis was bronchopulmonary dysplasia (BPD) requiring mechanical ventilation for approximately 10 weeks. He was slowly weaned to continuous positive airway pressure (CPAP) and eventually to a nasal canula for oxygen delivery.

SG was referred for physical therapy examination at 38 weeks PCA. Because he was on CPAP and quite medically fragile at the time, the initial examination was limited to assessment of his state regulation, postural control, positioning and tolerance for handling. Initially SG demonstrated limited ability to achieve and maintain a quiet alert state, poor tolerance for handling and position changes, jittery quality of active movement, and autonomic instability with frequent oxygen desaturation episodes. Due to SG's autonomic instability, his initial physical therapy and goals focused on parent education about BPD and understanding his behavioural signals. Once he was more medically stable and able to tolerate handling and position changes, however, he was an appropriate candidate for assessment with the TIMP.

At 3 weeks post-term AA, SG was assessed with the TIMP. His raw score was 80, placing him in the average range compared to similar-age peers (Fig. 13.4; Campbell 2001). This raw score of 80 yields a Z-score or standard score of .57 SD above the mean. Previous research on the TIMP has shown that test results at 1 month have a negative predictive value to 12-month performance of .91 and to preschool-age motor performance of .83, such that young infants who score well on the TIMP are highly likely to have a favourable motor outcome (Campbell et al 2002, Kolobe et al 2004). With a highly educated family such as SG's, the therapist shared the information with the parents that previous research on the TIMP suggests a high likelihood of continued typical development of gross motor milestones.

Although the overall score was in the typical performance range, the bidirectional TIMP items identified a marked asymmetry in performance. The therapist pointed out the asymmetry to SG's parents, who immediately enquired whether this might be indicative of CP. The therapist acknowledged the family's concerns and indicated that only repeated testing as SG continued to develop would reveal whether he would be able to recover from his adverse medical history to achieve typical motor development. She informed them that the fact that SG did receive credit for some of the quality of movement items on the Observed Items of the TIMP was a good sign, but reiterated that repeated testing over time was the best answer.

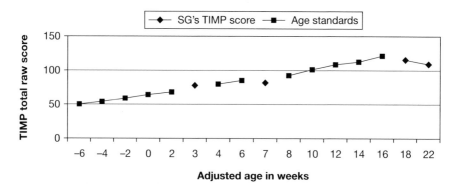

Fig. 13.4 Infant SG's TIMP raw scores compared to age standards.

In addition to providing an objective measurement of development of postural control, the TIMP provided other clinically useful information to help the therapist quantify the asymmetry and atypical movement patterns that she observed. The therapist noted that SG's scores were frequently lowered (per test scoring instructions) because his head was out of the midline, that he scored better to the right than to the left on all the bidirectional items, that he demonstrated neck hyperextension during prone items as well as an overall paucity of self-generated movement, and that he had poor endurance, requiring frequent rest breaks.

Even though SG scored in the average range on the TIMP, the therapist recommended home-based EI services as well as follow-up assessment in the hospital-based developmental follow-up clinic both because of his birth history and because of the asymmetry and atypical extension patterns observed during the TIMP examination. Results of studies documenting the developmental outcomes of infants with BPD also prompted the therapist to refer SG for services (O'Shea et al 1996, Gregoire et al 1998). SG's parents were given a home exercise programme (HEP) at the time of hospital discharge, as this has been shown in a controlled clinical trial to positively impact motor development of preterm infants in the first four months after discharge home (Lekskulchai and Cole 2001).

The pictorial format of the TIMP score sheet facilitates parent education and exercise prescription for infants. For example, SG needed to strengthen his anterior neck musculature to counteract the overuse of neck extension typical of infants with BPD (Georgieff and Bernbaum 1986). Items 17 (Head Control – Anterior Neck Muscles; Fig. 13.5a), 18 (Head Control – Lowered from Sitting; Fig. 13.5b) and 32 (Pull to Sit; Fig. 13.5c) on the TIMP score sheet were highlighted and demonstrated for his parents. The pull to sit item was modified to be administered with support more proximally around his rib cage and on his pectoral musculature, as he was too weak to perform the traditional pull to sit from the arms used during TIMP test administration. His parents provided a return demonstration to make sure the exercises were performed correctly.

On every bidirectional item on the TIMP, SG performed better to the right than to the left. His HEP was also designed to address this asymmetry. Items 14 (Visual Tracking to the Left; Fig. 13.5d), 24 (Supine Neck Rotation to the Left; Fig. 13.5e), 29 and 31 (Rolling Elicited from the Leg – Fig. 13.5f – and the Arm – Fig. 13.5g – to the Left), and 39 (Turn to Sound Toward the Left; Fig. 13.5h) all provided functional means of addressing the problem. Lastly, the therapist advised SG's parents of the importance of placing him in prone during his wakeful hours (Fig. 13.5i). There have been multiple reports in the literature recently indicating that infants who do not spend play time in prone can demonstrate delayed motor development (Monson et al 2003).

SG was assessed on two other occasions with the TIMP after he began EI services. At 7 weeks post-term AA, he achieved a raw score of 84 on the TIMP, again in the average performance range compared to same-age peers (Fig. 13.4). At 18 weeks AA he continued to perform in the average range with a raw score of 118. Over time and with intervention, the discrepancy in scores between the right and left sides diminished.

This case study demonstrates three common uses of the TIMP: assessment of motor performance to determine whether or not a delay exists; treatment planning including parent

239

Activities to strengthen anterior neck muscles and abdominals:

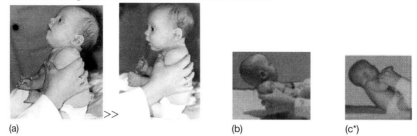

(a) (b) (c*)

Activities to address asymmetry:

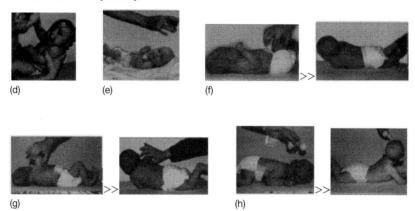

(d) (e) (f)

(g) (h)

Activities to improve prone skills:

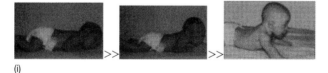

(i)

Fig. 13.5 SG's home exercise program based on TIMP findings. (a) = Anterior Neck Muscles, (b) = Lowered from Sitting, (c) = Pull to Sit (* this item was modified to be administered more proximally with support), (d) = Head Rotation to the Left, (e) = Supine Neck Rotation to the Left, (f) = Rolling Elicited from Leg to Left, (g) = Rolling Elicited from Arm to Left, (h) = Head Turn in Prone to Sound to Left, (i) = Head Lift in Prone.

Source: Photographs from the TIMP score sheet used with the permission of Infant Motor Performance Scales, LLC, 1301 W. Madison St. #526, Chicago, IL 60607-1953, USA, www.thetimp.com

education and exercise prescription; and assessment of change in motor performance over time. Although SG's overall TIMP score was age-appropriate, the test helped the therapist to identify problematic issues with the quality of SG's motor skills and to design a plan of care to address these issues. Furthermore, the pictorial score sheet provided a visual representation for his family of his asymmetry. It also yielded a professional, thorough, and immediately available HEP. Such efficiency in clinical practice is critical given the continually increasing time constraints on healthcare professionals. Most importantly, the TIMP provided evidence-based reassurance of overall motor competency for the concerned parents of a very sick infant.

Once SG was beyond the age range for the TIMP, his therapist began using the AIMS for assessment, treatment planning and parent education. Because the AIMS is so fast and easy to administer and score, and because it provides an excellent pictorial format for parent education, SG was reassessed on a monthly basis with this tool. His raw scores and percentile ranks are summarized in graphic form in Figs 13.6 and 13.7.

Treatment planning with the AIMS is very straightforward. The clinician simply identifies the items in the motor window that were scored as Not Observed and focuses intervention on achieving the missing components of movement required to achieve those skills. For example, at 6 months AA on the prone subscale of the AIMS SG was scored as Not Observed for Extended Arm Support and Rolling Prone to Supine without Rotation.

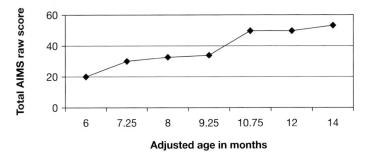

Fig. 13.6 Infant SG's AIMS raw scores.

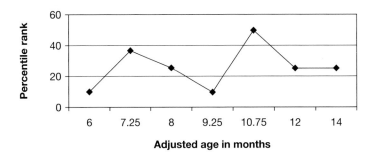

Fig. 13.7 Infant SG's AIMS percentile rankings.

241

For the supine subscale he did not receive credit for Hands to Feet or Rolling Supine to Prone. The only item scored as Not Observed within his motor window in the sitting subscale was Sitting with Arm Support. The acquisition of these gross motor milestones became short-term goals, and intervention included facilitation of these skills through handling and strategically placing toys to entice SG to move into or maintain these postures.

Home programme prescription with the AIMS is as easy as circling the items scored as Not Observed on the score sheet and teaching parents activities to help facilitate these skills. With monthly assessment on the AIMS, parents can clearly see the progress their infants are making as the skills that were previously not credited are achieved and the motor window moves further to the right on the score sheet to encompass more advanced motor skills. Another positive feature of the AIMS is that the item scoring format (Observed, Not Observed) facilitates its use with very delayed infants whose parents respond well to observations of performance versus the Pass/Fail scoring format of other tests.

Profiles of performance predicting high risk for CP

The potential value of the TIMP for predicting outcome and planning treatment programmes has recently been enhanced by the demonstration of differing profiles of development for typically developing infants versus those with delayed motor development or versus those with CP (Barbosa et al 2005).

In a longitudinal study of weekly performance on the TIMP of 85 infants with varying risk for impaired motor outcome, infants who were later diagnosed as having CP tended to differ from the other two groups in several ways: they performed *better* in the first month post-term on items involving neck extension and lateral head righting; however, they were unable to hold the head in midline in supine at about 20 days post-term; they demonstrated poor anti-gravity arm movements from 2–10 weeks AA; they had poor lateral hip abduction reactions when tilted in side-lying, and poor upright head control in supported sitting; they were unable to inhibit the neck righting reaction; and they demonstrated poor head righting during facilitated rolling to prone or when being pulled to sit from supine. The last item was particularly discriminating, because infants with CP showed virtually no development of the ability to right the head when pulled to sit, during the first several months of life. Children with delayed development showed fewer differences from typically developing children than did infants with CP, confirming the usual belief that these children show patterns of performance that are similar to typically developing children, but at a slower rate (Barbosa et al 2003).

Although there were only 10 infants with CP in this study, the clinical significance of this research should not be overlooked. Infants who will develop CP may appear *advanced* in neck extension activities during the first few weeks post-term but soon show delay or even regression in motor skills. Specifically, among the 10 infants with CP in Barbosa et al's study, five infants were unable to hold their head aligned in midline for two seconds at 20 days of age. Over the first four months post-term, eight could bring their head to vertical only when reaching 15 degrees from upright during pull to sit; seven had no head righting when rolled from supine to prone, and two did not even roll to prone with facilitation from the hip in the supine position. Six of the 10 lost the ability to hold both legs up in the air using anti-gravity muscles, so regression in previously acquired skills was also present.

In conjunction with general movement (GM) assessment to identify quality of movement concerns (see Chapter 5), the TIMP analysis of development in infants with CP offers a detailed description of how these infants move during functional activities at a very early age. Thus it might aid clinicians in identifying these infants earlier, rather than waiting until they fail to achieve gross motor milestones later in the first year of life. The period between 8 and 13 weeks seems to be particularly critical in making the transition to readiness for coming up against the force of gravity for sitting and other upright activities (Barbosa et al 2005).

Incorporating this research into clinical practice would entail identifying those infants at greatest risk for CP and performing repeated assessments over time with the TIMP while paying particular attention to the above-mentioned items. Although the TIMP is an assessment of the development of functional motor skills and not a diagnostic test for CP, early warning signs of CP captured by TIMP testing include excessive neck extension and inability to maintain the head in midline. Failure to progress to the higher performance levels on the pull to sit and upright head control items on the TIMP should also serve as a red flag for clinicians. Failure to achieve lateral head righting during facilitated rolling should raise suspicion as well and alert clinicians to the need to follow the infant closely.

In summary, both the TIMP and the AIMS offer clinicians research-based, psychometrically sound assessments of infant motor competency. Both tools have remarkable clinical utility in that a single assessment allows the therapist to determine whether a delay exists, to educate parents about motor development, to provide on-the-spot home exercise prescriptions, and to make evidence-based predictions about future motor performance. The TIMP should be the assessment of choice in infants under 4½ months adjusted age due to better precision of measurement and diagnostic sensitivity for detecting motor performance delay, while the AIMS ought to be the tool of choice from 5–6 months up to the acquisition of independent walking.

Although this chapter has presented clinical evidence-based use of these tools in patient case studies, further large-scale clinical trials of intervention effects are needed to guide the provision of therapy services. Topics for further research might include which types of interventions yield the best results, appropriate frequency, intensity and duration of services, and whether critical periods exist for the most effective provision of such services. Both the TIMP and the AIMS are ideally suited for daily clinical use as well as for research to help answer these and other questions in the developmental surveillance and treatment of high-risk neonates.

The primary focus of this chapter has been on the use of the TIMP and the AIMS by physical and occupational therapists working in NICUs and developmental follow-up clinics to diagnose delays in postural control and gross motor development. The concept, however, of using a standardized assessment to diagnose delay in any developmental domain, and planning interventions based on the delays identified, can be applied across all professional disciplines involved in the developmental follow-up of preterm infants. While a certain level of experience or expertise is imperative in order to work with this patient population, the objectivity and science of standardized testing are also critically important. Clinicians administering these tests should fully understand the meaning of the scores and should be able to interpret the scores in a way that is meaningful for parents. Successful developmental follow-up of high-risk neonates requires experienced clinicians, standardized testing, interpretation of test results with sensitivity, and parent education about the developmental domains assessed.

ACKNOWLEDGEMENTS

We are grateful to the parents of QA and SG for allowing their children's stories to be told. Unpublished research described in the chapter was funded by US National Institutes of Health grants R01 HD32567 and HD38867 to Suzann K Campbell, PT, PhD, and a fellowship for doctoral training from CAPES, Brazilian Ministry of Education, to Vanessa M Barbosa, OTR/L, PhD.

REFERENCES

Barbosa VM, Campbell SK, Sheftel D, Singh J, Beligere N (2003) Longitudinal performance of infants with cerebral palsy on the Test of Infant Motor Performance and on the Alberta Infant Motor Scale. *Phys Occup Ther Pediatr* 23(3): 7–20.

Barbosa VM, Campbell SK, Smith E, Berbaum M (2005) Comparison of Test of Infant Motor Performance (TIMP) item responses among children with cerebral palsy, children with developmental delay, and children with typical development. *Am J Occup Ther* 59: 446–456.

Bartlett DJ (2000) Comparison of 15 month motor and 18 month neurological outcomes of term infants with and without motor delays at 10 months of age. *Phys Occup Ther Pediatr* 19(3): 61–72.

Bayley N (1969) *Bayley Scales of Infant Development*. Berkeley, CA: Institute of Human Development, University of California.

Bayley N (1993) *Bayley II*. San Antonio, TX: Psychological Corporation.

Campbell SK (2001) *The Test of Infant Motor Performance. Test User's Manual Version 1.4*. Chicago: Infant Motor Performance Scales, LLC.

Campbell SK (2005) *The Test of Infant Motor Performance. Test User's Manual Version 2.0*. Chicago: Infant Motor Performance Scales, LLC.

Campbell SK, Hedeker D (2001) Validity of the Test of Infant Motor Performance for discriminating among infants with varying risk for poor motor outcome. *J Pediatr* 139: 546–551.

Campbell SK, Kolobe THA (2000) Concurrent validity of the Test of Infant Motor Performance with the Alberta Infant Motor Scale. *Pediatr Phys Ther* 12: 1–8.

Campbell SK, Kolobe THA, Osten ET, Lenke M, Girolami GL (1995) Construct validity of the Test of Infant Motor Performance. *Phys Ther* 75: 585–596.

Campbell SK, Kolobe THA, Wright BD, Linacre JM (2002) Validity of the Test of Infant Motor Performance for prediction of 6-, 9-, and 12-month scores on the Alberta Infant Motor Scale. *Dev Med Child Neurol* 44: 263–272.

Campbell SK, Levy P, Zawacki L, Liao P-J (2006) Population-based age standards for interpreting results on the Test of Infant Motor Performance. *Pediatr Phys Ther* 18: 119–125.

Chandler LS, Andrews MS, Swanson MW (1980) *Movement Assessment of Infants – A Manual*. Rolling Bay, WA: Movement Assessment of Infants.

Darrah J, Piper M, Watt MJ (1998a) Assessment of gross motor skills of at-risk infants: predictive validity of the Alberta Infant Motor Scale. *Dev Med Child Neurol* 40: 485–491.

Darrah J, Redfern L, Maguire TO, Beaulne AP, Watt J (1998b) Intra-individual stability of rate of gross motor development in full-term infants. *Early Hum Dev* 52: 169–179.

Fetters L, Tronick EZ (2000) Discriminate power of the Alberta Infant Motor Scale and the Movement Assessment of Infants for prediction of Peabody gross motor scale scores of infants exposed in utero to cocaine. *Pediatr Phys Ther* 12(1): 16–23

Flegel J, Kolobe THA (2002) Predictive validity of the Test of Infant Motor Performance as measured by the Bruininks-Oseretsky Test of Motor Proficiency at school age. *Phys Ther* 82: 762–771.

Folio MR, Fewell RR (1983) *Peabody Developmental Motor Scales and Activity Cards: A Manual*. Allen, TX: DLM Teaching Resources.

Folio MR, Fewell RR (2000) *Peabody Developmental Motor Scales Examiner's Manual*. Austin, TX: Pro-Ed.

Georgieff MK, Bernbaum JC (1986) Abnormal shoulder girdle muscle tone in premature infants during their first 18 months of life. *Pediatrics* 77: 664.

Girolami G, Campbell SK (1994) Efficacy of a Neuro-Developmental Treatment program to improve motor control of preterm infants. *Pediatr Phys Ther* 6: 175–184.

Gregoire MC, Lefebvre F, Glorieux J (1998) Health and developmental outcomes at 18 months in very preterm infants with bronchopulmonary dysplasia. *Pediatrics* 101: 856–860.

Kolobe THA, Bulanda M, Susman L (2004) Predicting motor outcome at preschool age for infants tested at 7, 30, 60, and 90 days after term age using the Test of Infant Motor Performance. *Phys Ther* 84: 1144–1156.

Lekskulchai R, Cole J (2001) Effect of a developmental program on motor performance in infants born preterm. *Aust J Physiother* 47: 169–176.

Liao P-JM, Campbell SK (2004) Examination of the item structure of the Alberta Infant Motor Scale (AIMS). *Pediatr Phys Ther* 16: 31–38.

Monson RM, Deitz, J, Kartin D (2003) The relationship between awake positioning and motor performance among infants who slept supine. *Pediatr Phys Ther* 15(4): 196–203.

Murney ME, Campbell SK (1998) The ecological relevance of the Test of Infant Motor Performance elicited scale items. *Phys Ther* 78: 479–489.

O'Shea TM, Goldstein DJ, de Regnier RA, Sheaffer CI, Roberts DD, Dillard RG (1996) Outcome at 4 to 5 years of age in children recovered from neonatal chronic lung disease. *Dev Med Child Neurol* 38: 830–839.

Piper MC, Darrah J (1994) *Motor Assessment of the Developing Infant*. Philadelphia: WB Saunders.

Piper MC, Pinnell LE, Darrah J, Maguire T, Byrne PJ (1992) Construction and validation of the Alberta Infant Motor Scale (AIMS). *Can J Public Health* 83(Suppl 2): S46–S50.

Provost B, Crowe TK, McClain C (2000) Concurrent validity of the Bayley Scales of Infant Development II Motor Scale and the Peabody Developmental Motor Scale in 2 year old children. *Phys Occup Ther Pediatr* 20(1): 5–18.

14

LONGITUDINAL MULTI-CENTRE FOLLOW-UP OF HIGH-RISK NEONATES: CURRENT STATUS AND FUTURE PROSPECTS

Michael Msall

Introduction

During the past 25 years, major advances in maternal-fetal medicine, neonatology, and translational developmental biology have resulted in survival rates exceeding 90 per cent among infants born with birthweights between 1000 grams (2.2 lbs) and 1499 grams (3.5 lbs) in centres of excellence for neonatal intensive care (Horbar et al 2002). In addition, combinations of maternal transport to advanced neonatal regional centres of excellence, use of prenatal maternal corticosteroids, and enhanced collaboration between obstetricians and neonatologists have resulted in survival rates exceeding 80 per cent for infants born with birthweights between 751 and 999 grams, and exceeding 60 per cent for infants born weighing 500–750 grams (Lemons et al 2001). These birthweight categories reflect appropriate weights for 28–30 weeks' (1000–1499g), 26–27 weeks' (751–999g), and 23–25 weeks' (500–750g) gestation approximately.

While there has been success in improving survival among these extremely low birthweight infants, preventing adverse neurodevelopmental outcomes in early childhood for these high risk survivors as well as other neonatal cohorts receiving new technologies remains a major challenge (Marlow 2004). However, with recent discoveries in brain structure and function, immunology, nutrition, early childhood learning, and developmental plasticity, the future holds promise.

The purpose of this chapter is to review model follow-up multi-centre or national studies from Europe, Canada, Australia, New Zealand, and the United States to understand developmental and functional pathways of risk and resiliency in early childhood, especially among neonates receiving new biomedical interventions. Although our focus will be on extremely low birthweight infants, we also acknowledge that neonates receiving cardiac, pulmonary, or neurological interventions require similar approaches which examine the impact of new technologies on survival, health, growth, development, functional disability, and family impact.

Models for understanding child health and well-being

The expansive concept of children's health encompasses measures of (1) neonatal status (live-born, gestational age, birthweight); (2) neonatal complications (neonatal resuscitation, respiratory distress, chronic lung disease, symptomatic patent ductus arteriosus, necrotizing enterocolitis, early and late onset sepsis); (3) postnatal growth (height, weight, head circumference); (4) genetic impairments (cleft lip and/or palate, congenital heart disease, omphalocele, inborn errors of metabolism); (5) neurological and sensory impairments (seizure disorders, cerebral palsy, microcephaly, hydrocephalus, blindness, deafness); (6) developmental brain injury (periventricular leukomalacia, grade 3–4 intraventricular hemorrhage, ventriculomegaly); (7) developmental disabilities (degrees of developmental cognitive disability, autistic spectrum disorders, communicative disorders); (8) complex physical impairments requiring medical technology (tracheostomy, gastrostomy, ventilator supports, central venous access); (9) chronic health impairments (asthma, gastroesophageal reflux, obesity, poor growth); (10) specific learning and attention disorders (dyslexia, dysgraphia, dyscalculia, impulsivity, hyperactivity, inattention); (11) injuries (fractures, lacerations, drowning, motor vehicle trauma); (12) behavioural and mental health disorders (self-regulation, aggression, hyperactivity, impulsivity, inattention, oppositionality, fearfulness, anxiety, and depression); (13) family impact; and (14) access to health, developmental, educational, and rehabilitation services.

A variety of frameworks have been used to describe the complex web of children's health and well-being. The first framework, the 'medical impairment model', focuses on medical diagnosis of impairments (pathophysiological processes affecting organ system performance). This clinical/medical tradition aims for accurate diagnosis, critical analysis of laboratory indicators, and use of optimal management strategies informed by intense medical cohort studies. For example, if a child has pre-threshold retinopathy of preterm birth, laser ablation of the proliferative retinal region is associated with significantly reducing retinal detachment and consequent blindness (Azad et al 2004). This framework is most useful in addressing impairments interfering with a child's daily health functioning, such as breathing, gaining weight, using basic senses, and being neurologically responsive.

The second framework, the 'developmental disability model', focuses on discrepancies between an individual child's performance and that of his/her peers, using appropriate psychometric tools. This tradition quantifies delays in development or intensity of clusters of behavioural states and establishes criteria for: (1) developmental motor, cognitive, social-emotional, or adaptive disorders; (2) communicative impairments; (3) coordination and perceptual impairments; (4) autistic spectrum disorders; (5) specific learning disabilities; and (6) attention deficit hyperactivity disorders.

The strength of the developmental disability model is the reliance upon comprehensive assessment of developmental and behavioural processes often involving several sessions of standardized interviewing and structured observation. The robust observational traditions of Gesell, Bayley, Illingworth, Griffiths, and Capute allow for descriptions of a child's movements and hand skills, and elicitation of problem-solving skills with blocks, toys, puzzles, crayons, and dolls – all of which are helpful in the assessment of young children (Neligan and Prudham 1969, Capute and Biehl 1973, Illingworth 1984). More recently, the MacArthur Communicative Development Inventories, the Communication and Symbolic Behavior Scales Developmental Profile, and the Capute Scales have demonstrated the value of gestures, non-verbal communication, and play as precursors of communicative and social skills (Capute and Accardo 1996, Fenson et al 2002, Wetherby and Prizant 2002).

Despite their relative strengths, both the medical impairment model and the developmental disability model focus on a child's deficits and do not adequately account for a child's skill in performing daily living activities in his/her natural environment (at home and in the community). For example, stating that a child has the medical impairment of diplegic cerebral palsy and does not perform the running task on the Gross Motor Function Measure does not acknowledge that the child may be able to execute many other important tasks, such as walking, dressing, and maintaining continency at kindergarten entry (Russell et al 2002). Similarly, describing a child with hemiplegic cerebral palsy and a Peabody Developmental Motor Scale Fine Motor Quotient of less than 70 as having a neuoromotor impairment because he or she does not perform bilateral manipulative and grasping tasks may obscure the child's functional strengths such as self-feeding, basic dressing without fasteners, and drawing with his or her dominant hand (Folio and Fewell 2000).

A shortcoming of both the medical impairment model and the developmental disability model is that a large number of children do not receive a combination of medical and developmental assessments over time which are informed by current best practices. Too often, explicit measures of spontaneous movements, postural skills, and adaptive and functional skills are not included, so that a child with cerebral palsy is only described with respect to his/her difficulty with motor skills that peers perform easily, and not with respect to self-mobility, postural control, manipulative hand skills, communicative understandings, and developmental style of curiosity, persistence, and problem-solving adaptability.

Most importantly, diagnosing a developmental disability does not necessarily mean that a child will not make progress in certain skills in the future. For example, most children with developmental language disorders (e.g. Preschool Language Scale 4 total score <80, with Bayley-II Mental Developmental Index >80) learn to adequately communicate in spoken sentences (Bayley 1993, Zimmerman et al 2002). However, these children often have mixed learning and behaviour disorders in elementary school which require additional resources and appropriate accommodations to allow them to keep up with the information requirements of their peers.

The third framework, the 'biopsychosocial model', combines biological, psychological and social perspectives on a child's health and well-being (Stein and Silver 1999). This model takes into account the child's physical, behavioural and developmental status, as well as increased use of the following services compared to his/her peers: medical services (glasses, hearing aids, inhalation medications for asthma, anticonvulsants, nutrition supports), rehabilitative and compensatory services (physical therapy, occupational therapy, speech-language therapy, alternative mobility supports, augmentative communication, robotic assistants), educational supports (Early Intervention and Special Education services), and behaviour supports (counselling, stimulant medication). This model also allows for descriptions of the child's developmental strengths as well as challenges with daily activities. In addition, it can be applied to a heterogeneous population of children with complex medical, developmental or behavioural impairments. The weakness of this model is that individuals with myopia, seasonal rhinitis, and eczema can be described as having multiple impairments because of repeated use of medications and health services, despite having readily controlled symptoms.

The fourth framework, the 'International Classification of Functioning (ICF) model', describes a child's health and well-being in terms of four components: (1) body structures, (2) body functions, (3) activities, and (4) participation. Body structures are anatomical parts of the body, such as organs and limbs, as well as structures of the nervous, sensory and musculoskeletal systems (World Health Organization 2001). Body functions are the physiological functions of body systems, including psychological functions, such as attending, remembering, and thinking. Activities are tasks, including learning, communicating, walking, carrying, feeding, dressing, toileting, bathing, reading, preparing meals, shopping, and washing clothes. Participation means involvement in community life, such as relationships, education, work, and recreational, religious, civic and social activities.

The ICF model also accounts for contextual factors in a child's life, including environmental and personal factors. Environmental factors, such as policy, social and physical facilitators and barriers, include positive and negative attitudes of others, legal protections, and discriminatory practices. Personal factors include age, gender, interests, and sense of self-efficacy. Fig. 14.1 illustrates how to apply the ICF model to a child with diplegia.

The strength of the ICF model is that it describes both functioning and enablement. Its weakness is that it has not been widely used with children and does not have explicit indicators for all the domains of the model. However, the model does offer the promise of a much broader perspective with respect to children's activities and participation (Simeonson et al 2000). To illustrate the potential of this model, a variety of scenarios are described in Table 14.1.

More recently, the Institute of Medicine proposed a 'Developmental Kaleidoscope Model of Children's Health' which includes biology and behaviour, physical and social

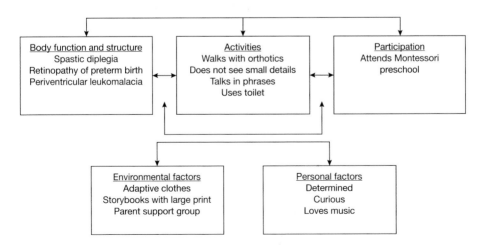

Fig. 14.1 Model for a 2.5-year-old boy with diplegia

environment, and policy and services. This is illustrated in Fig. 14.2 for a 2.5-year-old white male who weighed 750 grams at birth who is not yet communicating in words (National Research Council and Institute of Medicine 2004).

Measuring health and developmental status

Several tools are available to health professionals for early childhood assessment of health, development and behaviour (see Chapter 8 for a systematic review). These have

TABLE 14.1
ICF-model scenarios

Dimension	Definition	Girl, 2 years	Boy, 2.5 years	Girl, 3 years
Pathophysiology	Molecular/ biochemical mechanisms interfering with function	475 g birthweight, 26-week gestation, IUGR, developmental lung injury	750 g birthweight, 26-week gestation, periventricular white matter injury	900 g birthweight, 27-week gestation, grade 1 IVH
Body structures and body functions	Loss of organ structure or organ function	Growth delays, chronic lung disease, asthma, microcephaly	Threshold ROP, PVL with spastic diplegia, hyperactivity	Myopia, behaviour immaturity
Activity (functional) strengths	Ability to perform essential activities: feed, dress, toilet, walk, talk	Climbs, drinks from sippy cup, likes to pretend play with dolls	Ambulatory with AFOs, uses toilet, talks in phrases	Learning songs, playing with peers indoors
Activity (functional) limitations	Difficulty in performing essential activities	Difficulty chewing all textures, language and social delays	Difficulty with eye–hand coordination, seeing small details	Speech, perception and attention limitations
Participation	Involvement in community roles typical of peers	Plays indoors and outdoors with peers	Attends Montessori preschool	Attends YMCA swimming lessons
Participation restriction	Difficulty in assuming roles typical of peers	Misses daycare due to asthma flares, uses G tube for nutrition, enrolled in EI for language and peer interventions	Difficulty pedalling trike and climbing up slide on playground	Needs preschool supports including speech, perceptual and behavioural therapies
Contextual factors: environmental facilitators	Attitudinal, legal, policy and architectural facilitators	Good handwashing policies at daycare, asthma care plan	Adapted clothing to enhance dressing skills, story books with large print	Willing to understand her strengths and praise good behaviour
Contextual factors: environmental barriers	Attitudinal, legal, policy and architectural barriers	Quality paediatric nursing, respite daycare, and Hanen Language Intervention Program	Strategies to promote swimming, horseback riding, skating	Creative, holistic developmental curriculum with enhancement of play, communicative, adaptive and social skills

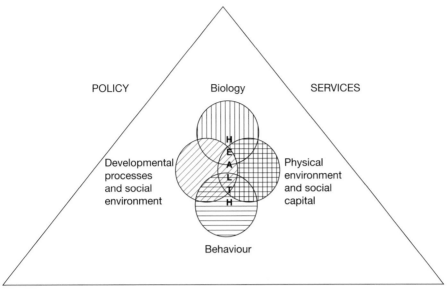

Fig. 14.2 Developmental kaleidoscope model for communicative and cognitive delays after 750 g birthweight

A 2-year-old boy who is not talking in words. He was born at 25 weeks' gestation and weighed 750 g.

- *Biology*: Vulnerability of extremely preterm infants to periventicular white matter injury.
- *Physical environment*: Home visitation reveals that he lives in substandard housing. There are no toddler toys or children's books. His mother did not finish high school and has limited family supports and financial resources.
- *Behaviour*: Child has a difficult temperament and intense tantrums to gain attention.
- *Policy*: Gaps in Early Intervention supports, skills of early childhood professionals and their ability to engage the family, prioritize interventions, and collaborate with medicine.
- *Services*: Quality early childhood development programs are scarce resources for children in poverty.
- *Child health*: Child with asthma as residual of chronic lung disease, shorter stature which makes adults relate to him as though he were younger, paediatrician frustrated in accessing childcare and speech therapy services despite repeated efforts. Waiting list is nine months for Hanen Speech Therapy Groups.
- *Potential*: If he accesses services that promote communication and adaptive skills, he will improve and learn.

been described in detail from several perspectives (Aylward 1994, Meisels and Fenichel 1996 Vohr and Msall 1997, Bracken 2000, Lidz 2003, Vohr et al 2004). I will describe several tools, with an emphasis on use in neonatal outcome studies.

The Child Health Questionnaires (CHQ) (Landgraf et al 1996) measure physical functioning, role and social limitations, general health perception, bodily pain, self-esteem, parental impact of time and emotions, mental health, general behaviour, family activities, family cohesion, and change in health among children aged 5 and older. The strength of this model is that it includes multiple domains of physical, behavioural and developmental health in middle childhood and adolescence, as well as impact on families, school functioning, and social functioning. Another strength of this model is that explicit parental interview formats are included and there is a checklist for identifying ongoing conditions such as anxiety, asthma, inattention, behavioural problems, chronic allergies and sinus disorders, chronic musculoskeletal problems, chronic respiratory disorders, chronic rheumatic disease, depression, developmental delay or learning disability, diabetes, epilepsy, hearing or visual impairments, learning problems, speech problems, and sleep disturbances. The weakness of this model is that there is not a preschool version.

To remedy this gap, Hogan and Msall developed the Preschool Child Health, Impairment, Functioning, Participation, and Supports Survey (Chi FPS). This multi-attribute tool includes descriptions of medical impairments, activity limitations, functional strengths and limitations, and ratings of physical, mental and developmental health status. In addition, for children aged 2 years and over, there are descriptions of health services, habilitative services, safety, and health status change. The overall goal of the CHi FPS is to capture key indicators of child well-being, non-categorical components of child disability, and serve as a bridge between validated survey questions and more detailed clinical assessments. The Preschool Child Health, Impairment, Functioning, Participation, and Supports Survey domains are listed in Table 14.2. Preliminary presentation of the domains occurred at the NIH-Casey Foundation Consensus Conference (Msall and Tremont 2002, Hogan and Msall 2007). This approach has also been used by Hogan and Park to link survey populations, family factors, and social support to developmental outcomes across very low, low, and normal birthweight survivors (Hogan and Park 2000).

Three additional measures have been developed to address the multi-attribute dimension of infant, toddler, and preschool parental perception of health status and health-related quality of life. Fekkes and colleagues, working in the Netherlands Office of Prevention, developed the Preschool Children Quality of Life Instrument (TAPQOL; Fekkes et al 2000). There are four subscales reflecting 12 domains. The physical functioning subscale includes sleeping, appetite (feeding), and problems with lungs, stomach and skin, as well as motor functioning (walking, running, balance). Social functioning includes play with peers, self-esteem, and social comfort, as well as problem behaviour (anger, irritability, short temper, aggression, restlessness, demand-making). Cognitive functioning includes understanding what others say, speech, and elaborating in expressive language. Emotional functioning includes mood, anxiety, and liveliness (energy and activity level).

The TAPQOL was used to assess 121 preterm children of whom over half were very preterm (<32 weeks' gestation) (Theunissen et al 2001). In addition, 362 term comparisons were seen, representing children seen in well child care between birth and age 5 years. Cronbach's alpha was very good in preterm, and adequate to very good in term. Concurrent validity included Stein and Jessop's Functional Status, 2nd edition-revised (FS-IIR), face validation with known chronic diseases, and both health and behavioural status Likert ratings by parents. The FS-IIR was designed to measure health status, compensatory modalities, and functional limitations in children with chronic illness aged from birth to 16 years (Stein and Jessop 1990). Correlations between total TAPQOL and FS-IIR were approximately .5 for both preterm children and controls, but lower across individual domains. Very preterm children, children with chronic medical impairments, children with lower parental rating of health status, and less happy children had significantly lower mean scores than comparison peers (Fekkes et al 2000).

Pregnancy
During what month of pregnancy did you first see a doctor? Did you take vitamins during your pregnancy? Did you smoke during your pregnancy? Did you have high blood pressure, diabetes, or require medications for a medical condition during your pregnancy? Were you supported by significant others during your pregnancy? What stressors arose or were preexisting during your pregnancy with respect to food, shelter, safety, emotional support, exposure to domestic violence, or income?

Birth
What was the child's birthweight and gestational age? What was your child's health status at birth? Did you have a multiple birth? Did you breastfeed your child? How long did you and your child stay in the hospital? Did your child have any medical complications during your stay in the hospital, such as respiratory assistance, requiring a breathing machine, feeding difficulties requiring feeding tubes/surgery, sepsis, seizures, meningitis, malformations, other?

Medical impairments
Has your child had any of the following: asthma, middle ear tubes, feeding (gastrostomy) tubes, heart disease requiring medication or surgery, cerebral palsy, developmental disabilities, seizure disorder, sleep disorder, sickle cell anemia, iron deficiency anemia, gastroesophageal reflux disease?

Participation
Does your child receive home nursing? Does your child have a home visitor? Is your child enrolled in Early Intervention?

Functioning
Does your child need more help than other children his/her age or have difficulty in completing the following activities due to an impairment or condition: eating, grasping objects, dressing, reaching overhead, bathing, lifting, toileting, bending, changing positions, walking, stooping, climbing stairs, standing indefinitely?

Multi-attribute status
Describe your child's vision: (1) Is blind; (2) Has difficulty seeing even with glasses; (3) Sees adequately with glasses; (4) Does not require correction.

Describe your child's hearing ability: (1) Is deaf; (2) Has difficulty hearing even with hearing aid; (3) Hears adequately with hearing aid; (4) Has no hearing problem.

Describe your child's ability to communicate: (1) Unable to communicate in words or gestures; (2) Unable to communicate in sentences or sign language; (3) Has difficulty being understood; (4) Has no problem communicating.

Describe your child's development: (1) Has some delay; (2) Has an emotional or behavioral problem lasting more than three months; (3) Has difficulty learning; (4) Has been seen by a doctor or counsellor for an emotional, developmental or behavioral problem.

Health status
How would you rate your child's physical health, mental health, and developmental status on a scale of Excellent, Very good, Good, Fair, and Poor? How would you rate your own physical and mental health?

Building on Landgraf's CHQ, Klassen and colleagues developed and validated a 103-item Infant and Toddler Quality of Life Questionnaire (ITQOL) for children aged 2 months to 5 years. Domains include physical abilities, growth and development, pain and discomfort, temperament and mood, general behaviour, getting along with others, general health perception, and change in health (Klassen et al 2003). There are also five parental categories, including anxiety and worry about child's health, limitations in time to meet parental needs because of child's health, general health perception, and family cohesion.

This instrument was used to assess 1140 neonatal intensive care survivors and 393 healthy term infants. Children who were in the NICU differed from healthy children in physical abilities, growth, development, temperament, mood, behaviour, general health perceptions, and caregivers' burden.

Using the Health Classification System Preschool Version (HSCS-PS) – a multi-attribute assessment of hearing, speaking, mobility, use of hands and fingers, self-care, feelings, learning and remembering, thinking and solving problems, pain and discomfort, general health, and behaviour – in a British Columbia cohort of neonatal intensive care survivors, both very low birthweight and extremely low birthweight children had more problems with sight, speech, mobility, manipulative skills, self-care, learning, remembering, thinking, problem solving, pain, general health and behaviour than term healthy neonates (Klassen et al 2004). Subsequent studies by Klassen and colleagues at age 3–4 years used the Child Behavioral Checklist (CBCL/1.5–5; Achenbach and Rescorla 2000), the Medical Outcomes Study Short Form 36 (MOS SF36) for parental physical and mental health, and an assessment of family functioning . These studies confirmed good reliability and construct validity in a sample of healthy and at-risk children who had survived neonatal intensive care (Klassen et al 2003).

The Capute Scales consist of the Clinical Adaptive Test (CAT) and the Clinical Linguistic and Auditory Milestone Scale (CLAMS) and have established reliability and validity (Accardo and Capute 2005). This assessment tool for children aged from birth to 36 months gives the examiner age equivalent scores and developmental quotient scores for visual-motor problem-solving skills and pre-linguistic receptive- expressive language skills. The Capute Scales with the CAT and CLAMS subscales have been used with a normative population as well as with children with motor delay, preterm birth, prenatal drug exposure, chronic illness, developmental delay, and those receiving Early Intervention services (Wachtel et al 1994, Capute and Accardo 1996, Belcher et al 1997 Voigt et al 2003). The Capute Scales were recently re-normed and now include a Spanish and Russian version (Accardo and Capute 2005).

The Ages and Stages Questionnaire (ASQ) is a parent-completed child monitoring system for preschool-aged children (Squires et al 1999). Dimensions include gross and fine motor, communication, problem-solving, and personal-social skills. Validation studies have involved over 7000 children, with overall agreement between parents and discriminative assessment measures of 83 per cent. The ASQ was used in 177 former preterm survivors at ages 12, 18, 24, and 48 months and compared to the Griffiths Mental Developmental Scales, the Bayley-II Scales, and the McCarthy Scales. Using a cut-off point of 2 standard deviations below the mean in an ASQ domain resulted in over-referral in 20 per cent of children, under-referral in 1 per cent, and agreement between screening and developmental assessments in 79 per cent. Though the ASQ negative predictive value is very high at 98 per cent, the positive predictive value of 40 per cent requires that this screening tool not be used alone to assess child disability status (Skellern et al 2001).

The Functional Independence Measure for Children (WeeFIM-TM) consists of 18 items encompassing three subscales. There are eight items for self-care activities of daily living and continence: five items for changing positions, indoor and outdoor mobility, and negotiating stairs; and five items for cognitive functioning, including understanding verbal and nonverbal communication, use of language and gestures, social interaction, play, and memory of routines. The WeeFIM instrument has been normed on a population of over 500 non-disabled children aged 1–7 years and has a robust correlation with chronological age between 18 and 48 months (Msall et al 1994a, 1994b). Initial validation studies included over 700 children with neurodevelopmental disabilities, including extreme preterm birth (N = 200), cerebral palsy (N = 100), and genetic disorders (N = 150) (Msall et al 1994a, 1994b).

In preschool children with evolving motor, communicative and developmental impairment, the WeeFIM proves to have excellent test–retest reliability, excellent equivalence reliability for face-to-face or telephone interviews, as well as concurrent validity with psychological and educational measures of adaptive functioning (Ottenbacher et al 1996, 1997, 1999, 2000a). Most importantly, the WeeFIM demonstrated responsiveness to change over time in the preschool years in a diverse cohort of children with motor, communicative, health and developmental challenges (Ottenbacher et al 2000b).

The WeeFIM has been used in the longitudinal study of developmental, health and functional outcomes in children with severe congenital heart disease (Limperopoulos et al 2001), in children with spinal muscle atrophy (Chung et al 2004), in girls with severe disabilities as a result of Rett syndrome (Colvin et al 2003), and in survivors of shaken baby-inflicted head trauma. The WeeFIM has been translated into Japanese, Chinese and Thai, with both norms generated and application to children with disability in these diverse cultures (Tsuji et al 1999, Jongjit et al 2002, Wong et al 2002).

Because of problems with aggregated skills in the WeeFIM, Msall and colleagues have developed the Warner Initial Developmental Evaluation of Adaptive and Functional Skills (WIDEA-FS™). The WIDEA-FS is a 50-item inventory encompassing domains of self-care (eating, dressing, and diaper awareness), motor tasks, communication, and social cognition. Initial standardization involved over 300 children aged 2–30 months seen in paediatric primary care during well child visits. Robust construct validity was demonstrated between the WIDEA-FS and Capute Scales and between child age and progression of adaptive skills (Msall et al 2001).

The Pediatric Evaluation of Disability Inventory (PEDI) assesses skills, caregiver assistance, and modification of environment for self-care, mobility, and social functioning of children aged 6 months to 7.5 years (Feldman et al 1990). Social functioning includes communication, problem solving, play, peer and adult interaction, memory, household chores, self-protection, and community safety. The PEDI has been used in children with traumatic brain injury, children with cerebral palsy, children with spina bifida, and children in preschool programs because of physical or developmental impairments (Kothari et al 2003, Haley et al 2004).

The PEDI Caregiver Assistance and Modification Scale includes eight self-care, seven mobility, and five social interaction items. These categories directly overlap with the WeeFIM. Correlations between the WeeFIM and PEDI Caregiver Assistance are excellent (Ziviani et al 2001). Thus one can use either the WeeFIM or PEDI if one wishes to measure functional strengths and limitations in toddlers and preschoolers.

255

The strength of the WeeFIM and PEDI is that they reflect a rich tradition of basic activities of daily living. Additional benefits of the PEDI are that there is a computer-assisted testing format, it has been widely translated into European languages, and it has been widely used among paediatric rehabilitation professionals in hospital and community settings. The weaknesses of the WeeFIM are that it was not designed by the distributors for outpatient surveillance and its US norms are from only one US region.

In England, Jones and colleagues developed the Health Status Questionnaire as an alternative method for assessing outcome in neonatology (Jones et al 2002). Key domain questions include malformation, neuromotor function (walk, sit, use hands, control head), seizures, auditory and visual function, communication (sounds, words, understanding of language), cognitive function on developmental assessment, and physical disability (respiratory, gastrointestinal, renal, and growth). Jones and colleagues applied this measure to 297 survivors of gestational ages less than 31 weeks or birthweights less than 1500 grams born in Wales in 1994. They compared their disability severity classification with that of Victoria, Australia and the Mersey area in the UK.

These criteria often differ in the use of cognitive cut-off points. Severe disability may be defined as a developmental quotient (DQ) of: (1) less than 70, reflecting standard scores more than 2 standard deviations below the mean; (2) less than 55, reflecting standard scores more than 3 standard deviations below the mean; or (3) less than 50, reflecting developmental performance at less than half the typical rate. The cut-off point in intellectual disability discriminates between those classified as mild and those classified as severe. Impairment without disability may defined as a DQ of 70–79 or a DQ of 50–69. Overall, once growth was removed as a variable, severe disability rates ranged between 8 and 9 per cent. In comparison with the Mersey Criteria, the Health Status Questionnaire correctly identified 88 per cent of the children with normal developmental status and 96 per cent of the children classified as severely disabled. This questionnaire has the potential to enhance systematic follow-up using survey indicators in high-risk populations (Jones et al 2002).

The Parent Stress Index – 3rd edition (PSI 3) is a screening tool which examines the relationship between a parent's level of stress and the impact that stress has on the child (Abidin 1995). The PSI 3 is a 101-item scale divided into three domains: child domain (47 items), parent domain (54 items), and the optional Life Stress Scale (19 items). The PSI 3 has demonstrated good-to-excellent concurrent and discriminate validity with respect to children who are at risk for emotional or behavioural problems, as well as parents who may be in need of parenting education and supports. There is a 36-item short form (PSI-SF). Three important factors captured in this scale are: maternal self-esteem, parent–child inter-action, and child self-regulation. It has been used in Scandinavia including recently on a Norwegian cohort of preterm survivors.

The Impact on the Family Scale includes 15 items for the assessment of the social and family impact of a child's disability. As an assessment of parental perception of the impact of a child's illness on family life, it measures psychological outcomes, social outcomes, and health service use. It also includes changes in family life and parental attributions of the impact of the child's illness on that change (Stein and Jessop 2003).

The Family Resource Scale (FRS) measures the adequacy of various resources in households with young children (Dunst and Leet 1987). It includes 31 items rated on a five-point scale ranging from not at all adequate to almost always adequate. The hierarchy is derived from a conceptual framework which predicts that inadequacy of resources necessary to meet individually identified needs will negatively affect both personal well-being and parental commitment to carrying out professionally prescribed regimes unrelated to identified needs.

The Home Observation for Measurement of the Environment (HOME) was developed by Caldwell and Bradley to link environmental components of social disadvantage to practices that promote early childhood development. The Home Inventory for Families of Infants and Toddlers has six subscales for ages from birth to 3 years: responsivity, acceptance, organization, learning material, involvement, and enrichment. HOME scores at 24 months correlate highly with 3-year Binet IQ scores and substantially contribute to 54-month Binet IQ variance. The domains of appropriate play material and maternal involvement are highly predictive of cognitive performance, and identified children with developmental cognitive disability at age 3 more than two-thirds of the time and those with IQs of more than 90 at age 3 more than 60 per cent of the time. It can be a useful tool for support within high risk environments for developmental cognitive disability (Bradley et al 1995). It was also recently used in the Maternal Lifestyle Study of prospectively followed infants who were prenatally exposed to licit and illicit drugs (Messinger et al 2004).

Given the multiple risks of preterm infants who are at highest biological, developmental and social risk, the HOME combined with explicit parenting supports (Portage Program in the Avon Premature Infant Project, Learningames in the Infant Health and Development Programs (IHDP)) is required so that proactive supports rather than deficit remediation become the emphasis of follow-up programs (Avon Premature Infant Project 1998, McCormick et al 1998).

Though there are gaps in the literature with respect to the role of comprehensive preventive supports versus periodic screening and referral supports for survivors of very low birthweight (VLBW) and extremely low birthweight (ELBW), the Avon Project, which includes a maternal and child health nurse visitation, an explicit child development curriculum, and parenting supports, had a positive outcome effect at age 2 years for children who had been born under 1250 grams. These children scored over 5 points higher on the Griffiths Scale, and those children with abnormal cranial ultrasounds scored over 7 points higher (Avon Premature Infant Project 1998).

Among the 280 VLBW and 80 ELBW children in the Infant Health and Development Program, the group who received the child development and parent-focused activity curricula had Stanford Binet IQs that were 7–10 points higher than those in the comparison group. The group with the highest social disadvantage combined with the best program attendance benefited the most. It should be noted that both these programs had comprehensive interventions with health, developmental, and social supports.

Model multi-centre studies

Despite advances in postnatal surfactant replacement, more physiological ventilation techniques, improved nutrition, and management strategies that decrease the risks of grade 3 and 4 intraventricular hemorrhage, the increased survival of infants with birthweights of 501–1000 grams has not been associated with decreases in major neurodevelopmental impairments in the first two years of life. As multi-centre trials took place during the 1990s, concerns were raised about increasing survival without decreasing rates of disability. In this section I will review several studies in order to suggest how we might frame our outcomes to address the impact of our interventions on child disability. I will also emphasize that understanding a child's functioning with respect to daily activities and community participation provides important indicators of supports that will be required.

Jacobs and colleagues described the developmental outcomes of 274 survivors of 23–26 weeks gestation age. These neonates had received surfactant in 1990–1994 in the two largest nurseries in Toronto. Overall, 65 per cent of survivors were without neurodevelopmental impairments, at ages 18–24 months, 23 per cent had some neurodevelopmental impairments of mild (e.g. abnormal gait) to moderate (e.g. sitting but not walking) motor disability with concurrent cognitive impairments reflected in MDI scores of 70–84. Twelve per cent were severely disabled, characterized by an inability to sit, blindness, sensorineural hearing loss requiring amplification, cognitive disability (MDI scores <70), and/or shunted hydrocephalus (Jacobs et al 2000).

Both the Jacobs study and several multi-centre studies which examined 18–24-month outcomes in extremely preterm infants are illustrated in Table 14.3. In the three largest studies, Schmidt, Vohr, and Wood (Schmidt et al 2003, Vohr et al 2000, Wood et al 2000) found rates of cerebral palsy syndromes in 13–17 per cent of the children, developmental cognitive disability (Bayley Scores of Infant Development-II more than 2 standard deviations below the mean for corrected age) in 26–37 per cent, sensorineural hearing impairment requiring amplification in 2 per cent, and visual impairment worse than 20/200 in 2–3 per cent. For perspective, the rate of these impairments in term children is 0.2 per cent for cerebral palsy, 2–3 per cent for developmental cognitive disability, 0.1–0.3 per cent for hearing loss, and 0.1 per cent for severe visual impairment (Msall et al 2001).

A different strategy was undertaken by Doyle who examined 2-year outcomes for ELBW infants born in 1997 in the Victorian Infant Collaborative Group. Overall, in comparing survivors in the 1979–1980 group to those in the 1985–1987, 1991–1992, and 1997 groups, rates of early child disability initially decreased from 61 per cent to 45 per cent, but then plateaued at 45 per cent and 49 per cent (Doyle 2001a, 2001b, 2004).

Tommiska and colleagues examined all 211 surviving ELBW infants born in Finland in 1996–1997. Cerebral palsy occurred in 11 per cent, blindness in 0.5 per cent, hearing impairment in 3 per cent, and severe developmental delay in 6 per cent of the study population. In addition, 36 per cent had mild communicative cognitive developmental delay, 13 per cent had minor motor delay, and 3 per cent had recurrent seizures. Overall, 18 per cent were considered severely disabled with a major neurodevelopmental impairment (Tommiska et al 2003).

In the Leiden follow-up of very preterm infants at 18–24 months who were born in 1996–1997, Stoelhorst and colleagues followed 168 (71 per cent) survivors (n = 235) at 18

TABLE 14.3
Multi-centre model extremely low birthweight short-term outcome studies

Study	Sample	CP %	DD %	HI %	VI %
Schmidt 1996–1998	N = 910 500–999 g	13	26	2	2
Jacobs 1990–1994	N = 274 23–26 wks	15	26	4	4
Vohr 1993–1994	N = 1151 400–999 g	17	37	2	3
Wood 1995	N = 283 22–25 wks	16	30	2	2
Doyle 1997	N = 233 500–999 g	11	22	2.4	1.5
Finnstrom 1998	N = 362 500–999 g	7	15	1	4
Stoll (A) 1993–2001	N = 2161 400–999 g No infection	8	22	1	5
Stoll (B) 1993–2001	N = 3460 400–999 g Sepsis	16	35	2.5	15
Stoll (C) 1993–2001	N = 392 400–999 g Nec/Men	20	40	3.2	16

Nec = necrotizing enterolitis
Men = meningitis
CP = cerebral palsy
DD = developmental disability: MDI/PDI <70
HI = hearing impairment requiring aids
VI = visual impairment worse than 20/200 corrected

months and 151 (64 per cent) at 24 months. Six to 7 per cent of children had severe neurodevelopmental impairment at 18–24 months, and 33–34 per cent had mild–moderate neurodevelopmental impairment. The mean Performance Developmental Index subscore of the Bayley-II was more than one standard deviation lower at 18 months for those infants who had received postnatal dexamethasone for bronchopulmonary dysplasia (BPD). Overall, BPD, ethnicity, birthweight, and gender were predictive of developmental outcome (Stoelhorst et al 2003).

Several strategies have been used to examine functional disability. Elbourne et al evaluated the impact of ethamsylate to prevent IVH in VLBW infants born under 33 weeks' gestation. Severe functional disability at age 2 was present in 8.3 per cent and included the inability to sit, see, use hands, or perform developmental skills typical of a 1-year-old (Elbourne et al 2001). In the Vohr 12-centre 1993–1994 neonatal network study, 7 per cent could not sit, 17 per cent could not walk, and 14 per cent could not finger feed (Vohr et al 2000). In the Epicure study, functional observations at 30 months revealed that 10 per

TABLE 14.4
Key mobility, manipulative and cognitive functioning indicators

Moving about and manipulating objects
Does the child: (1) walk without help; (2) stack two blocks; (3) mark on paper with a crayon or pencil; (4) walk up stairs putting both feet on each step; (5) walk down stairs putting both feet on each step; (6) kick a ball; (7) run smoothly and change direction; (8) open a door by turning and pulling the doorknob or handle; (9) open a jar by unscrewing the lid; (10) jump over a small object; (11) throw a ball several feet; (12) unbutton the buttons on clothing; (13) catch a ball thrown from several feet away?

Caring for self
Does the child: (1) drink from an open cup or glass; (2) use a straw for drinking; (3) understand that hot things are dangerous; (4) use a spoon to feed him/herself; (5) take off clothes; (6) ask to use the toilet/bathroom; (7) urinate ('pee') in toilet or potty chair; (8) have bowel movements ('poop') in toilet or potty chair; (9) put on underpants, shorts, pants with elastic waistband; (10) wash his/her hands?

Acquiring and using information
Does the child: (1) follow simple directions ('Come here.' 'Sit down.'); (2) say 1–10 words; (3) use gestures such as waving 'hi' and 'bye' or shaking head for 'no'; (4) respond to the request to 'give me' an object; (5) point to a few pictures that someone names; (6) name a few pictures; (7) point to or name a few body parts on self or doll; (8) put two words together; (9) use own name to talk about him/herself; (10) use action words ending in 'ing' ('sleeping', 'eating'); (11) answer 'yes' and 'no' correctly when asked a question; (12) understand and use words meaning more than one thing ('cats', 'toys')?

Attending to and completing tasks
Does the child: (1) look at someone who speaks to him/her; (2) listen and pay attention to a simple story being read; (3) play with toys for a few minutes; (4) change activities without getting upset?

Interacting and relating to others
Does the child: (1) give objects or point to objects to show them to others; (2) use names for at least two people; (3) smile or laugh when others say something funny or nice ('Good work.' 'That's a pretty hat.'); (4) try to please other people; (5) play a simple game with another person (hiding, chasing); (6) play 'make believe' (feed dolls, put dolls to bed, pretend to go shopping)?

cent were unable to walk, 3 per cent were unable to sit, 4 per cent were unable to feed self a cracker, and 6 per cent could not communicate in speech. Overall, 50 per cent were free of disability, 26 per cent had mild–moderate disability, and 24 per cent had severe disability (Wood et al 2000). Table 14.4 provides additional indictors that would help define dimensions of functional skills in children receiving new technologies.

Using large multi-centre studies to understand pathways in multiple disabilities
The most recent study to examine post-neonatal processes that might be amenable to intervention has been by Stoll and colleagues (Stoll et al 2004). These investigators examined the role of postnatal infection on neurodevelopmental impairments among 6093 survivors who weighed between 401 and 1000 grams and were born between 1993 and 2001. In this study, five subgroups of infants were identified: (1) infants without infection during their hospital stay (n = 2161); (2) infants with clinical infection who received parental antibiotics for at least five days (n = 1538); (3) infants with sepsis (n = 1922); (4) infants with sepsis and necrotizing enterocolitis (n = 279); and (5) infants with meningitis (n = 193). In Table 14.3, we have combined categories 2 and 3 and categories 4 and 5.

Almost two-thirds of survivors had postnatal infections, the overwhelming majority of which were late-onset. Among those without infection, 29 per cent had neurodevelopmental impairments. Approximately 50 per cent of infants with sepsis, sepsis and necrotizing enterocolitis, or meningitis had neurodevelopmental impairments. One of the disquieting outcomes of the Stoll study was the high rate of cognitive developmental disability. This occurred in 22 per cent of infants without infection and in 35–40 per cent of those with infection. One mediator of this effect was brain growth at 36 weeks postmenstrual age. In children with infection, 41–60 per cent had acquired microcephaly (e.g. head circumference of less than 10 per cent on standardized preterm infant charts). In contrast, only 25 per cent of children without infection had acquired microcephaly. The relationship between infection status and neurodevelopmental impairment held when adjusting for bronchopulmonary dysplasia, postnatal steroids, and sonographic parenchymal brain injury – three major determinants of adverse outcomes in ELBW survivors (Ment et al 2000, Schmidt et al 2003).

To date, no multi-centre interventional study has been able to reduce the rates of cerebral palsy, deafness, blindness, and multiple neurodevelopmental disabilities to less than 5 per cent of ELBW survivors. Attempts at decreasing BPD have not met with success in ELBW cohorts. The TIPP study and the New England IVH prevention study demonstrated that even when one decreases IVH grade 3 and 4, neurodevelopmental impairments do not decrease and rates of cognitive disability are similar between groups (Ment et al 2000, Schmidt et al 2003). This suggests that different mechanisms determine cognitive disability besides IVH.

An important lesson can be learned from a multi-centre study which examined the impact of an early marker and its relationship to longer-term outcomes. In the croyosurgery for retinopathy of preterm birth cooperative group, the infants who weighed <1250 grams had sequential ophthalmological examinations. At age 5.5 years, the WeeFIM was administered and recognition acuity was measured using Teller Acuity Cards (Msall et al 2000). The cohort included 1063 survivors from the five-centre Extended Natural History Cohort and 223 survivors from all 23 centres who reached threshold retinopathy of preterm birth (ROP). In this latter group, infants were enrolled in a randomized clinical trial of cryosurgery. Eighty-seven per cent of these children had globally normal functional skills, defined as a WeeFIM rating of within 2 standard deviations of peers without disability (WeeFIM' Manual, version 5, 1998). Severe functional disability was defined as a WeeFIM score of more than 4 standard deviations below the mean and was equivalent to a child of age 2 years without disabilities. Among those with threshold ROP, 26 per cent had a severe functional disability, while only 11 per cent with pre-threshold ROP and 3.7 per cent without any ROP had a severe functional disability.

In analysing the outcomes for children with threshold ROP who had favourable visual status at 5.5 years, the following functional disabilities were found: self-care (25 per cent), motor (5 per cent), continence (5 per cent), and communicative-cognitive (22 per cent). In contrast, children with threshold ROP and unfavourable visual status had higher rates of functional disability: self-care (77 per cent), motor (43 per cent), continence (50 per cent), and communicative-cognitive (66 per cent). Both the pathways that lead to more severe ROP and the processes that allow for preservation of some visual functioning after threshold ROP are involved in the severity of disability at kindergarten entry.

Similar efforts will be required in examining interventions to decrease both parenchymal brain injury and severity of cerebral palsy. Most importantly, strategies to optimize growth, decrease bronchopulmonary dysplasia severity, and decrease rates of postnatal infections should be examined with respect to their impact on reducing degrees of developmental cognitive and communicative impairments (i.e. Standard Scores (SS) ≥80, 65–79, 50–64 and <50). This will also require developmental examinations beyond 2 years, with a focus on 30, 42 and 54 months.

If we are to move beyond strategies for increasing survival and develop strategies for optimizing health, development and family supports, then five important challenges must be addressed.

First, we need to develop explicit hypotheses about inflammatory mediators, disruption of the blood-brain barrier, and mechanisms impairing cranial growth and their impact on emerging developmental processes of sensory, hand skill, mobility, communicative, and problem-solving skills (Dammann and Leviton 2004).

Second, we need to define developmental variables and their severity and functional outcomes a priori so that the effects of new interventions on severe multiple disability can be measured consistently. It is very different to be legally blind yet able to read large print, run in the playground with peers, and do all self-care, compared with being unable to walk, say words, and feed oneself despite normal vision.

Third, we need to analyse the impact of neonatal interventions to decrease BPD, IVH grade 3–4, PVL, and threshold ROP, and to assess their impact on degrees of neuro-developmental impairments and functional skills in self-care, mobility, communication, learning, and behaviour regulation. It is in the latter two categories where both biological and environmental risks operate that we need to creatively examine our impact so that combinations of minor impairments in learning, attention and perception do not lead to non-competitive academic and vocational careers.

Fourth, we need to link survey data to comprehensive developmental process assessments so that we can better understand how specific neonatal populations are faring compared to their peers and to other preterm weight groups (e.g. infants born at 1001–1500 grams, 1501–2000 grams, and 2001–2500 grams, and children receiving cardiopulmonary technologies who weigh >2500 grams).

Fifth, by understanding the mechanisms whereby short-term neonatal morbidities increase developmental cognitive disability, additional developmental supports and family interventions after discharge can be promoted. Long-term outcomes are often compromised by adverse family and community factors, such as parental poverty, inadequate housing, low parental education attainment, and family stressors. By combining biomedical risk reduction strategies and explicitly designing, prioritizing and evaluating our biopsychosocial interventions, further progress can be made toward enhancing survival and optimizing developmental outcomes.

Until preterm birth can be prevented, it is both our obligation and our challenge to systematically create mechanisms to analyse the impact of current practices on health, developmental, behavioural and family outcomes in the preschool years. Children aged 18–24 months are at a critical phase in laying the foundation for future developmental, communicative and perceptual abilities. Neonatology has a long tradition of systematically evaluating past and new interventions so that we do not do harm. The challenge for the next decade is to begin to address more comprehensively our secondary and tertiary prevention efforts for all children with preterm birth and biomedical and social risk, especially those who are most vulnerable.

ACKNOWLEDGEMENTS

This research was supported by 1U01 HD37614 entitled 'NICHD Family and Child Well Being Network: Child Disability'. This chapter is dedicated to Irving Harris for his lifelong commitment to enhancing health and developmental outcomes of vulnerable populations. Herb Abelson, Paula Jaudes and Steve Goldstein provided ongoing support and a shared vision of biopsychosocial commitments to children at risk medically or socially. Shelly Field was invaluable in editing and technical assistance.

REFERENCES

Accardo PJ, Capute AJ (2005) *The Capute Scales: Cognitive Adaptive Test/Clinical Linguistic and Auditory Milestone Scale*. Baltimore, MD: Paul H Brookes Publishing Co.

Abidin RR, editor (1995) *Parenting Stress Index, 3rd edn*. Odessa, FL: Psychological Assessment Resources.

Achenbach TM, Rescorla MA, editors (2000) *Manual for the ASEBA Preschool Forms and Profiles*. Burlington, VT: University of Vermont Department of Psychiatry.

Avon Premature Infant Project (1998) Randomized trial of parental support for families with very preterm children. *Arch Dis Child Fetal Neonatal Ed* 79: F4–F11.

Aylward GP, editor (1994) *Practitioner's Guide to Developmental and Psychological Testing*. New York: Plenum.

Azad RV, Pasumala L, Kumar H, Talwar D, Pal R, Paul VK, Chandra P (2004) Prospective randomized evaluation of diode-laser and cryotherapy in prethreshold retinopathy of prematurity. *Clin Exp Ophthalmol* 32(3): 251–254.

Bayley N (1993) *Bayley Scales of Infant Development-II*. San Antonio, TX: Psychological Corporation.

Belcher HM, Gittlesohn A, Capute AJ, Allen MC (1997) Using the clinical linguistic and auditory milestone scale for developmental screening in high-risk preterm infants *Clin Pediatr* (Phila) 36(11): 635–642.

Bracken BA, editor (2000) *The Psychoeducational Assessment of Preschool Children, 3rd edition*. Needham Heights, MA: Allyn & Bacon.

Bradley RH, Whiteside L, Mundfrom DJ, Blevins-Knabe B, Casey PH, Caldwell BM, Kelleher KH, Pope S, Barrett K (1995) Home environment and adaptive social behavior among premature, low birth weight children: alternative models of environmental action. *J Pediatr Psychol* 20(3): 347–362.

Capute AJ, Accardo PJ (1996) The infant neurodevelopmental assessment: a clinical interpretive manual for CAT-CLAMS in the first two years of life. *Curr Probl Pediatr* 26: 238–257(part 1); 279–306 (part 2).

Capute AJ, Biehl RF (1973) Functional developmental evaluation: prerequisite to habilitation. *Pediatr Clin N Am* 20: 3–26.

Chung BH, Wong VC, Ip P (2004) Spinal muscular atrophy: survival pattern and functional status. *Pediatrics* 114(5): e548–e553. Epub 18 Oct.

Colvin L, Fyfe S, Leonard S, Schiavello T, Ellaway C, De Klerk N, Christodoulou J, Msall M, Leonard H (2003) Describing the phenotype in Rett Syndrome using a population database. *Arch Dis Child* 88(1): 38–43.

Dammann O, Leviton A (2004) Inflammatory brain damage in preterm newborns – dry numbers, wet lab, and causal inferences. *Early Hum Dev* 79(1): 1–15.

Doyle LW (2001a) Outcome at 14 years of extremely low birthweight infants: a regional study. *Arch Dis Child Fetal Neonatal Ed* 85: F159–F164.

Doyle LW (2001b) Outcome at 5 years of age of children 23 to 27 weeks gestation: refining the prognosis. *Pediatrics* 108(1): 134–141.

Doyle LW (2004) Evaluation of neonatal intensive care for extremely low birthweight infants in Victoria over two decades: I. effectiveness. *Pediatrics* 113: 505–509.

Dunst CJ, Leet HE (1987) Measuring the adequacy of resources in households with young children. *Child Care Health Dev* 13(2): 111–125.

Elbourne D, Ayers S, Dellagrammaticas H, Johnson A, Leloup M, Lenoir-Piat S, EC Ethamsylate Trial Group (2001) Randomised controlled trial of prophylactic ethamsylate: follow up at 2 years of age. *Arch Dis Child Fetal Neonatal Ed* 84(3): F183–F187.

Fekkes M, Theunissen NC, Brugman E, Veen S, Verrips EG, Koopman HM, Vogels T, Wit JM, Verloove-Vanhorick SP (2000) Development and psychometric evaluation of the TAPQOL: a health-related quality of life instrument for 1-5-year-old children. *Qual Life Res* 9(8): 961–972.

Feldman AB, Haley SM, Coryell J (1990) Concurrent and construct validity of the Pediatric Evaluation of Disability Inventory. *Phys Ther* 70(10): 602–610.

Fenson L, Dale PS, Reznick JS, Thal D, Bates E, Hartung JP, Pethick S, Reilly JS, editors (2002) *MacArthur Communicative Development Inventories: User's Guide and Technical Manual*. Baltimore, MD: Paul H Brookes Publishing Co.

Finnstrom O, Otterblad Olausson P, Sedin G, Serenius F, Svenningsen N, Thiringer K, Tunnell R, Wesstrom G (1998) Neurosensory outcome and growth at three years in extremely low birthweight infants: follow-up results from the Swedish national prospective study. *Acta Paediiatr* 87(10): 1055–1060.

Folio MR, Fewell RR, editors (2000) *Peabody Developmental Motor Scale, 2nd edition*. Austin, TX: ProEd.

Haley SM, Fragala-Pinkham MA, Ni PS, Skrinar AM, Kaye EM (2004) Pediatric physical functioning reference curves. *Pediatr Neurol* 31(5): 333–341.

Hogan DP, Msall ME (2007) Key indicators of health and safety: infancy, preschool and middle childhood. In: Brown B, editor. *Indicators of Child and Youth Well-being: Completing the Picture*. New York: Lawrence Erlbaum Associates.

Hogan DP, Park JM (2000) Family factors and social support in the developmental outcomes of very low-birth weight children *Clin Perinatol* 27: 433–459.

Horbar JD, Badger GJ, Carpenter JH, Fanaroff AA, Kilpatrick S, LaCorte M, Phibbs R, Sol RF, for the Members of the Vermont Oxford Network (2002) Trends in mortality and morbidity for very low birth weight infants, 1991–1999. *Pediatrics* 110: 143–151.

Illingworth RS (1984) *The Development of the Infant and Young Child: Normal and Abnormal, 8th edition*. London: Churchill Livingstone.

Jacobs SE, O'Brien KO, Inwood S, Kelly EN, Whyte HE (2000) Outcome of infants 23–26 weeks' gestation pre and post surfactant. *Acta Paediatr* 89: 959–965.

Jones HP, Guildea ZES, Stewart JH, Cartlidge PHT (2002) The Health Status Questionnaire: achieving concordance with published disability criteria. *Arch Dis Child* 86: 15–20.

Jongjit J, Komsopapong L, Chira-Adisai W (2002) Measuring functional status in Thai children with disabilities. *J Med Assoc Thai* 85: 446–454.

Klassen, AF, Landgraf JM, Lee SK, Barer M, Raina P, Chan HP, Matthew D, Brabyn D (2003) Health related quality of life in 3 and 4 year old children and their parents: preliminary findings about a new questionnaire. *Health Qual Life Outcomes* 1: 1–12.

Klassen AF, Lee SK, Raina P, Chan HWP, Matthew D, Brabyn D (2004) Health status and health-related quality of life in a population-based sample of neonatal intensive care unit graduates. *Pediatrics* 113: 594–600.

Kothari DH, Haley SM, Gill-Body KM, Dumas HM (2003) Measuring functional change in children with acquired brain injury (ABI): comparison of generic and ABI-specific scales using the Pediatric Evaluation of Disability Inventory (PEDI). *Phys Ther* 83(9): 776–785.

Landgraf JM, Abetz L, Ware JE, editors (1996) *Child Health Questionnaire (CHQ): A User's Manual, 1st edition*. Boston, MA: Health Institute, New England Medical Center.

Lemons JA, Bauer CR, Oh W, Korones SB, Papile LA, Stoll BJ, Verter J, Temprosa M, Wright LL, Ehrenkranz RA, Fanaroff AA, Stark A, Carlo W, Tyson JE, Donovan EF, Shankaran S, Stevenson DK (2001) Very low birth weight outcomes of the national institute of child health and human development neonatal research network. January 1995 through December 1996. *Pediatrics* 107(1): e1.

264

Lidz CS, editor (2003) *Early Childhood Assessment*. Hoboken, NJ: John Wiley.

Limperopoulos C, Majnemer A, Shevell MI, Rosenblatt B, Rohlicek C, Tchervenkov C, Darwish HZ (2001) Functional limitations in young children with congenital heart defects after cardiac surgery. *Pediatrics* 108(6): 1325–1331.

McCormick MC, McCarton C, Brooks-Gunn J, Belt P, Gross RT (1998) The Infant Health and Development Program: interim summary. *J Dev Behav Pediatr* 19: 359–370.

Marlow N (2004) Neurocognitive outcome after very preterm birth. *Arch Dis Child Fetal Neonatal Ed* 89: F224–F228.

Meisels SJ, Fenichel ES, editors (1996) *New Visions for the Developmental Assessment of Infants and Young Children. Zero to Three*. Herndon, VA: National Center for Infants.

Ment L, Vohr B, Allan W (2000) Outcome of children in the indomethacin intraventricular hemorrhage prevention trial. *Pediatrics* 105(3 Pt 1): 485–491.

Messinger DS, Bauer CR, Das A (2004) The Maternal Lifestyle Study: cognitive, motor, and behavioral outcomes of cocaine-exposed and opiate-exposed infants through three years of age. *Pediatrics* 113: 1677–1685.

Msall ME, Tremont MR (2002) Measuring functional outcomes after prematurity: developmental impact of very low birth weight and extremely low birth weight status on childhood disability. *Ment Retard Dev Disabil Res Rev* 8: 258–272.

Msall ME, DiGaudio K, Rogers BT, LaForest S, Lyon N, Campbell J, Wilczenski F, Duffy L (1994a) The Functional Independence Measure for Children (WeeFIM): conceptual basis and pilot use in children with developmental disabilities. *Clin Pediatr* 33: 421–430.

Msall ME, Di Gaudio K, Duffy LC, La Forest S, Braun, S, Granger CV (1994b) WeeFIM: normative sample of an instrument for tracking functional independence in children. *Clin Pediatr* 33: 431–438.

Msall M, Phelps DL, DiGaudio KM, Dobson V, Tung B, McClead RE, Quinn GE, Reynolds JD, Hardy RJ, Palmer EA (2000) Severity of neonatal retinopathy of prematurity is predictive of neurodevelopmental functional outcome at age 5.5 years. *Pediatrics* 106(5): 998–1005.

Msall M, Tremont MR, Ottenbacher KJ (2001) Functional assessment of preschool children: optimizing developmental and family supports in early intervention. *Infants Young Child* 14(1): 46–66.

National Research Council and Institute of Medicine (2004) *Children's Health, the Nation's Wealth: Assessing and Improving Child Health*. Committee on Evaluation of Children's Health. Board on Children, Youth, and Families, Division of Behavioral and Social Sciences and Education. Washington, DC: National Academies Press.

Neligan G, Prudham D (1969) Norms for four standard developmental milestones by sex, social class and place in family. *Dev Med Child Neurol* 11: 413–422.

Ottenbacher KJ, Taylor ET, Msall ME, Braun S, Lane SJ, Granger CV, Lyons N, Duffy LC (1996) The stability and equivalence reliability of the Functional Independence Measure for Children (WeeFIM·). *Dev Med Child Neurol* 38: 907–916.

Ottenbacher KJ, Msall ME, Lyon NR, Duffy LC, Granger CV, Braun S (1997). Interrater agreement and stability of the Functional Independence Measure for Children (WeeFIM): use in children with developmental disabilities. *Arch Phys Med Rehabil* 78: 1309–1315.

Ottenbacher KJ, Msall ME, Lyon N, Duffy LC, Granger CV, Braun S (1999) Measuring developmental and functional status in children with disabilities. *Dev Med Child Neurol* 41:186–194.

Ottenbacher KJ, Msall ME, Lyon N, Duffy LC, Ziviani J, Granger CV, Braun S (2000a) Functional assessment and care of children with neurodevelopmental disabilities. *Am J Phys Med Rehabil* 79:114–123.

Ottenbacher KJ, Msall ME, Lyon NR, Duffy LC, Ziviani J, Granger CV, Braun S, Feidler RC (2000b) The WeeFIM instrument: its utility in detecting change in children with developmental disabilities. *Arch Phys Med Rehabil* 81: 1317–1326.

Russell DJ, Rosenbaum PL, Avery LM, Lane M, editors (2002) *Gross Motor Function Measure (6MFM-66 and 6MFM-88) User's Manual*. London: Mac Keith Press.

Schmidt B, Asztalos EV, Roberts RS, Robertson CM, Sauve RS, Whitfield MF, Trial of Indomethacin Prophylaxis in Preterms (TIPP) Investigators (2003) Impact of bronchopulmonary dysplasia, brain injury, and severe retinopathy on the outcome of extremely low-birth-weight infants at 18 months: results from the trail of indomethacin prophylaxis in preterms. *JAMA* 289(9): 1124–1129.

Simeonson RJ, Lollar DJ, Hollowell J, Adams M (2000) Revision of the international classification of impairments, disabilities and handicaps: developmental issues. *J Clin Exp* 53: 113–124.

Skellern CY, Rogers Y, O'Callaghan MJ (2001) A parent-completed developmental questionnaire: follow up of ex-premature infants. *J Paediatr Child Health* 37: 125–129.

Squires J, Bricker D, Potter L (1997) Revision of a parent-completed development screening tool: Ages and Stages Questionnaires. *J Pediatr Psychol* 22(3): 313–328.

Stein RE, Jessop DJ (1990) Functional Status IIR: a measure of child health status. *Med Care* 28: 1041–1055.

Stein RE, Jessop DJ (2003) The impact on family scale revisited: further psychometric data. *J Dev Behav Pediatr* 24(1): 9–16.

Stein RE, Silver EJ (1999) Operationalizing a conceptually based noncategorical definition: a first look at US children with chronic conditions. *Arch Pediatr Adolesc Med* 153: 68–74.

Stoelhorst GM, Rijken M, Martens SE, van Zwieten PH, Feenstra J, Zwinderman AH, Wit JM, Veen S, Leiden Follow-Up Project on Prematurity (2003) Developmental outcome at 18 and 24 months of age in very preterm children: a cohort study from 1996 to 1997. *Early Hum Dev* 72(2): 83–95.

Stoll BJ, Hansen NI, Adams-Chapman I, Fanaroff AA, Hintz SR, Vohr B, Higgins RD, for the National Institute of Child Health and Human Development Neonatal Research Network (2004) Neurodevelopmental and growth impairment among extremely low-birth-weight infants with neonatal infection. *JAMA* 292(19): 2357–2365.

Theunissen NC, Veen S, Fekkes M, Koopman HM, Zwinderman KA, Brugman E, Wit JM (2001) Quality of life in preschool children born preterm. *Dev Med Child Neurol* 43(7): 460–465.

Tommiska V, Heinonen K, Kero P, Pokela M-L, Tammela O, Jarvenpaa AL, Salokorpi T, Virtanen M, Fellman V (2003) A national two year follow up study of extremely low birthweight infants born in 1996–1997. *Arch Dis Child Fetal Neonatal Ed* 88: F29–F35.

Tsuji T, Liu M, Toikawa H, Hanayama K, Sonoda S, Chino N (1999) ADL structure for nondisabled Japanese children based on the Functional Independence Measure for Children (WeeFIM). *Am J Phys Med Rehabil* 78(3): 208–212.

Vohr B, Msall M (1997) Neuropsychological and functional outcomes of very low birth weight infants. *Semin Perinatol* 21: 202–220.

Vohr BR, Wright LL, Dusick AM, Mele L, Verter J, Steichen JJ, Simon NP, Wilson DC, Broyles S, Bauer CR, Delaney-Black V, Yolton KA, Fleisher BE, Papile LA, Kaplan MD (2000) Neurodevelopmental and functional outcome of extremely low birth weight (ELBW) infants in the National Institute of Child Health and Human Development Neonatal Research Network 1993–94. *Pediatrics* 105: 1216–1226.

Vohr B, Wright LL, Hack M, Aylward G, Hirtz D (2004) Follow-up care of high-risk infants. *Pediatrics* 114: 1377–1397.

Voigt RG, Brown FR, Fraley JK, Llorente AM, Rozelle J, Turcich, M, Jensen CL, Heird WC (2003) Cognitive adaptive test/clinical linguistic and auditory milestone scale (CAT/CLAMS) and the mental developmental index of the Bayley scale of infant development. *Clin Pediatr* 42: 427–432.

Wachtel RC, Shapiro BK, Palmer FB, Allen MC, Capute AJ (1994) CAT/CLAMS: a tool for the pediatric evaluation of infants and young children with developmental delay *Clin Pediatr* (Phila) 33(7): 410–415.

Wetherby AM, Prizant BM, editors (2002) *Communication and Symbolic Behavior Scales Developmental Profile-TM*. Baltimore, MD: Paul H Brookes Publishing Co.

Wong V, Wong S, Chan K, Wong W (2002) Functional Independence Measure (WeeFIM) for Chinese children: Hong Kong cohort. *Pediatrics* 109(2): E36.

Wood NS, Marlow N, Costeloe K, Gibson AT, Wilkinson AR (2000) Neurologic and developmental disability after extreme preterm birth. *New Engl J Med* 343: 378–384.

World Health Organization, editor (2001) *International Classification of Functioning Disability and Health*. Geneva: WHO.

Zimmerman IL, Steiner VG, Pond NE, editors (2002) *Preschool Language Scale-4*. San Antonio, TX: Harcourt Assessment.

Ziviani J, Ottenbacher KJ, Shephard K, Foreman S, Astbury W, Ireland P, et al (2001) Concurrent validity of the Functional Independence Measure for Children (WeeFIM) and the Pediatric Evaluation of Disabilities Inventory in children with developmental disabilities and acquired brain injuries. *Phys Occup Ther Pediatr* 21: 91–101.

INDEX

272

274